1

STEROID RECEPTORS IN HEALTH AND DISEASE

SERONO SYMPOSIA, USA

Series Editor: James Posillico

ACROMEGALY: A Century of Scientific and Clinical Progress
Edited by Richard J. Robbins and Shlomo Melmed

BASIC AND CLINICAL ASPECTS OF GROWTH HORMONE
Edited by Barry B. Bercu

THE PRIMATE OVARY
Edited by Richard L. Stouffer

SOMATOSTATIN: Basic and Clinical Status
Edited by Seymour Reichlin

STEROID RECEPTORS IN HEALTH AND DISEASE
Edited by Virinder K. Moudgil

A Continuation Order Plan is available for this series. A continuation order will bring delivery of each new volume immediately upon publication. Volumes are billed only upon actual shipment. For further information please contact the publisher.

STEROID RECEPTORS IN HEALTH AND DISEASE

Edited by
Virinder K. Moudgil

Oakland University
Rochester, Michigan

PLENUM PRESS • NEW YORK AND LONDON

Library of Congress Cataloging in Publication Data

Meadow Brook Conference on Steroid Receptors in Health and Disease (1st: 1987: Rochester, Mich.)
  Steroid receptors in health and disease / edited by Virinder K. Moudgil.
    p.   cm.
  "Proceedings of the Meadow Brook Conference on Steroid Receptors in Health and Disease, spon-
sored by Serono Symposia, USA and Oakland University, held September 20–23, 1987, in Rochester,
Michigan"—T.p. verso.
  Includes bibliographies and indexes.
  ISBN 0-306-42987-X
  1. Steroid hormones—Receptors—Congresses. I. Moudgil, V. K. (Virinder K.), 1945–   . II.
Serono Symposia, USA. III. Oakland University. IV. Title.
  [DNLM: 1. Receptors, Steroid—congresses. W3 ME378 1st 1987s / WK 150 M482 1987s]
QP571.7.M42 1987
612'.405—dc19
DNLM/DLC   88-22477
for Library of Congress   CIP

The views expressed in this volume are the responsibility of the named authors. Great care has been taken to maintain the accuracy of the information contained in the volume. However, neither Plenum Press, Serono Symposia, USA, nor the editors can be held responsible for errors or any consequences arising from the use of information contained herein.

Some of the names of products referred to in this book may be registered trademarks or proprietary names, although specific references to this fact may not be made; however, the use of a name without designations is not to be construed as a representation by the publisher or editors that it is in the public domain. In addition, the mention of specific companies or of their products or proprietary names does not imply any endorsement or recommendation on the part of the publisher or editors.

Proceedings of the Meadow Brook Conference on Steroid Receptors in Health and Disease,
sponsored by Serono Symposia, USA and Oakland University, held September 20–23, 1987,
in Rochester, Michigan

© 1988 Plenum Press, New York
A Division of Plenum Publishing Corporation
233 Spring Street, New York, N.Y. 10013

Printed in the United States of America

SCIENTIFIC COMMITTEE

Virinder Moudgil, Chairman
Rochester, MI

Etienne-Emile Baulieu
Paris, France

Jack Gorski
Madison, WI

Benita Katzenellenbogen
Urbana, IL

David Toft
Rochester, MN

James Wittliff
Louisville, KY

ORGANIZING SECRETARY

Dr. James T. Posillico
Serono Symposia, USA
Randolph, Massachusetts

PREFACE

During the last two decades, progress in steroid hormone research has resulted in the development of new approaches to contraception as well as diagnosis and treatment of endocrine disorders and cancers. Although significant advances have been made in the purification, characterization, immunochemistry and molecular biology of steroid receptors, the precise molecular mechanism of steroid hormone action has remained obscure. This book captures the detailed presentations made at the first conference on Steroid Receptors in Health and Disease held at Meadow Brook Hall, Oakland University in the fall of 1987. The purpose of this international conference was to facilitate scientific exchange toward a better understanding of the mode of action of steroid hormones. The scientific sessions consisted of poster presentations and state-of-the-art lectures, the latter of which make up this volume. The first chapter is meant to provide the reader with a more general background of the topics covered in the book, as well as to discuss certain theme-related issues that are either not yet well-established or accepted or are in the stage of infancy. It is hoped that this volume will serve as a useful treatise for students and investigators interested in basic and clinical aspects of biological regulation by steroid hormones.

A task of this magnitude could not have been undertaken without the encouragement, advice and continued generous assistance of the members of the scientific committee. I am gratefully indebted to Drs. Etienne Baulieu, Jack Gorski, Benita Katzenellenbogen, David Toft, and James Wittliff for providing guidance and direction in the planning and execution of the scientific program. The stimulating and relaxed ambiance was provided by the venue of the conference, Meadow Brook Hall, a national treasure and designated historic site in the State of Michigan. Thanks are due to Drs. Joanne Williams, Theodore Landau, and Naomi Eliezer, Mr. John Shiff, Mr. Cliff Hurd, Ms. Rita Perris, and many of our students and colleagues whose invaluable help in the planning and operation of the conference made it a successful and memorable event.

The conference was made possible through generous financial support from Serono Symposia, USA, Oakland University and Meadow Brook Hall. Local arrangements were facilitated by thoughtful contributions from William Beaumont Hospital, Schering Corporation, The Squibb Institute for Medical Research, Oxford Biomedical Research and Protein International. The excellent cooperation from the authors and the timely and skillful assistance from the publications and editorial staff of Serono Symposia, USA and Plenum Press has made the job of editing this volume an enjoyable experience. I am particularly indebted to Dr. James Posillico and his staff for the support and encouragement received from the time of planning the conference to the compilation of this volume.

Virinder K. Moudgil

CONTENTS

IV.   RECEPTOR GENE STRUCTURE AND FUNCTION

V.   BIOCHEMICAL ACTIONS AND ANTIHORMONES

VI.   PHARMACOLOGICAL AND CLINICAL CORRELATIONS

I. INTRODUCTION AND KEYNOTE ADDRESS

STEROID RECEPTORS IN HEALTH AND DISEASE

Virinder K. Moudgil

Department of Biological Sciences, Oakland University
Rochester, Michigan 48309-4401, U.S.A.

The influence of steroid hormones on various complex physiological and developmental processes is well known. Their role in the fetal brain development, attainment of puberty, sexual differentiation, regulation of reproductive function, normal and tumor cell proliferation, and maintenance of mineral balance has long been recognized. During the past twenty years, progress in research on the effects and mode of action of steroid hormones has resulted in the development of new approaches to contraception as well as diagnosis and treatment of endocrine disorders and cancers. It is now known that proliferation of almost one-third of reported breast and uterine cancers is influenced by circulating hormones: a high percentage of these cancers respond favorably to endocrine manipulations.

The actions of steroid hormones are mediated by their initial interaction with specific intracellular "receptor" proteins in the target cells. Although significant advances have been made in the purification, characterization, immunology and molecular biology of steroid hormone receptors (SRs), the precise molecular mechanism of steroid hormone action is incompletely understood. In this review, an attempt is made to discuss some recent developments in the field which bring to focus major issues and hypotheses concerning the mode of action of steroid hormones. The reader is referred to a recently compiled treatise for a more complete and comprehensive treatment of the subject (1).

SUBCELLULAR LOCALIZATION OF STEROID RECEPTORS

Availability of radioisotopic estrogen in the early 1960s accelerated the progress in its cellular localization in various target tissues. Subsequently, an initial characterization of [^{3}H]estradiol binding in the rat uterus was accomplished (2). Ever since, it had been believed that the effects of steroid hormones on specific protein synthesis were mediated via specific receptor proteins which exist in the cytoplasm of target cells. To explain the sequence of events in the course of a steroid hormone action, a two-step model was proposed (3,4). Accordingly, a steroid hormone may enter a target cell via passive diffusion to bind its receptor in the cytoplasm. The binding of steroid to its cytoplasmic receptor in vivo results in some conformational changes (activation/transformation) in the steroid-receptor complex (SRc) leading to its translocation into the nucleus. Once in the nucleus, the translocated SRc interacts with DNA and chromatin to influence cellular protein synthesis. In the past few years, this model has undergone reevaluation and some of its fundamental assumptions have been challenged.

Biochemical fractionation and autoradiography techniques employed in most of the early work in the field helped develop the concept of the presence of unoccupied receptor in the cytoplasm. Essentially all unoccupied receptors were isolated in the high-speed supernatant (cytosol) of the target tissues. Following an administration of a steroid in vivo, or uptake of the hormone in intact tissue slices, a majority of the receptors were obtained in the nuclear fraction. When cells were exposed to radioligand and incubated at 4°C, autoradiography demonstrated the presence of radioactivity in the cytoplasm. Consequently, it was concluded that incubation of cells at elevated temperatures caused the radioactive ligands to appear in the nucleus. Although these observations met with general acceptance for nearly two decades, the interpretation of the results of these studies was not uniformly adopted.

Unoccupied estrogen receptors (ER) may appear variably in the nucleus or cytoplasm depending upon whether the tissue extracts are concentrated or diluted with buffer (5). This suggests that the localization of receptors in cellular compartments may be influenced by many factors. These important observations called into question the results of analysis of SRs localized in cells where membranes were still intact. The laboratories of Gorski and Greene employed cell enucleation and immunocytochemistry to avoid contamination of cellular compartments that may normally occur during tissue preparation. Welshons et al. (6) demonstrated that 90% of the unoccupied ER in GH_3 cells could be found in the nucleoplasts of the enucleated cells. Homogenization of intact nucleoplasts in dilute buffer and subsequent centrifugation showed the presence of unoccupied receptors in the nucleosol. Using anti-ER monoclonal antibodies, King and Greene (7) also demonstrated nuclear localization of ER in a number of target cells. The nuclear localization of unoccupied receptors for other steroids has also been reported (8-13). The receptor recovered in the cytosol fraction of homogenates may, therefore, represent that population of receptor which is loosely associated with the nucleus, and its binding with the hormone may lead to a tighter association of the SRc with the nuclear sites. Should these postulations prove to be correct, the conformational changes, which were collectively referred to as activation or transformation and were thought to be necessary for nuclear translocation of SRc, would simply represent intranuclear event(s).

Gasc and Baulieu (chapter 3) have presented evidence that, under a variety of experimental conditions, antibodies to chick progesterone receptor (PR) reveal the presence of receptor molecules in the cell nuclei independent of receptor occupancy by ligand. The authors have proposed that the occurrence of PR in the cytosol could be due to a loss or leak of nuclear receptor during homogenization. Results presented by Brenner et al. (chapter 4) show that in the target cells of estrogen in spayed monkeys, the majority of ER is cytosolic. However, immunocytochemical analysis indicated that all of the specific staining was nuclear. These findings support the view that in the absence of hormone, the unoccupied, nontransformed ER can be easily stripped from the nucleus during homogenization to become detectable in the cytosolic fraction. Sequential progesterone treatment for two weeks lowers both cytosolic and nuclear ER below the level achieved with estrogen administration.

In contrast to the above observations, glucocorticoid receptor (GR) was revealed by immunostaining in both the cytoplasmic and the nuclear compartments. It was observed that ligand administration leads to intensification of immunostaining in the nucleus, as is also reported by

Carlstedt-Duke et al. and Brenner and co-workers in this volume. Although these latter observations lend support to the nuclear translocation hypothesis, intensified nuclear staining of GR following hormone administration could also suggest that steroid binding allows a better and prolonged nuclear retention during experimental processing.

The question of subcellular localization of SRs in the presence or absence of hormone is still a subject of some debate (14-16), although there is overwhelming evidence in support of nuclear localization of unoccupied receptors. The fundamental tenets of the two-step hypothesis are: the phenomena of ligand binding and subsequent alterations (activation/transformation) of SRs, appear unchanged in the proposed revised model based on the data from exclusive nuclear localization of SRc (17). Furthermore, SRs have always been recognized as nuclear regulatory elements regardless of their location in the cell. A model that represents our current thinking about steroid receptor action has been presented in this volume by Gorski, who has also provided a historic perspective of the investigations involving SRs.

LIGAND-FREE STEROID RECEPTORS: PROPERTIES AND STRUCTURE

The physicochemical properties of unoccupied receptors had remained unexplored due to the nonavailability of adequately sensitive in vitro techniques. Virtually all the data on the structure and composition of SRs has been obtained from studies on receptor molecules and their binding to the corresponding steroids or hormonal ligands. The ligand binding itself may induce alterations in receptor structure, which may precede other modifications prior to a final cellular response to the hormone (4).

Exposure of unoccupied SRs to elevated temperatures is known to result in the loss of cytosol steroid binding sites. The presence of ligand may protect or stabilize these binding sites (1), and influence affinity of receptor for DNA (18). In addition, the physicochemical properties of unoccupied receptor have been shown to be different from occupied SRc (19). Previous work from this laboratory demonstrated that although transformation in vitro of chicken oviduct or calf uterine progesterone receptor (PR) could be accomplished in the absence of added ligand, the extent of transformation was lower (20-23). A clearer picture has emerged from a recent study which demonstrated that the 9S (untransformed) to 4S (transformed) conversion of rat liver GR was absolutely dependent on the occupancy of steroid binding site by ligand (24). These observations suggest that the conformation and properties of SRs are influenced by their interaction with ligands.

In order to probe the molecular properties of the surface of the estrogen receptor (ER), Hansen and Gorski (25,26, and chapter 7 in this volume) employed the technique of aqueous two-phase partitioning (ATPP) to characterize conformational and electrostatic properties of unoccupied and liganded rat uterine ER. The technique allows a quantitative assessment of the behavior of both unoccupied and liganded receptors under identical conditions. Using ATPP, it was possible to demonstrate the occurrence of a ligand-induced change in the properties of the unoccupied receptor, which precedes the process of heat-transformation in vitro. Both unoccupied and nontransformed ER were shown to have the same PI but a significantly different partition coefficient. This suggested that these ER forms differed in conformation but not in electrostatic properties. Furthermore, the binding of estradiol to its receptor makes the complex less hydrophobic and causes a change in its surface properties which is independent of receptor transformation. Moudgil et al. (27) have recently reported ligand-dependent structural change in the rat liver GR at 0°C that is distinct from those caused by receptor transformation. Ligand binding may, therefore, independently induce conformational changes in the receptor which precede or accompany other changes in receptor conformation (28).

TRANSFORMATION OF STEROID RECEPTORS

Regardless of their cellular location, upon homogenization, the SRs are recovered in the high speed supernatant fraction where they can be incubated at 0-4°C with the hormone to form "nontransformed" complexes. SRs in such complexes are believed to occur in an oligomeric form which sediments as 7-9S molecules and exhibit very little affinity for nuclear sites (29-32). Increased nuclear binding capacity can be induced in vitro by increasing the ionic strength of the medium, by incubating the receptor preparations at elevated temperatures in the presence of hormone, and by incubation of the cytosol at 0-4°C with 10 mM ATP and other agents (22-24,27,32-34). The above treatments are thought to induce some alterations in the physicochemical properties of the SRs collectively known as activation or transformation (both terms have been used to describe the same process). The term transformation has also been used to refer to an in vitro alteration of the cytosol receptor involving a change from its oligomeric 8-10S form to a monomeric form that sediments as a 4-5S species. The transformed 4-5S receptor exhibits increased affinity for isolated nuclei, chromatin, DNA-cellulose, phosphocellulose, and ATP-Sepharose. It also shows an alteration in the dissociation kinetics of the SRc (31,32). Although knowledge about the process of receptor transformation has been accumulating from studies performed in cell-free systems, the transformation of SRc in intact target cells has also been described under physiological conditions (35). The following discussion will focus on recent developments which implicate roles for RNA, heat-shock proteins and phosphorylation in the transformation of SRs.

Role of RNA

Many published reports have implicated a role for RNA in the structure and function of SRs (36-54). Liao and co-workers originally suggested that androgen and estrogen receptors may exist as complexes of protein and RNA (37,44). It has also been shown that the structure of SRs could be altered by a heat-stable RNase-labile factor in the cytosol. The initial studies employed crude cytosol receptor preparations that were incubated with exogenous ribonuclease. Such treatments resulted in changes in the physicochemical properties of SRs leading to their increased DNA binding ability and slower sedimentation rate. Association of RNA with purified GR has also been reported recently (47). Results of some of these studies (45,47,48,50) suggested that ribonuclease treatment caused transformation of receptor by hydrolyzing RNA. Anderson and Tymoczko have identified a low molecular weight factor which inhibits the effects of RNase on GR thus stabilizing the 9-10S form and inhibiting its binding to DNA (54). Accordingly, the 9-10S hepatic GR is believed to be a hetero-oligomeric structure composed of this low molecular weight factor, a chymotrypsin-sensitive factor, RNA and the monomeric 4S receptor itself. Rowley et al. (48) have identified a 7.7S androgen receptor (AR) which reportedly contains ribonucleoprotein; the RNA component of the complex is thought to be important for maintaining the structural integrity of the receptor. The SR-RNA interaction may be involved in the stabilization of SRc, its transfer into the nucleus or nuclear retention, or it may influence turnover of specific RNA or regulation of gene expression (49,50).

A MW 36,000 RNA, later identified as a transfer RNA (tRNA), was initially suggested to be an integral component of the 5.2S oligomeric transformed mouse GR (50,51). Recent work from this laboratory indicates that purified untransformed mouse GR preparation from the AtT-20 pituitary tumor cell line does not contain RNA (55). Accordingly, RNA binding to SRc may occur after dissociation of the oligomeric untransformed GR-complex into monomers. If RNA association occurs subsequent to receptor activation, the polyribonucleotide may still play an important role in the effective functioning of the transformed receptor preceding its alteration of the expression of SR-responsive genes.

Involvement of Heat-Shock Proteins

In the absence of steroids, SRs can be extracted from target tissue cytosols as large protein complexes of MW 300,000 and a sedimentation coefficient of 8-10S. In their native hetero-oligomeric structure SRs can be stabilized in the presence of molybdate, an agent shown to block transformation of SRc to the slower sedimenting, DNA binding form (56,57). Consequently the laboratories of Baulieu and Toft had isolated avian PR in the 8S, molybdate-stabilized forms (58,59). These preparations contained a major 90K peptide. Toft's laboratory further demonstrated the existence of two 8S receptor forms: type I which contained the 90K peptide and the A receptor (MW 79K), and type II which contained the 90K peptide and the B receptor (MW 110K) (60). Birnbaumer et al. (61) attempted purification of avian PR using methods employed by Baulieu and Toft and reported that the 90K peptide in their preparation did not bind progesterone and was not associated with PR. Subsequently, Dougherty et al. (62) obtained highly purified preparations of PR that contained the type I 8S complex composed of the hormone binding A peptide plus a 90K peptide which did not bind the steroid; and the type II 8S complex that contained the B peptide plus the 90K nonsteroid binding peptide. Furthermore, all three peptides were reported to exist as phosphoproteins. Joab et al. (63) extended these observations to other systems and reported the presence of the 90K peptide as a common, nonhormone binding component of the nontransformed chick oviduct receptors of four steroid hormones. Additional evidence has accumulated, suggesting that the nonhormone binding component of SRs exists in a wide range of receptor systems, tissues and species (64-68).

The relationship between the steroid binding subunits and the non-steroid binding 90K peptide is not yet clear but the 90K peptide appears to be present in excess over the hormone-binding peptides (61,62). Although the involvement of 90K peptide in the process of receptor trans-formation has not been directly demonstrated, it is widely known that the 90K peptide is absent from receptor preparations purified in the absence of molybdate and exists only as a component of the 8-10S SR forms. Many indirect clues, including the reported size and molecular abundance of 90K peptide, have led to the identification of 90K peptide of SRs as a major heat-shock protein (hsp) (69-72). Although the 90K hsp (hsp90), like other such proteins, increases in abundance when cells are stressed by elevated temperature or by certain cytotoxic agents, it is also a major ubiquitous cytosolic protein in unstressed cells (69,73).

Baulieu has proposed (chapter 18) that hsp90 is involved in the oligomeric structure of SRs. The latter caps the DNA binding site of the receptor to prevent it from binding to hormone regulatory elements (HREs) to increase the transcription of regulatory genes. A hormone agonist may, according to Baulieu, induce the dissociation of the receptor oligomer to unmask the functional DNA binding domain. RU 486, a recently synthesized progestin antagonist, may stabilize the 8S form of PR that is unable to dissociate from hsp90 to elicit a hormonal response. This suggestion is consistent with the recent findings of Moudgil and Hurd (20) that the ability of calf uterine PR to undergo 8S to 4S transformation in vitro is impaired when the receptor is occupied by RU 486. Horwitz (chapter 8) has presented a model for the structure of native human PR (hPR) proposing two classes of 8S PR, each associated with nonsteroid binding peptides of 72K and 90K. Accordingly, transformation results from dissociation of the 90K protein exposing DNA binding site masked in the 8S receptor form. These observations appear to represent a general phenomenon. Mendel et al. (68) recently reported that molybdate-stabilized nontransformed GRc contain a 90K nonsteroid binding phosphoprotein that is lost on transformation. These investigators also suggest that nontransformed complexes and heteromeric structures containing steroid binding and 90K nonsteroid binding proteins are phosphoproteins which dissociate during thermal activation in intact cells as well as under cell-free conditions (68).

Because of its relation to SRs and other proteins, hsp90 has become a subject of many further investigations. Catelli et al. (72) have cloned a short cDNA segment for the gene encoding hsp90. As to its significance, hsp90 is known to form complexes with a number of tyrosine protein kinases which are products of viral oncogenes, including the Rous Sarcoma virus-transforming tyrosine protein kinase (70,74). The role of hsp90 may be to associate with both viral tyrosine kinases and SRs to form inactive complexes. Dissociation or separation of hsp90 from these complexes may, therefore, transform the complexes to their active DNA binding forms (74,75). Attempts to recombine 4S, transformed DNA binding forms of SRs with the hsp90 to generate inactive non-DNA binding 8-10S receptors are in progress. Success in this effort will clarify the role of hsp90 in the cell-free transformation of SRs, and in the regulation of equilibrium between active and inactive receptors in intact cells.

Receptor Phosphorylation vs. Transformation

Many hypotheses have been proposed to explain the process of receptor transformation (31). These include: proteolysis of receptor, subunit aggregation and dissociation, and conformational alterations in receptor. A hypothesis that has attracted considerable attention suggests that phosphorylation-dephosphorylation reactions modulate transformation of SRs in vitro, or perhaps in the intact cells. The origin of this hypothesis has roots in the initial observations made on the effects of molybdate on transformation of SRs.

It is now widely believed that phosphatase inhibitors such as molybdate, tungstate, and vanadate stabilize SRc and blocked their thermal activation to a DNA or ATP-Sepharose binding form(s) (56,76). These compounds were initially shown to have no effect on the activated SRc. Furthermore, the rate of transformation of GR was reported to be stimulated by incubation with calf uterine alkaline phosphatase (77). Based on these observations, it was suggested that transformation of SRc involves a dephosphorylation of the receptor itself or of some regulatory component(s) (77,78). Alternatively, other studies have proposed that molybdate actions on SRs are direct and may not involve phosphorylation-dephosphorylation mechanisms (79-82). The latter view was supported by observations that other phosphatase inhibitors, such as levamisole or fluoride, failed to block receptor transformation, and that high concentrations of alkaline phophatase converted nontransformed receptor to a transformed form (56,76,77). Results from this author's laboratory provided the first clues that molybdate and tungstate had a direct effect on SRc (80,81). In these studies, DNA binding of activated GR was inhibited by preincubation of receptor with these transition metal ions; the latter were also effective in extraction of DNA-cellulose-bound or nuclear-bound receptors. The question as to whether receptor dephosphorylation is a pre- or corequisite to transformation of SRs is still open. Recent developments in this field suggest that phosphorylation of

SR may occur in a multiple sequential manner, or may be involved in the action of steroid hormones in other ways such as processing or down-regulation of receptors.

HORMONE ACTION WITHOUT HORMONE?

As a result of the recent employment of the tools of molecular biology, the functional domains of SRs have been shown to be highly conserved (83). The primary amino acid sequence of human and chicken ER appears to contain six distinct regions; region E is hydrophobic in char-acter and is thought to contain the hormone binding domain between amino acids 301 and 552 (84). Occupancy of the hormone binding domain under physiologic conditions is thought to induce the receptor to bind DNA. Using a series of human ER deletion mutants, Chambon's group found that receptors containing large deletions within the hormone binding domain failed to activate transcription (85). This suggested that the hormone binding domain was indispensable for gene activation, and that the func-tion of an unoccupied hormone binding domain may be to discourage receptor binding to the estrogen-responsive element, thereby preventing transcrip-tion.

The presence of hormone appears to be essential for gene activation in vivo (86), although the mechanism by which binding of hormone leads to activation of SRc and stimulation of gene transcription is unclear. The latter view, however, is not supported by recent findings suggesting that hormone plays no role in determining the specificity of GR and PR binding to DNA in vitro (87,88). Results of Giuere et al. (89) raised the pos-sibility that the regions in the GR which are necessary for full trans-criptional activation are not specifically involved in steroid or DNA binding. Willman and Beato (87) have reported that steroid-free GR binds specifically to MMTV DNA, and that the function of hormone in vivo could be to modulate nuclear partitioning of the receptor. However, in vivo, protein-DNA interaction in glucocorticoid response elements appears to require the presence of the hormone, and the hormone-free GR appears to be unable to recognize specific response elements of a target gene in vivo (90). The role of hormone in vivo may, therefore, be to unmask a pre-formed DNA binding domain eclipsed in the unoccupied receptor, probably by a nonhormone binding subunit of SR hetero-oligomer, such as hsp90. Chambon's group has shown that mutants, deleted of the hormone binding domain, are unable to stimulate gene transcription (83). At least for ER, occupancy of the steroid binding domain appears to be indispensable for transcription. Truncated GR, however, differs in that it is possible to stimulate transcription without the presence of the hormone binding domain (91,92).

In cell-free systems, many of the structural changes related to transformation of SR can occur with the unoccupied receptor subjected to transforming conditions (23,24,28). The 8S chick oviduct PR can be transformed by salt and ATP, and to a lesser extent by heat, to a 4S form in the absence of an added ligand (23). Rat liver GR, however, shows an exclusive hormone-dependency for the 9S to 4S transformation (24).

The demonstrated translational efficiency achieved in vitro by receptor mutants lacking the hormone binding domain, and ability of the unoccupied receptor to undergo transformation to a DNA binding state, undermine the central role of the steroid hormone in this process (hormone action). Alternatively, the results of several studies performed in vivo strongly endorse a crucial role for steroids in triggering a hormonal response. If a receptor-mediated process were shown to occur in the absence of the hormone, this would raise the question of its physiologic relevance. However, to date, hormone-independent processes have been observed in cell-free systems, which can be explained by the lack of certain cellular regulatory mechanisms operating in vivo. Taken together, the above discussion points to the distinct structural and compositional aspects of SRc and their hormone requirement for performing various functions.

INTERACTION OF STEROID RECEPTORS WITH NUCLEAR COMPONENTS

Chromatin Acceptor Sites

Interaction of SRc with nuclear components of target cells is required in order to observe a hormonal response. Spelsberg and colleagues (93) have recently reviewed the general properties of the chromatin acceptor sites which possess specific DNA sequences to which SRc are thought to bind. For characterizing the chromatin acceptor sites of chick oviduct PR, the authors have developed a cell-free binding assay utilizing both partially and highly purified receptor and chromatin preparations. The assay depended on intact and functional PR whose binding to native or deproteinized chromatin was saturable, of high affinity, and mimicked the in vivo pattern of nuclear binding. The capacity of PR to interact with nuclear sites in vivo was altered as a function of age, season and physiologic status of the animal. The Ruhs have studied antiestrogen interaction with ER, which is reported to alter the receptor in a manner such that its properties become distinct from ERc, and the anti-ERc showed altered interaction with chromatin acceptor sites (94). These observations were consistent when chromatin rather than pure DNA was used as an acceptor. Whereas the total genomic DNA may display nonsaturable binding of SRc to acceptor-protein DNA complexes, the latter are considered different from "acceptor sites" which consist of DNA sequences flanking the 5' end of steroid-regulated structural genes (93).

Only a limited number of specific DNA sequences in the avian genome may contribute to the regeneration of acceptor sites and these sequences do not reside in or near the ovalbumin gene (93). The existence of genes whose transcriptions are more rapidly regulated by steroids than by some secretory proteins has been recently documented (93). The mRNA levels of c-myc gene in the avian oviduct can be seen to rise within 5-10 min after progesterone administration. Since the c-myc protein is known to be an intranuclear gene regulator, it has been suggested that the regulation of c-myc gene expression may be an important step in the general steroid regulation of cell division and cytodifferentiation (93).

The Nuclear Matrix

The organization of nuclear components may play a crucial role in the regulation of hormonal responses. Association of AR and ER with the nuclear matrix has been recently reviewed by Barrack (95). This work has provided insights into the probable role of the nuclear matrix in the regulation of steroid hormone action. The nuclear matrix is an insoluble component of the eukaryotic nuclei, lacking nuclear envelope phospholipid and chromatin. It serves as an anchor for eukaryotic DNA which is organized into supercoiled loops, and is a major site of SR localization following hormone administration. The specific activity of receptors in the nuclear matrix is higher than that in intact nuclei and nuclear salt extract (95). Administration of physiological doses of steroid hormones leads to biochemical and immunochemical detection of receptors in the nuclear matrix of the target cell nuclei. The matrix-associated ER possess properties similar to those exhibited in the cytosol preparations (95).

A major portion of nuclear receptors are associated with DNase-resistant and salt-resistant nuclear matrix, although a portion of the receptor population may not be tightly associated. This raises the question of whether heterogeneity of functional nuclear receptors is responsible for their incomplete extraction. The extraction of nuclear receptors may be influenced by sulfhydryl reducing agents, which play a role in nuclear matrix integrity (95). The proportion of extracted AR goes up from 0-50% in the absence of dithiothreitol, and to 80-90% in its presence. Sulfhydryl modifying agents are generally known to interfere with the steroid and DNA-binding properties of SRs. Other factors which may influence extraction of nuclear matrix-bound receptor include proteolysis and phosphorylation of nuclear receptors which affect the solubility and compartmentalization of receptors.

RECEPTOR INTERACTION WITH DNA: CLONING AND EXPRESSION OF RECEPTOR GENES

Hormonal ligands can confer on SRs the ability to act as trans-acting regulatory proteins that are capable of modulating gene expression. The SRc have been reported to interact specifically with promotor "enhancer" elements of target cell genes (83,96). The hormone-responsive DNA sequences (enhancers) are located in the 5'-flanking region (97-99). The DNA binding site(s) have also been localized far upstream from the initiation site and within introns of the transcription unit (97,100,101).

Preferential binding of the transformed SRc to specific DNA sequences in regions upstream from the transcriptional start site of steroid regulated genes has been described (102-107). In order to elucidate the role of SR binding to DNA sequences, hybrid genes have been constructed and used to transfect SR-containing target cells. Results of these experimental manipulations indicate that the promotor region of a steroid-controlled gene containing DNA binding site(s) is sufficient to confer hormone inducibility on heterologous gene (101,108-110).

Investigations of SRs at the molecular level (83-86,89,111-115) have allowed mapping of the putative DNA binding domain (region C), which is a highly conserved region of 66 amino acids capable of forming two DNA-binding "fingers" (97). Carlstedt-Duke et al. (chapter 5) have purified GR in its activated DNA binding form. Limited proteolysis revealed that GR consists of three functional domains. The DNA-binding domain is hydrophilic and rich in Cys, Lys and Arg. The region corresponds to residues 414-517, which corresponds well with the functional domain defined on the basis of mutational data.

Gronemeyer et al. (chapter 11) have presented functional characterization of the estrogen and progesterone receptors. Analysis of the amino acid sequence of ER from human and chicken reveals three highly conserved regions: A (AA 1-38), C (AA 180-263) and E (AA 302-553). All SRs and v-erbA/thyroid receptors contain sequences homologous to regions C and E. Region E represents the steroid binding domain located in the C-terminal half of each of the receptors (83), while region C constitutes the DNA-binding domain. Both regions C and E are required for efficient activation of the HREs of various genes. However, the question as to whether the efficiency of SR binding to responsive elements is influenced by or dependent on the presence of hormone remains unresolved. Although it may be possible to trigger transcriptional activation by SR in the absence of a hormonal ligand in vitro, presence of hormone appears to be essential for specific DNA-binding in vivo.

The data on the cloning and sequencing of the cPR has led Gronemeyer and coauthors to conclude that it follows a structural organization characteristic of the steroid/thyroid hormone receptor supergene family. The domains responsible for tight nuclear binding and progestin binding were found to correlate with regions C and E, respectively. Since chick PR has been described to be composed of two forms, A and B, with apparent different functional characteristics, the cloning of the cPR cDNA and gene excluded that the two forms are the products of different genes. Since both PR forms bind hormone in the c-terminus, the differences between A and B may be a consequence of different lengths of the N-terminal region. The authors conclude that the appearance of form A is a chick oviduct cell-specific characteristic generated by proteolysis of form B or due to initiation of translation at an internal AUG.

Rosenfeld and colleagues (chapter 12) have reviewed regulation of rat prolactin (PRL) and growth hormone gene expression by estrogen and thyroid hormone receptors. Estrogen directly increases PRL gene transcription, raising the transcription rate by four- to fivefold to suggest that ER directly interacts with a DNA element(s) near or within the PRL gene. The estrogen-regulated element (ERE) identified in rPRL gene lies 1.5 kb upstream from PRL transcriptional start site. Consistent with results of some other studies, the c-terminal ligand-binding domain of steroid receptor gene family appears to exert a regulatory function and is itself not required for transcriptional activation. Further, the properties of DNA binding and transcriptional activation reside within the ER region containing basic amino acids and the conserved cysteines and histidines. The negative regulation of PRL gene is exercised by glucocorticoids and the high levels of ER following removal of ERE. Some evidence suggests that two different domains are responsible for positive and negative regulation of PRL gene transcription.

Savouret et al. (chapter 13) have presented data on the cloning of rabbit and human PR genes. Using electron microscopy to observe PR binding to regulatory regions of uteroglobin and mouse mammary tumor virus genes, these investigators demonstrated the binding of PR oligomers at two DNA sites. The interaction results in DNA-loops when the HREs were at a distance from one another. The data suggested high-affinity interaction between steroid receptors and discrete regions of DNA.

The preceding discussion has emphasized the importance of an inter-action of SRc with enhancer-like DNA regions for the modulation of gene expression but the involvement of chromatin structure in this process cannot be undermined. The two phenomena, interaction of SRc with chromatin component(s) and binding of SRc to DNA sequences, may actually operate sequentially to induce alterations in expression of hormonally controlled genes in target cells. According to Gorski (chapter 2), chromatin proteins as well as DNA are critical for the estrogen response and an interaction between SR and chromatin proteins is likely to contribute to this phenomenon.

In an attempt to define functional domains of the human AR involved in gene regulation, Govindan (chapter 14) has reported isolation of cDNA clones encoding AR from human testis λ-gt-11 cDNA library. The cDNA clones were inserted into a bacterial expression vector. The protein product of the clones bound [^{3}H]DHT with high affinity and specificity. To elucidate mechanisms by which steroids control target tissue gene expression, Janne (chapter 9) has discussed AR-mediated androgenic regulation of the ornithine decarboxylase (ODC) genes. Androgen treatment of female mice increased ODC mRNA accumulation and ODC protein concentration. Although antiandrogens exhibited a dose-dependent accumulation of androgen receptors in the renal nuclei, receptor-antagonist complexes failed to influence gene expression.

CLINICAL CONSIDERATIONS OF STEROID RECEPTORS

Detection and quantitation of both ER and PR are now used routinely in the clinical management of breast and endometrial cancers as predictive indices of a patient's response to endocrine therapy, and as prognostic indicators of a patient's clinical course. The origin and physiological significance of receptor heterogeneity observed with breast cancer patients is the focus of the review by Wittliff et al. (chapter 21). Posttranscriptional modifications, such as receptor phosphorylation and association of steroid binding peptide(s) with nonhormone binding peptides or protein kinases, may contribute to the polymorphism. Gurpide and co-workers (chapter 20) have suggested that the presence of receptors in breast cancer or endometrial adenocarcinoma reveals cellular properties that make the tumor more responsive, without implying receptor-mediated effects of drugs with hormonal action. Accordingly, the presence of SRs characterizes a physiological state of the cancer cell and is associated with, rather than responsible for, responses to therapy. It was shown that receptor levels correlate with DNA polymerase and ornithine decarboxylase activities in certain endometrial cancer cell lines and that in non-estrogen responsive tumor cells, the ability of ER to interact with a monoclonal anti-ER antibody is impaired.

Rochefort and colleagues have described how in ER-positive human breast cancer cell line, MCF-7, estrogens specifically increase the secretion into the culture medium of a 52,000 dalton (52K) glycoprotein and stimulate cell proliferation (chapter 16). The 52K protein has been identified as a secreted precursor of a cathepsin D, and is mitogenic in vitro in estrogen-deprived MCF-7 cells. The concentration of total cellular cathepsin D is related to the proliferation of mammary ducts and to the prognosis of breast cancer. The 52K protease, according to Rochefort, appears to be useful as a tissue marker for predicting high-risk mastopathies and invasive breast cancers.

The transforming genes (oncogenes), and their cellular homologues, termed proto-oncogenes, have the ability to induce neoplastic growth. Specific mechanisms have been proposed in which proto-oncogenes cause cellular transformation, e.g., point mutation, gene truncation, transcriptional activation, and gene amplification. To date more than 20 proto-oncogenes have been identified and grouped into various categories. There are at least four ras genes in the human genome. Proto-oncogene ras^H, which is involved in tumorigenesis of human breast cancer cells, is the subject of discussion by Gelmann and co-workers (chapter 22). They investigated the influences of ras^H expression levels and activating mutations on tumorigenesis by these cells by transfecting into MCF-7 cells isogenic constructs of the ras^H gene with only single point mutations. Of the ras^H gene mutants, only the v-ras^H homologue conferred an increased incidence of tumor formation on the MCF-7 cells in the absence of estrogen, but estrogen was required for maximal tumor growth. The results of transgenic experiments described by the authors suggest that a mutated ras^H oncogene can contribute to the development of mammary carcinoma, but expression of the oncogenic transgene must be accompanied by other somatic events to generate tumors.

ANTIHORMONES AND MODE OF ACTION

Antisteroid hormones compete for hormone binding at the receptor level to prevent a hormonal response. Investigations with antiestrogens in human breast cancer cells in culture indicate that antiestrogens (e.g., tamoxifen) preferentially inhibit the proliferation of ER-containing breast cancer cells. Elucidation of the mechanisms by which antiestrogens inhibit proliferation and specific protein synthesis in target cells is the theme of chapter 15 by Katzenellenbogen and colleagues. It has been demonstrated that MCF-7 cells increase their proliferation rate and grow rapidly in the long-term absence of estrogen while showing high levels of ER, sensitivity to antiestrogens as measured by suppression of growth, and sensitivity to estrogen as measured by stimulation of cellular PR. Antiestrogens may suppress the proliferation of cancer cells by decreasing constitutive growth factor production or increasing growth inhibitors.

Antisteroid hormones appear to favor maintenance of SRs in larger aggregate forms, which afford less effective interaction with chromatin binding sites (20). Ruh et al. (chapter 17) have presented data to reveal that ER bound by antiestrogen, H1285, interacts with antiestrogen specific sites but binds poorly to some chromatin sites which preferentially bind ER complexes. The authors have suggested that distinct nonhistone chromosomal proteins may play a role in biological actions induced by estrogens and antiestrogens. In addition, Janne (115a) has provided evidence that although antiandrogens cause accumulation of AR in the renal nuclei, anti-ARc is unable to induce a hormonal response.

HORMONES AND BEHAVIOR

Gonadal steroids are secreted in response to signals emanating from the brain and are known to influence animal behavior. The actions of gonadal hormones on the reproductive tract and the brain influence synchronization of events related to successful reproduction. McEwen (chapter 19) has described his studies on the mechanism by which steroids regulate lardosis (mating) behavior of female rats in response to estradiol and progesterone. Induction of lardosis involves hormonal activation of the genome of a small group of neurons in the ventromedial hypothalamus (VMN). Exposure of the VMN to testosterone early in life renders the animal defeminized. McEwen demonstrated that since the VMN contains the same density of ER in male and female rats, factors other than receptor must contribute to sex differences.

COVALENT MODIFICATIONS OF STEROID RECEPTORS

Results of many published studies suggest that steroid binding as well as transformation of SRc may be influenced by phosphorylation-dephosphorylation reactions. As a result, there is a growing consensus that SRs are phosphoproteins. During the past five years, phosphorylation of various SRs has been reported both under physiological conditions and in cell-free systems. The physiological role of phosphorylation in receptor function, however, is still far from completely understood.

Identification and characterization of different protein kinases (PKs), which employ SRs as substrates, is being carried out in many laboratories. Weigel et al. (116) initially reported that the two known subunits of chicken PR, A and B (117), are substrates for cAMP-dependent PK (cAMP-PK) in vitro. The rapidity and the relative ease with which cAMP-PK could phosphorylate the receptor subunits at physiologic concentrations of the enzyme led Weigel et al. (118) to suggest that phosphorylation of receptor may be involved in the regulation of its function. Singh et al. (67) demonstrated that incubation of purified nontransformed chicken oviduct PR preparations with $[\gamma-^{32}P]ATP$ and cAMP-PK led to incorporation of radioactivity on serine residues in all three major peptides of PR. Isolation of PKs from the chicken oviduct which phosphorylate PR in vitro has also been reported (118). Recent results from Weigel's laboratory (personal communication) indicate chick PR is a good substrate for several kinases, including the catalytic subunit of the cAMP-PK, and a polypeptide-dependent PK. Phosphorylation by cAMP-PK results in an apparent increase in the molecular weight of the receptor (119). This is consistent with the finding that administration of progesterone results in increased phosphorylation of rabbit PR and an apparent increase in its molecular weight (120).

Sullivan et al. (chapter 6) present immunochemical analysis of avian PR, which demonstrates its existence in two forms, A (79K) and B (110K), both of which exist as phosphoproteins and whose origin and significance remain unclear. Excessive homogenization, storage of tissue and exposure to elevated temperature are conditions detrimental to the receptor's ability to bind steroid in target tissue cytosols. Within a 5-min period of progesterone administration, a time-dependent increase in receptor phosphorylation was evident, implying that receptor phosphorylation occurs very early in progesterone action.

Isolation of multiple phosphopeptides from tryptic digests of chicken oviduct PR-B phosphorylated in vivo has also been reported recently (121). This suggests that the receptor protein has multiple phosphorylation sites and may be phosphorylated under physiologic conditions by more than one enzyme (121). The 90K protein, which is now being recognized as a non-hormone binding subunit of the hetero-oligomeric nontransformed SR (63), was shown to be a substrate for a partially purified preparation of the nuclear type II casein kinase (122). Dougherty and co-workers (73) have also identified a 90K peptide which binds SR and serves as a substrate for rat liver type II casein kinase.

Chicken PR is phosphorylated in vitro by the epidermal growth factor (EGF) receptor, which is a tyrosine kinase (123). In another study, both the insulin and EGF receptors phosphorylated PR exclusively at tyrosine residues with maximal stoichiometries that were near unity (124). The substrate activity of PR for EGF and insulin receptor kinase may be a mechanism by which peptide hormones, including growth factors, could influence steroid hormone action at the level of a SR.

Steroid binding ability of uterine ER may be reversibly altered upon phosphorylation on tyrosine. Castoria et al. (chapter 10) have discussed identification of (i) a ca^{++}-stimulated kinase that phosphorylates ER on tyrosine and confers on it a hormone binding ability and (ii) a phosphotyrosine phosphatase whose action causes loss of hormone binding (125). Furthermore, phosphorylation on tyrosine is not a phenomenon unique to ER. Antiphosphotyrosine antibodies were shown to recognize both ER and rat liver GR.

Purified rat liver GR is a good substrate for phosphorylation in vitro by cAMP-PK (79). The process was exclusively dependent on exogenous kinase and Mg^{++} ions. Many Mg^{++}-dependent kinases are known to co-purify with SRs (126-128). Isolation and characterization of these protein kinases should provide information on the physiologic role of receptor phosphorylation. Phosphorylation of GR has been reported under physiological conditions (79). GR phosphorylated in these preparations represents a nontransformed receptor (79). Nontransformed GRc are heteromeric structures containing 100K steroid binding proteins and 90K nonsteroid binding proteins, both of which are phosphoproteins (68). The 90K non-steroid binding phosphoprotein is lost during thermal transformation in the intact cell(s) as well as under cell-free conditions.

In an effort to seek a possible role of phosphorylation in GR function, Gruol et al. (129) inquired whether murine lymphoma cells containing defective kinase activity would exhibit variants with an additional defect in steroid responsiveness. Using a WEHI-7 cell line, which contains two functional GR alleles, a new class of dexamethasone-resistant variants was identified from a cAMP-resistant population of WEHI-7 cells. The decreased levels of steroid binding observed in the dexamethasone resistant lines indicate that steroid resistance may involve alterations in functions which regulate receptor activity rather than mutations in the structural genes for receptor synthesis.

STEROID RECEPTORS AND PROTEIN KINASE ACTIVITIES

Receptors for various peptide hormones exhibit intrinsic PK activity that is considered important in the function-receptor structure relationship (130). There is, however, considerable disagreement over whether receptors for steroid hormones possess enzyme activity. Garcia et al. (131) were the first to report that highly purified avian PR contained PK activity. These investigators, however, have recently reported separation of PK activity from PR preparations (128). Kurl and Jacob (132) initially suggested that the dexamethasone affinity column-purified 90K GR from rat liver possessed Mg^{++}-dependent endogenous PK activity capable of phosphorylating the receptor molecule. Singh and Moudgil (133) obtained purified molybdate-stabilized rat liver GR preparations that exhibited PK activity, the extent of which was increased in the presence of exogenously added steroid. Litwack and co-workers have also described a PK activity associated with the purified, activated rat hepatic GR (134). Although it has been suggested that these observations do not unequivocally prove that GR displays PK activity, some recent reports have shown that kinase activity can be separated from the receptor (126,127). Physiologic relevance of SR-associated PK activity is, therefore, under close examination in many laboratories. Previous reports have also suggested an interaction between immobilized nucleotides and steroid receptors but it is not certain whether these results imply the presence of a nucleotide binding site on receptors that is characteristic of protein kinases (22,34,135-141).

Lack of unanimity in the results published on the potential PK activity of SR suggests that biological implications of these observations must be considered. If the recent reports, which indicate that SRs are localized in the nucleus, even in the absence of ligand, are correct, then receptors might exert their action by phosphorylating chromatin proteins, thereby modulating transcription of specific genes (131,133). This postulation is relevant to the widely accepted view that SRs function as regulators of gene expression. Autokinase activity of receptor or phosphorylation of other substrates by receptor may also influence the modulation of steroid binding and regulation of receptor conformation.

SUMMARY, CONCLUSION AND FUTURE DIRECTIONS

The recent anatomical analysis of the structure of SRs and their genes has brought us into a new era of investigations on hormone action. These developments will allow a close examination and scrutiny of receptor structure, the gene(s) responsible for their synthesis, and the cellular factor(s) which would potentially modulate both the gene expression and receptor activity. Among the fundamental questions that need answering is one that addresses clearly the role of hormone in target cell responses. Is hormone limited merely to binding to the receptor, or is it involved in exposing certain domains of ligand-free receptor which are eclipsed by cellular components? Does it merely navigate the SRs to select sequences on the hormone-responsive genome? Modifications of receptor structure that influence its cellular regulation should also be examined to learn more about the flexibility of the target cell response to reversibly controlled hormone-dependent alterations. Future work in the molecular biology of steroid receptors should aid in understanding the precise structure-functional relationship, and allow in vitro mutagenesis to locate the inter-receptor binding regions and correlate them with a function or biological activity.

The observations on the modifications of receptor structure and function via phosphorylation require delineation of its significance. Which particular aspects or cellular components of a receptor system are influenced by phosphorylation and can also be associated with a biological function? For example, which of the functions of SRs is primarily influenced by phosphorylation: hormone binding, receptor transformation, nuclear binding or interaction of receptor with nuclear components such as acceptor sites? The identity of the activities which co-purify with receptor, and whether these are intrinsic to receptors or are separable from it, is an important question. If certain enzymes co-purify with the receptor, are these associated with the receptor physiologically? Various aspects of steroid hormone action discussed in this article and the related work presented in this volume will aid in arriving at a better understanding of the structure and function of SRs. As the mysteries of hormone action are unveiled, society will benefit distinctly from the clinical applications of these scientific revelations.

ACKNOWLEDGEMENTS

The work in the author's laboratory is supported by National Institutes of Health grant DK-20893. The critical reading of the manuscript by Cliff Hurd and the valuable editorial assistance provided by Deborah Szobel are gratefully appreciated.

REFERENCES

1. Moudgil VK, ed. Recent advances in steroid hormone action. Berlin: Walter de Gruyter, 1987.
2. Toft D, Gorski J. A receptor molecule for estrogens: isolation from the rat uterus and preliminary characterization. Proc Natl Acad Sci USA 1966; 55:1574-81.
3. Jensen EV, Suzuki T, Kawashima T, Stumpf WE, Jungblut PW, DeSombre ER. A two-step mechanism for the interaction of estradiol with rat uterus. Proc Natl Acad Sci USA 1968; 59:632-8.
4. Gorski J, Toft DO, Shyamala G, Smith D, Notides A. Hormone receptors: studies on the interaction of estrogen with the uterus. Recent Prog Horm Res 1968; 24:45-80.
5. Sheridan PJ, Buchanan JM, Anselmo VC, Martin PM. Equilibrium: the intracellular distribution of steroid receptors. Nature 1979; 282:579-82.
6. Welshons WV, Lieberman ME, Gorski J. Nuclear localization of unoccupied oestrogen receptors. Nature 1984; 307:747-9.
7. King WJ, Greene GL. Monoclonal antibodies localize oestrogen receptor in the nuclei of target cells. Nature 1984; 307:745-7.
8. Welshons WV, Krummel BM, Gorski J. Nuclear localization of unoccupied receptors for glucocorticoids, estrogens, and progesterone in GH$_3$ cells. Endocrinology 1985; 117:2140-7.
9. Shull JD, Welshons WA, Lieberman ME, Gorski J. The rat pituitary estrogen receptor: role of the nuclear receptor in the regulation of transcription of the prolactin gene and the nuclear localization of the unoccupied receptor. In Moudgil VK, ed. Molecular mechanism of steroid hormone action: recent advances. Berlin: Walter de Gruyter, 1985:539-62.

10. Perrot-Applanat M, Logeat F, Groyer-Picard MT, Milgrom E. Immunocyt-ochemical study of mammalian progesterone receptor using monoclonal antibodies. Endocrinology 1985; 116:1473-84.

11. Callard GV, Mak P. Exclusive nuclear location of estrogen receptors in Squilus testis. Proc Natl Acad Sci USA 1985; 82:1336-40.

12. Walters SN, Reinhardt TA, Domonick MA, Horst RL, Littledike ET. Intracellular location of unoccupied 1, 25-dihydroxyvitamin D recep-tors: a nuclear-cytoplasmic equilibrium. Arch Biochem Biophys 1985; 262:366-73.

13. Gasc JM, Renoir JM, Radanyi C, Joab I, Tuohimaa P, Baulieu EE. Pro-gesterone receptor in the chick oviduct: an immunohistochemical study with antibodies to distinct receptor components. J Cell Biol 1984; 99:1193-201.

14. Szego CM, Pietras RJ. Subcellular distribution of oestrogen recep-tors. Nature 1985; 317:88-9.

15. Jensen EV. Intracellular localization of estrogen receptors: Implications for interaction mechanism. Lab Invest 1984; 51:487-8.

16. Schrader WT. New model for steroid hormone receptors? Nature 1984; 308:17-8.

17. Gorski J, Welshons W, Sakai D. Review: remodeling the estrogen receptor model. Mol Cell Endocrinol 1984; 36:11-5.

18. Skafar DF, Notides AC. Modulation of the estrogen receptor's affin-ity for DNA by estradiol. J Biol Chem 1985; 22:12208-13.

19. Hansen JC. Characterization of the conformational transitions of the estrogen receptor monomer by partition in aqueous two-phase systems [Dissertation]. University of Wisconsin-Madison, 1986.

20. Moudgil VK, Hurd C. Transformation of calf uterine progesterone receptor: analysis of the process when receptor is bound to proges-terone and RU 38486. Biochemistry 1987; 26:4993-5001.

21. Hurd C, Moudgil VK. Impaired transformation of mammalian proges-terone receptor bound to progesterone antagonist RU486 [Abstract]. Proc Endo Soc, Anaheim, 1986; 1008.

22. Moudgil VK, Eessalu TE, Paulose CS, Taylor MG, Hansen JC. Activation of progesterone receptor by ATP. Eur J Biochem 1981; 118:547-55.

23. Moudgil VK, Eessalu TE, Buchou T, Renoir JM, Mester J, Baulieu EE. Transformation of chick oviduct progesterone receptor in vitro: effects of hormone, salt, heat and adenosine triphosphate. Endo-crinology 1985; 116:1267-74.

24. Moudgil VK, Lombardo G, Eessalu T, Eliezer N. Hormone dependency of transformation of rat liver glucocorticoid receptor in vitro: effects of heat, salt and nucleotides. J Biochem 1986; 99:1005-16.

25. Hansen JC, Gorski J. Conformational and electrostatic properties of unoccupied and liganded estrogen receptors determined by aqueous two-phase partitioning. Biochemistry 1985; 24:6078-85.

26. Andreasen PA, Junker K. Specific effects of monovalent cations and of adenine nucleotides on glucocorticoid receptor activation, as studied by aqueous two-phase partitioning. In: Moudgil VK, ed. Molecular mechanism of steroid hormone action: recent advances. Berlin: Walter de Gruyter, 1985; 199-224.

27. Moudgil VK, Vandenheede L, Hurd C, Eliezer N, Lombardo G. In vitro modulation of rat liver glucocorticoid receptor by urea. J Biol Chem 1987; 262:5180-7.

28. Hansen JC, Gorski J. Conformational transitions of the estrogen receptor monomer. Effects of estrogens, antiestrogen, and tem-perature. J Biol Chem 1986; 261:13990-6.

29. Jensen EV, DeSombre ER. Estrogen-receptor interaction. Science 1973; 182;126-34.

30. Moudgil VK. Progesterone receptor. In: Agarwal MK, ed. Principles of recepterology. Berlin: Walter de Gruyter, 1983:273-381.

31. Moudgil VK. Interaction of nucleotides with steroid receptors. In:

Moudgil VK, ed. Molecular mechanism of steroid hormone action: recent advances. Berlin: Walter de Gruyter, 1985:351-76.

32. Milgrom E, Atger M, Baulieu EE. Acidophilic activation of steroid hormone receptors. Biochemistry 1973; 12:5198-205.

33. John JK, Moudgil VK. Activation of glucocorticoid receptor by ATP. Biochem Biophys Res Commun 1979; 90:1242-8.

34. Moudgil VK, John JK. Interaction of rat liver glucocorticoid receptor with adenosine 5'-triphosphate. Characterization of interaction by use of ATP-Sepharose affinity chromatography. Biochem J 1980; 190:809-18.

35. Munck A, Foley R. Activation of steroid hormone-receptor complexes in intact cells in physiological conditions. Nature 1979; 278:752-4.

36. Liao S, Liang T, Tymoczko JL. Ribonucleoprotein binding of steroid receptor complexes. Nature New Biol 1973; 241:211-3.

37. Liao S, Smythe S, Tymoczko JL, et al. RNA-dependent release of androgen- and other steroid-receptor complexes from DNA. J Biol Chem 1980; 255:5545-51.

38. Rossini GP. Molybdate inhibits glucocorticoid receptor complex binding to DNA. Mol Cell Endocrinol 1987; 49:129-35.

39. Schmidt TJ, Diehl EE, Davidson CJ, et al. Effects of bovine pancreatic ribonuclease A, S protein, and S peptide on activation of purified rat hepatic glucocorticoid receptor complexes. Biochemistry 1986; 25:5955-61.

40. Rossini GP. RNA containing nuclear sites for glucocorticoid receptor complexes. Biochem Biophys Res Commun 1984; 123:78-83.

41. Tymoczko JL, Phillips MM. The effects of ribonuclease on rat liver dexamethasone receptor: increased affinity for deoxyribonucleic acid and altered sedimentation profile. Endocrinology 1983; 112:142-9.

42. Tymoczko JL, Phillips MM, Vernon SS. Binding of the rat liver 7-8 S dexamethasone receptor to deoxyribonucleic acid. Arch Biochem Biophys 1984; 230:345-54.

43. Economidis IV, Rousseau GG. Association of the glucocorticoid hormone receptor with ribonucleic acid. FEBS Lett 1985; 181:47-52.

44. Liang T, Liao S. Association of the uterine 17β-estradiol receptor complex with ribonucleic-protein in vitro and in vivo. J Biol Chem 1974; 249:4671-78.

45. Thomas T, Kiang DT. Ribonuclease-induced transformation of progesterone receptor from rabbit uterus. J Steroid Biochem 1986; 24:505-11.

46. Tymoczko JL, Anderson EE, Lee JH, Unger AL. Studies with chymotrypsin and RNAs showing a hetero-oligomeric structure of the glucocorticoid receptor complex from rat liver which is stabilized by a low molecular weight factor. Biochem Biophys Acta 1986; 888:296-305.

47. Webb ML, Schmidt TJ, Robertson NM, Litwack G. Evidence for an association of a ribonucleic acid with purified, unactivated glucocorticoid receptor. Biochem Biophys Res Commun 1986; 140:204-11.

48. Rowley DR, Premont RT, Johnson MP, Young CYF, Tindall DJ. Properties of an intermediate-sized androgen receptor: association with RNA. Biochemistry 1986; 25:6988-95.

49. Lamb DJ, Kima PE, Bullock DW. Occurrence of a 6S intermediate form of the progesterone receptor that is sensitive to ribonuclease. Mol Cell Biochem 1987; 73:77-84.

50. Kovacic-Milivojevic BK, LaPointe MC, Reker CE, Vedeckis WV. Ribonucleic acid is a component of the oligomeric, transformed mouse AtT-20 cell glucocorticoid receptor. Biochemistry 1985; 24:7357-66.

51. Ali M, Vedeckis WV. The glucocorticoid receptor protein binds to transfer RNA. Science 1987; 235:467-70.

52. Ali M, Vedeckis WV. Interaction of RNA with transformed glucocorticoid receptor. J Biol Chem 1987; 262:2671-7.

53. Reker CE, Kovacic-Milivojevic B, Eastman-Rekers SB, Vedeckis WV. Transformed mouse glucocorticoid receptor: generation and intercon-

version of the 3.8S monomeric, and 5.2S oligomeric species. Biochemistry 1985; 24:196-204.

54. Anderson EE, Tymoczko JL. Stabilization of glucocorticoid receptor association with RNA by a low molecular weight factor from rat liver cytosol. J Steroid Biochem 1985; 23:299-306.

55. Kovacic-Milivojevic B, Vedeckis WV. Absence of detectable ribonucleic acid in the purified untransformed mouse glucocorticoid receptor. Biochemistry 1986; 25:8266-73.

56. Nishigori H, Toft DO. Inhibition of progesterone receptor activation by sodium molybdate. Biochemistry 1980; 19:77-83.

57. Toft DO, Nishigori H. Stabilization of the avian progesterone receptor by inhibitors. J Steroid Biochem 1979; 11:413-16.

58. Puri RK, Grandics P, Dougherty JJ, Toft DO. Purification of nontransformed avian progesterone receptor and preliminary characterization. J Biol Chem 1982; 257:10831-7.

59. Renoir JM, Yang CR, Formstecher P, et al. Progesterone receptor from chick oviduct: purification of molybdate-stabilized form and preliminary characterization. Eur J Biochem 1982; 127:71-9.

60. Dougherty JJ, Puri RK, Toft DO. Phosphorylation in vivo of chicken oviduct progesterone receptor. J Biol Chem 1982; 257:14226-30.

61. Birnbaumer M, Bell RC, Schrader WT, O'Malley BW. The putative molybdate-stabilized progesterone receptor subunit is not a steroid-binding protein. J Biol Chem 1984; 259:1091-8.

62. Dougherty JJ, Toft DO. Characterization of two 8S forms of chick oviduct progesterone receptor. J Biol Chem 1982; 257:3113-9.

63. Joab I, Radanyi C, Renoir JM, et al. Common non-hormone binding component in nontransformed chick oviduct receptors of four steroid hormones. Nature 1984; 308:850-3.

64. Riehl RM, Sullivan WP, Vroman BT, Bauer VT, Pearson GR, Toft DO. Immunological evidence that the non-hormone binding component of avian steroid receptors exists in a wide range of tissues and species. Biochemistry 1985; 24:6586-91.

65. Renoir JM, Buchou T, Baulieu EE. Involvement of a non-hormone binding 90-kilodalton protein in the nontransformed 8S form of the rabbit uterus progesterone receptor. Biochemistry 1986; 25:6405-13.

66. Housley PR, Sanchez ER, Westphal HH, Beato M, Pratt WB. The molybdate-stabilized L-cell glucocorticoid receptor isolated by affinity chromatography or with a monoclonal antibody is associated with a 90-92K nonsteroid binding phosphoprotein. J Biol Chem 1985; 260:13810-7.

67. Singh VB, Eliezer N, Moudgil VK. Transformation and phosphorylation of purified molybdate stabilized chicken oviduct progesterone receptor. Biochim Biophys Acta 1986; 888:237-48.

68. Mendel DB, Bodwell JE, Gametchu B, Harrison RW, Munck A. Molybdate-stabilized nonactivated glucocorticoid-receptor complexes contain a 90K-Da steroid binding phosphoprotein that is lost on activation. J Biol Chem 1986; 261;3758-63.

69. Schlesinger MJ, Ashburner M, Tissieres A, eds. Heat shock: from bacteria to man. New York: Cold Spring Harbor Laboratory, Cold Spring Harbor, 1982.

70. Schuh SS, Yonemoto W, Brugge J, Bauer VJ, Riehl RM, Sullivan WP, Toft DO. A 90,000-dalton binding protein common to both steroid receptors and the Rouse Sarcoma Virus transforming protein pp60^{v-src}. J Biol Chem 1985; 26:14292-6.

71. Sanchez ER, Toft DO, Schlesinger MJ, Pratt WB. Evidence that the 90-kDa phosphoprotein associated with the untransformed L-cell glucocorticoid receptor is a murine heat shock protein. J Biol Chem 1985; 260:12398-401.

72. Catelli MG, Binart N, Feramisco JR, Helfman DM. Cloning of the chick hsp 90 cDNA in expression vector. Nucleic Acids Res 1985; 13:6035-47.

73. Dougherty JJ, Rabideau DA, Iannotti AM, Sullivan WP, Toft DO. Identification of the 90-kDa substrate of rat liver type II casein kinase with the heat shock protein which binds steroid receptors. Biochim Biophys Acta 1987; 927:74-80.

74. Renoir JM, Radanyi C, Devin J, Baulieu EE. Cytosol rabbit progesterone receptor-RU486 complex is not readily activated because the antagonist does not promote dissociation of hsp90 from the steroid binding protein [Abstract]. Proceedings of the Meadow Brook Conference on Steroid Receptors in Health and Disease. Rochester, Michigan, 1987:23.

75. Lefebvre P, Formstecher P, Dautrevaux M. Correlation between antiglucocorticoid activity and ability to stabilize the interaction between the glucocorticoid receptor and the 90k non steroid binding protein [Abstract]. Proceedings of the Meadow Brook Conference on Steroid Receptors in Health and Disease. Rochester, Michigan, 1987:7.

76. Moudgil VK, Nishigori H, Eessalu TE, Toft DO. Analysis of the avian progesterone receptor with inhibitors. In: Roy A, Clark JH, eds. Gene regulation by steroid hormones. New York: Springer-Verlag, 1980:103-19.

77. Barnett CA, Schmidt TJ, Litwack G. Effects of calf intestinal alkaline phosphatase, phosphatase inhibitors and phosphorylated compounds on the rate of activation of glucocorticoid-receptor complexes. Biochemistry 1980; 19:5446-55.

78. Leach KL, Dahmer MK, Hammond ND, Sando JJ, Pratt WB. Molybdate inhibition of glucocorticoid receptor inactivation and transformation. J Biol Chem 1979; 254:11884-90.

79. Singh VB, Moudgil VK. Phosphorylation of rat liver glucocorticoid receptor. J Biol Chem 1985; 260:3684-90.

80. Murakami N, Moudgil VK. Inactivation of rat liver glucocorticoid receptor by molybdate. Biochem J 1981; 198:447-55.

81. Murakami N, Moudgil VK. Interaction of rat liver glucocorticoid receptor with sodium tungstate. Biochem J 1982; 204:777-86.

82. Housley PR, Dahmer MK, Pratt WB. Inactivation of glucocorticoid-binding capacity by protein phosphatases in the presence of molybdate and complete reactivation by dithiothreitol. J Biol Chem 1982; 257:8615-8.

83. Green S, Chambon P. A superfamily of potentially oncogenic hormone receptors. Nature 1986; 324:615-7.

84. Green S, Walter P, Kumar V, Krust A, Bornet JM, Argos P, Chambon P. Human oestrogen receptor cDNA: sequence expression and homology to v-erb-A. Nature 1986; 320:134-9.

85. Kumar V, Green S, Staub A, Chambon P. Localization of the oestradiol-binding and putative DNA-binding domains of the human oestrogen receptor. EMBO J 1986; 5:2231-6.

86. Green S, Kumar V, Krust A, Chambon P. The oestrogen receptor: structure and function. In: Moudgil VK, ed. Recent advances in steroid hormone action. Berlin: Walter de Gruyter, 1987:161-83.

87. Willmann T, Beato M. Steroid-free glucocorticoid receptor binds specifically to mouse mammary tumor virus DNA. Nature 1986; 324:688-91.

88. Bailly A, Le Page C, Rauch M, Milgrom E. Sequence-specific DNA binding of the progesterone receptor to the uteroglobin gene: effects of hormone, antihormone and receptor phosphorylation. EMBO J 1986; 5:3235-41.

89. Giguere S, Hollenberg SM, Rosenfeld MG, Evans RM. Functional domains of the human glucocorticoid receptor. Cell 1986; 46:645-52.

90. Becker PB, Gloss B, Schmid W, Strahle U, Schutz G. In vivo protein-DNA interactions in a glucocorticoid response element require the presence of the hormone. Nature 1986; 326:686-8.

91. Godowski PJ, Rusconi S, Miesfeld R, Yamamoto KR. Glucocorticoid

receptor mutants that are constitutive activators of transcriptional enhancement. Nature 1987; 325:365-8.

92. Hollenberg SM, Giguere V, Sequi P, Evans RM. Colocalization of DNA binding and transcriptional activation functions in the human glucocorticoid receptor. Cell 1987; 49:39-46.

93. Spelsberg TC, Horton M, Fink K, et al. A new model for steroid regulation of gene transcription using acceptor sites and regulatory genes and their products. In: Moudgil VK, ed. Recent advances in steroid hormone action. Berlin: Walter de Gruyter, 1987:59-83.

94. Ruh MF, Ruh TS. Antiestrogen action: properties of the estrogen receptor and chromatin acceptor sites. In: Moudgil VK, ed. Recent advances in steroid hormone action. Berlin: Walter de Gruyter, 1987:109-31.

95. Barrack ER. Specific association of androgen receptors and estrogen receptors with the nuclear matrix: summary and perspectives. In: Moudgil VK, ed. Recent advances in steroid hormone action. Berlin: Walter de Gruyter, 1987:85-107.

96. Yamamoto KR. Steroid receptor regulated transcription of specific genes and gene networks. Annu Rev Genet 1985; 19:209-52.

97. Payvar F, Wrange O, Carlstedt-Duke J, Okret S, Gustafsson JA, Yamamoto KR. Purified glucocorticoid receptors bind selectively in vitro to a cloned DNA fragment whose transcription is regulated by glucocorticoids in vivo. Proc Natl Acad Sci USA 1981; 78:6628-32.

98. Pfahl M. Specific binding of the glucocorticoid-receptor complex to the mouse mammary tumor proviral promotor region. Cell 1982; 31: 475-82.

99. Govindan MV, Spiess E, Majors J. Purified glucocorticoid receptor-hormone complex from rat liver cytosol binds specifically to cloned mouse mammary tumor virus long terminal repeats in vitro. Proc Natl Acad Sci USA 1982; 79:5157-61.

100. Moore DD, Marks AR, Buckley DI, Kapler G, Payvar F, Goodman HM. The first intron of the human growth hormone gene contains a binding site for glucocorticoid receptor. Proc Natl Acad Sci USA 1985; 82:699-702.

101. Bechet D. Control of gene expression by steroid hormones. Reprod Nutr Develop 1986; 26:1025-55.

102. Mulvihill ER, Le Pennee JP, Chambon P. Chicken oviduct progesterone receptor: location of specific regions of high affinity binding in cloned DNA fragments of hormone-responsive genes. Cell 1982; 24:621-32.

103. Compton JG, Schrader WT, O'Malley BW. DNA sequence preference of the progesterone receptor. Proc Natl Acad Sci USA 1983; 80:16-20.

104. Karin M, Haslinger A, Holtgreve H, Richards RI, Krauter P, Westphal HM, Beato M. Characterization of DNA sequences through which cadmium and glucocorticoid hormones induce human metaollthionine in-11A gene. Nature 1984; 308:513-9.

105. Groner B, Kennedy N, Skroch P, Hynes NE, Ponta H. DNA sequences involved in the regulation of gene expression by glucocorticoid hormones. Biochim Biophys Acta 1984; 781:1-6.

106. Scheidereit C, Beato M. Contacts between hormone receptor and DNA double helix within a glucocorticoid regulating element of mouse mammary tumor virus. Proc Natl Acad Sci USA 1984; 81:3029-33.

107. Jost JP, Seldran M, Geiser M. Preferential binding of estrogen-receptor complex to a region containing the estrogen-dependent hypomethylation site preceding the chicken vitellogenin II gene. Proc Natl Acad Sci USA 1984; 81:429-33.

108. Lee F, Mulligan R, Berg P, Ringold G. Glucocorticoids regulate expression of dehydrofolate reductase cDNA in mouse mammary tumor virus chimeric plasmids. Nature 1981; 294:228-32.

109. Renkawitz R, Beng H, Graf T, Matthias P, Grez M, Schutz G. Expression of a chicken lysozome recombinant gene is regulated by proges-

terone and dexamethasone after microinjection into oviduct cells. Cell 1982; 31:168-76.

110. Dean DC, Knoll BJ, Riser ME, O'Malley BW. A 5'-flanking sequence essential for progesterone regulation of an ovalbumin fusion gene. Nature 1983; 305:551-4.

111. Miesfeld R, Okret S, Wikstrom A, et al. Characterization of a steroid hormone receptor gene and mRNA in wild type and mutant cells. Nature 1984; 312:779-81.

112. Hollenberg SM, Weinberger C, Ong ES, et al. Primary structure and expression of a functional human glucocorticoid receptor cDNA. Nature 1985; 318:635-41.

113. Krust A, Green S, Argos P, et al. The chicken estrogen receptor sequence: homology with v-erb A and the human oestrogen and glucocorticoid receptors. EMBO J 1986; 5:891-7.

114. Jeltsch JM, Krozowski Z, Quirin-Stricker C, et al. Cloning of the chicken progesterone receptor. Proc Natl Acad Sci USA 1986; 83: 5424-8.

115. Conneely DM, Sullivan WP, Toft DO, et al. Molecular cloning of the chicken progesterone receptor. Science 1986; 233:767-70.

115a. Janne OA. Androgen regulation of gene expression [Abstract]. Program of the Meadow Brook Conference on Steroid Receptors in Health and Disease, Rochester, Michigan, 1987.

116. Weigel NL, Tash JS, Means AR, Schrader WT, O'Malley BW. Phosphorylation of hen progesterone receptor by cAMP dependent protein kinase. Biochem Biophys Res Commun 1981; 102:513-9.

117. Schrader WT, Birnbaumer ME, Hughes MR, Weigel NL, Grody WW, O'Malley RW. Studies on the structure and function of the chicken progesterone receptor. Recent Prog Horm Res 1981; 37;583-633.

118. Weigel NL. Isolation of protein kinase from chicken oviduct which phosphorylate the progesterone receptor in vitro [Abstract]. In: Excerpta Medica, Abstracts of the 7th International Cong Endocrinol. New York: Elsevier Science Publishers, 1984:2710.

119. Denner LA, Bingman WE, Weigel NL. Phosphorylation of the chicken progesterone receptor [Abstract]. Proc VII Internatl Cong Horm Steroids, Madrid, 1986.

120. Logeat F, LeCunff M, Pamphile R, Milgrom E. The nuclear-bound form of the progesterone receptor is generated through a hormone-dependent phosphorylation. Biochem Biophys Res Commun 1985; 131:421-7.

121. Puri RK, Toft DO. Peptide mapping analysis of the avian progesterone receptor. J Biol Chem 1986; 260:5651-7.

122. Dougherty JJ. Phosphorylation of progesterone receptor. In: Moudgil VK, ed. Molecular mechanism of steroid hormone action: recent advances. Berlin: Walter de Gruyter, 1985:299-308.

123. Ghosh-Dastidar P, Coty WA, Griest RE, Woo DDL, Fox CF. Progesterone receptor subunits are high-affinity substrates for phosphorylation by epidermal growth factor receptor. Proc Natl Acad Sci USA 1984; 81:1654-8.

124. Woo DDL, Fay SP, Griest R, Coty W, Goldfine I, Fox CF. Differential phosphorylation of the progesterone receptor by insulin epidermal growth factor, and platelet-derived growth factor receptor tyrosine protein kinases. J Biol Chem 1986; 261:460-7.

125. Auricchio F, Migliaccio A, Rotondi A, Castoria G. Phosphorylation of tyrosine of the 17-beta estradiol. In: Moudgil VK, ed. Molecular mechanism of steroid hormone action: recent advances. Berlin: Walter de Gruyter, 1985:279-98.

126. Sanchez ER, Pratt WB. Phosphorylation of L-cell glucocorticoid receptors in immune complexes: evidence that the receptor is not a protein kinase. Biochemistry 1986; 25:1378-82.

127. Hapgood JP, Sabbatini GP, Holt CV. Rat liver glucocorticoid receptor isolated by affinity chromatography is not a Mg^{2+}- or Ca^{2+}- dependent protein kinase. Biochemistry 1986; 25:7529-34.

128. Garcia T, Buchou T, Renoir JM, Mester J, Baulieu EE. A protein kinase copurified with chick oviduct. Biochemistry 1986; 25:7937-42.

129. Gruol DJ, Campbell NF, Bourgeois S. Cyclic AMP-dependent protein kinase promotes glucocorticoid receptor function. J Biol Chem 1986; 261:4909-14.

130. Carter-Su C, Pratt WB. Receptor phosphorylation. In: Conn PM, ed. The receptors; vol I. New York: Academic Press, 1984:541-85.

131. Garcia T, Tuohimaa P, Mester J, Buchou T, Renoir JM, Baulieu EE. Protein kinase activity of purified components of the chicken oviduct progesterone receptor. Biochem Biophys Res Commun 1983; 113:960-6.

132. Kurl RN, Jacob ST. Phosphorylation of purified glucocorticoid receptor from rat liver by an endogenous protein kinase. Biochem Biophys Res Commun 1984; 119:700-5.

133. Singh VB, Moudgil VK. Protein kinase activity of purified rat liver glucocorticoid receptor. Biochem Biophys Res Commun 1984; 125:1067-73.

134. Miller-Diener A, Schmidt TJ, Litwack G. Protein kinase activity associated with the purified rat hepatic glucocorticoid receptor. Proc Natl Acad Sci USA 1985; 82;4003-7.

135. Moudgil VK, Toft DO. Binding of ATP to progesterone receptors. Proc Natl Acad Sci USA 1975; 72:901-5.

136. Moudgil VK, Toft, DO. Binding of progesterone receptors to immobilized adenosine triphosphate. Biochim Biophys Acta 1977; 490:477-88.

137. Moudgil VK, John JK. ATP-dependent activation of glucocorticoid receptor from rat liver cytosol. Biochem J 1980; 190:799-808.

138. Moudgil VK, Eessalu TE. Activation of estradiol receptor complex by ATP in vitro. FEBS Lett 1980; 122:189-92.

139. Miller JB, Toft DO. Requirement for activation in the binding of progesterone receptor to ATP-Sepharose. Biochemistry 1978; 17:173-77.

140. Moudgil VK. Interaction of nucleotides with steroid hormone receptors. In: Moudgil VK, ed. Molecular mechanism of steroid hormone action: recent advances. Berlin: Walter de Gruyter, 1985:351-76.

141. McBlain WA, Toft DO. Interaction of chick oviduct progesterone receptor with the 2',3'-dialdehyde derivative of adenosine 5'-triphosphate. Biochemistry 1983; 22:2262-70.

2

STEROID RECEPTORS: A HISTORICAL PERSPECTIVE

Jack Gorski

Department of Biochemistry
University of Wisconsin, 420 Henry Mall
Madison, WI 53706

Receptor theory got its start over a century ago when Langley (1) proposed that tissues contained specific substances that combined with drugs to produce their effects. However, it was not until 1959 that the direct demonstration of tissue binding of a cell regulator was reported. Jensen and associates (2) and Glascock and Hoekstra (3) observed that target organs of the estrogens retained more labeled estrogen than non-target organs after systemic administration of the labeled hormone. Thus was born the concept of the estrogen receptor and the whole field of experimental receptorology.

The years between 1879 and 1959 were important in the elucidation of the structure of the steroid hormones, the enzymes, the genetic apparatus and many of the other cell components. Information concerning regulatory mechanisms lagged, however, and was often negatively influenced by the focus of investigators on metabolism, enzymes and enzyme cofactors.

The study of regulatory biology in animal systems in the 1950s was dominated by the impact of biochemists who had worked out the details of intermediary metabolism, including the enzymes and cofactors required for each step. The vitamins, which like the hormones are found in very small amounts, were shown to be cofactors in the metabolic reactions of the enzymes. The vitamins took part in the reactions and were themselves reversibly metabolized. It had been predicted by enzymologists (4) that hormones would also turn out to be associated with enzymes as cofactors. I can remember attending a symposium in the early 1960s along with neuro-biologists who still were studying acetylcholinesterase as a model system for neurotransmitter receptors.

The focus on metabolism had a great impact on studies of steroid hormone action. The bulk of the work in the 1950s concerned the metab-olism of the steroids in various target and non-target tissues. The search for new metabolites was in vogue with the goal being to find the key metabolite involved in the action of a particular steroid hormone. The culmination of the metabolic period of steroid hormone action studies was the development of the transhydrogenase theory which was based on observations that in the human placenta estradiol metabolism was asso-ciated with both the pyridine nucleotide cofactors, NADP and NAD (Fig. 1) (5). Furthermore, it was noted that at low concentrations of estradiol or estrone, reduced NAD (NADH) could transfer reducing equivalents to NADP.

This reaction was thought to involve an estrogen dependent transhydrogenase in which the estradiol/estrone acted as an oxidation/reduction cofactor. The resulting reduced NADP (NADPH) was thought to stimulate biosynthetic reactions that require this pyridine nucleotide. The transhydrogenase theory was widely accepted and was noted in biochemistry texts of that era. Its acceptance was dictated by the widespread interest and knowledge about metabolism that pervaded biology and biochemistry at that time. An anecdote that illustrates this was told to me by Elwood Jensen. Jensen made the first report of his work on tissue retention of estrogens at the 1958 International Congress of Biochemistry in Vienna. To an audience of 5, he presented the data that were to drastically change all of endocrinology. Ironically, at the same time a large audience was in attendance at a symposium about transhydrogenases. The widespread acceptance of the now defunct transhydrogenase theory should remind us that even good scientists can be misled by preconceived ideas or wishful thinking. Working in the current era of molecular biology presents similar dangers.

Even in the 1950s, careful examination of the data supporting the transhydrogenase theory raised serious questions about its physiological relevance. For example, diethylstilbestrol, a very potent estrogen, has phenolic hydroxyls that would be unlikely to be metabolized by the same enzyme that metabolizes the 17-hydroxyl of estradiol. In addition, the transhydrogenase was found principally in the placenta, which is not generally considered to be an estrogen target tissue, whereas it was not found in uterine tissue, which is very responsive to estrogens.

The 1950s also gave birth to the new field that we now call molecular biology. The concept that DNA coded for RNA that in turn coded for proteins was established at this time with the operon theory of gene regulation in bacteria presented by Jacob and Monod in 1961 (6). These concepts would have a great impact on all of biology including the study of hormone action.

In 1953 Szego and Roberts (7) presented a summary of their work including a model of estrogen action that is surprisingly similar to current models. They suggested that the steroid hormones interacted with specific proteins in target tissues resulting in the synthesis of new proteins. Mueller and his associates (1985) (8) were the first investigators in the steroid action area to develop a model that made use of concepts arising from studies of bacterial gene regulation. In 1957 at the Laurentian Hormone Conference, Mueller presented the model shown in Figure 2. While some of the terminology differs, it is apparent that there are many similarities with current models of steroid hormone action. Mueller's group initiated studies and presented data indicating that estrogen had a marked influence on several components of the protein and RNA synthesis systems. Thus the concept that nuclear events might be associated with estrogen action had already been introduced in the 1950s before the steroid receptor was actually discovered. This set the stage for the work of the next decade.

The discovery of the steroid receptors, like many other breakthroughs in biology, was due to an advance in methodology. Jensen and associates as well as Glascock and Hoekstra made use of new methods of tritium labeling that resulted for the first time in steroids with very high specific activity. These high specific activities were required for physiological concentrations of the labeled steroid to be administered. Earlier studies using low specific activity steroids had revealed nothing about target tissues to distinguish them from non-target tissues. Figure 3 shows some of the original data of Jensen and Jacobson (2) demonstrating that the uterus retains the administered estrogen differentially when compared to liver or muscle. When the radioactive estrogen from the

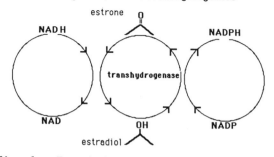

Fig. 1. Transhydrogenase model of estrogen action circa 1958.

uterus was examined by chromatography and other separation techniques, it showed no signs of any metabolism. Because of the widespread belief in the transhydrogenase theory, Jensen went to great lengths to prove that metabolism of the estrogen was not occurring. A particularly elegant study compared tritium labeling at the 17 to the 6,7 positions of estradiol to ensure that a recycling equilibrium between estrone and estradiol did not occur. The data were all consistent in showing that estrogen was not metabolized during the time it was bringing about its tissue response. That was the end of the transhydrogenase theory.

After the initial breakthrough by Jensen et al. and Glascock and Hoekstra, high specific activity steroids became generally available and studies of steroid receptors were carried out in a number of laboratories. This led to the isolation of the receptors and to the determination of their subcellular localization and differential affinity for various steroids (9,10). It also meant that running sucrose gradients became a way of life for certain graduate students and postdoctoral fellows.

A complementary development in studies of steroid hormone action was the use of inhibitors of protein and RNA synthesis to demonstrate the essential role of macromolecular synthesis. Mueller et al. (11) were first to use this approach by showing that puromycin, a protein synthesis

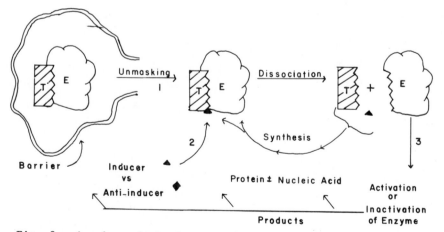

Fig. 2. A scheme depicting possible sites of hormonal regulation of induced biosynthesis. T = template; E = enzyme; 1, 2, or 3 = possible sites of hormone action (8).

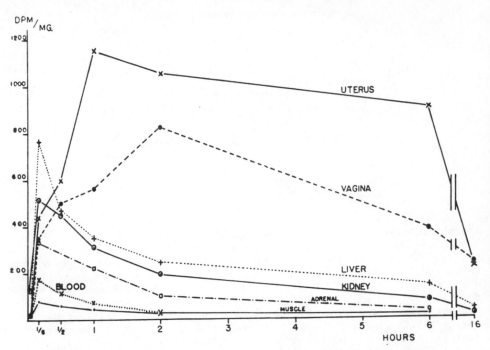

Fig. 3. Concentration of radioactivity in rat tissues after a single subcutaneous injection of approximately 0.01 μg of estradiol (specific activity 195 μCi/μg) in saline. Liver and kidney points are mean values of 4 aliquots of dried pooled tissue; other points are median values of individual samples from 6 animals (2).

inhibitor, blocked all the uterine responses to estrogen. Actinomycin D, an inhibitor of RNA synthesis, was later shown to block the estrogen response, also. These observations provided the basis for the early interest in the role that protein and RNA synthesis played in steroid hormone action and led to the eager acceptance of molecular biological approaches to study specific gene expression.

Estrogen binding was observed in both nuclear and cytoplasmic compartments and some of the physical characteristics of the binding entities were different enough to indicate that two or more receptors might be involved. However, studies in the 1960s determined that only one receptor was probably involved and this led to the translocation or two-step model of 1968 which is shown in Figure 4 (12,13). This model appeared to account for the data on a number of the steroid hormones and was widely accepted. With time many details were added to the model, in particular regarding receptor interaction with the nucleus. A variety of these have been discussed at great length elsewhere (14-16).

It is relevant to the historical perspective to note that almost all nuclear components have been shown to bind steroid receptors yet most models and discussions of the mechanism of steroid hormone action focus on DNA binding. I believe that this is due as much to the popularity of molecular biology theory as it is to convincing data. A variety of data that are in conflict or are difficult to explain by receptor binding to DNA are generally ignored. The concept of receptor binding to DNA has been around for some time but has not been conclusively demonstrated. We need to avoid the mistakes made by supporters of the transhydrogenase

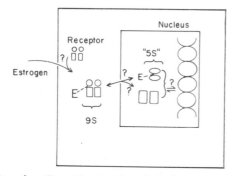

Fig. 4. Hypothetical model for estrogen
interaction with uterine cell (13).

theory who ignored the inconsistencies and focused only on the data
supportive of their position.

The translocation model was in vogue until the 1980s with a minimum
of conflicting results. Again, a few people pointed out problems with
some of the data. Peter Sheridan (17), for example, pointed out that
autoradiography indicated that at least some of the unoccupied receptor
was in nucleus. Again it was the introduction of new technology that
permitted a new look at the translocation model. The use of enucleation
of intact cells (18) and immunocytochemistry (19,20) independently showed
that the unoccupied as well as the occupied receptors were located mainly
in the nucleus and not in the cytoplasm. It was obvious that the translocation model for the steroid hormone receptors was probably incorrect
and would need revising.

The model shown in Figure 5 presents our current thinking about
estrogen receptor action. This is a very low resolution model in which a
great deal of information on the structure of the receptor has been
omitted. The model also does not address the problem of the nature of the
receptor-nuclear interaction or even which nuclear components are
involved. It is in this area of investigation that we have the most
doubts and see the most inconsistencies. The attractiveness of the
hypothesis that specific DNA sequences (response elements) bind the
receptor is reminiscent of the attractiveness of the transhydrogenase
theory 30 years ago. This is not to say such studies are unimportant but
rather that they should be carefully criticized and inconsistencies, such
as low affinity interactions between receptors and DNA or the low level of
homology between response elements for the same receptor, should be
recognized and investigated to determine the nature of these interactions.
It is my belief that chromatin proteins as well as DNA are critical for
the estrogen response and that essential receptor interaction with
chromatin proteins is very likely.

Whether history, as it applies to science, repeats itself or not, it
is interesting to look back through several decades of research on the
steroid hormones to see the trends, waves and high points. While progress
in this field has been astounding, it must be pointed out that we are
still unable to present a cogent and detailed model of steroid hormone
action at the molecular level.

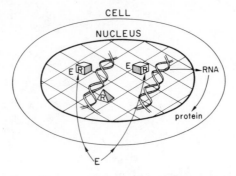

Fig. 5. Current model of estrogen receptor action. E, estrogen; R, receptor (14).

ACKNOWLEDGEMENTS

This work was supported in part by National Institutes of Health grants CA18110, HD08192, training grant HD07259 and by the National Foundation for Cancer Research. The author would also like to thank Diana Metcalf for her editorial assistance.

REFERENCES

1. Langley JN. On the physiology of the salivary secretion. J Physiol (London) 1879; 1:339-69.
2. Jensen EV, Jacobson HI. Fate of steroid estrogens in target tissues. In: Pincus G, Vollmer E, eds. Biological activities of steroids in relation to cancer. New York: Academic Press, 1960:161-78.
3. Glascock RF, Hoekstra WG. Selective accumulation of tritium-labelled hexoestrol by the reproductive organs of immature female goats and sheep. Biochem J 1959; 72:673-82.
4. Green DE. Enzymes and trace substances. In: Nord FF, ed. Advances in enzymology. New York: Interscience Publishers, Inc., 1941:177-98.
5. Villee CA, Hagerman DD, Joel PB. An enzymatic basis for the physiologic functions of estrogens. Recent Prog Horm Res 1960; 16:49-77.
6. Jacob F, Monod J. Genetic regulatory mechanisms in the synthesis of proteins. J Mol Biol 1961; 3:318-56.
7. Szego CM, Roberts S. Steroid action and interaction in uterine metabolism. Recent Prog Horm Res 1953; 8:419-69.
8. Mueller CC, Herranen AM, Jervell KF. Studies on the mechanism of action of estrogens. Recent Prog Horm Res 1958; 14:95-139.
9. Toft D, Gorski J. A receptor molecule for estrogen: isolation from the rat uterus and preliminary characterization. Proc Natl Acad Sci USA 1966; 55:1574-80.
10. Gorski J, Toft D, Shyamala G, et al. Studies on the interaction of estrogen with the uterus. Recent Prog Horm Res 1968; 24:45-80.
11. Mueller GC, Gorski J, Aisawa Y. The role of protein synthesis in the early estrogen response. Proc Natl Acad Sci USA 1961; 47:164-9.
12. Jensen EV, Suzuki T, Kawashima T, et al. A two-step mechanism for the interaction of estradiol with rat uterus. Proc Natl Acad Sci USA 1968; 59:632-8.

13. Gorski J, Toft D, Shyamala G, et al. Hormone receptors: studies on the interaction of estrogen with the uterus. Recent Prog Horm Res 1968; 24:45-80.

14. Gorski J, Welshons W, Sakai D, et al. Evolution of a model of estrogen action. Recent Prog Horm Res 1986; 42:297-329.

15. Gorski J, Hansen J. The one and only step model of estrogen action. Steroids (in press).

16. Yamamoto KR. Steroid receptor regulated transcription of the specific genes and gene networks. Annu Rev Genet 1985; 19:209-52.

17. Sheridan PJ, Buchanan JM, Anselmo VC, et al. Equilibrium: the intracellular distribution of steroid receptors. Nature 1979; 282:579-82.

18. Welshons WV, Lieberman ME, Gorski J. Nuclear localization of unoccupied oestrogen receptors. Nature 1984; 307:747-9.

19. King WJ, Greene GL. Monoclonal antibodies localize oestrogen receptor in the nuclei of target cells. Nature 1984; 307:745-7.

20. McClellan MC, West NB, Tacha DE, et al. Immunocytochemical localization of estrogen receptors in the Macaque reproductive tract with monoclonal antiestrophilins. Endocrinology 1984; 114:2002-14.

II. RECEPTOR STRUCTURE AND MOLECULAR ORGANIZATION

3

INTRACELLULAR LOCALIZATION OF STEROID HORMONE RECEPTORS: IMMUNOCYTOCHEMICAL ANALYSIS

Jean-Marie Gasc and Etienne-Emile Baulieu

INSERM U 33
Lab Hormones 94275 Bicetre Cedex, France

INTRODUCTION

The development of antibodies to steroid hormone receptors consecutively to their purification, represents an important improvement to label and localize receptor molecules inside the target cells. Antibodies recognize various small epitopes on the large receptor molecules, and therefore receptors can be detected independently of the occupancy of the binding site by the hormonal ligand. Unlike radioactive ligands, antibodies reveal hormone-free as well as occupied receptors, thus providing the first direct specific means to localize unoccupied receptor molecules. Although other techniques were proposed in the past, based on the binding of a label to the receptor molecule (1,2), none of them met the criteria necessary to conclude to the specific detection of steroid hormone receptors as defined by their well established physicochemical characteristics (3). Morphological techniques are particularly well suited to address the question of the intracellular distribution of the receptors. They imply no disruption of the cells and little disturbance of the two major cellular compartments: cytoplasm and nuclei. However, although less dramatic to the cell integrity than tissue homogenization, histological procedures may induce alterations and movements of the intracellular material which must not be ignored in the interpretation of the observations.

The immunohistochemical studies with antibodies to steroid receptors have, in the past few years, raised numerous comments and criticisms. This new approach made possible the first verifications, with a methodology different from that used previously, of the hypothesis proposed in 1968 to explain the intracellular distribution of the steroid hormones and their receptors (4,5). The first observations published were sometimes contradictory, and a growing number contradicted the concept of nuclear translocation which was commonly accepted until then. Although some aspects of the controversy remain obscure, the new data are now strongly validated and they lead to modify the general mechanism of action of steroid hormones. In this article, based on our experience with the progesterone (PR) and glucocorticosteroid receptors (GR), we summarize the main acquisitions of this new methodology, particularly the aspects related to cellular biology. We examine the discrepancy between PR and GR and discuss whether it is accounted for by a true difference in the mechanism of action of the two receptors, or rather by technical artifacts.

The first indication of nuclear PR in absence of ligand was obtained with frozen sections of chick oviduct (6), and then confirmed with paraffin sections of the same target organ (7), and also various other tissues and organs (see review in reference 8). Under all experimental conditions with different types of fixative solutions PR immunostaining was found exclusively in the cell nuclei in young sexually immature animals. Biochemical studies with the same biological material constantly led to the recovery of the progesterone binding sites in the cytosolic fraction of tissue homogenates. Furthermore, when progesterone was administered to the animals, the intracellular distribution and the intensity of immunostaining were not modified. These observations are in complete disagreement with a process of receptor nuclear translocation, since there is no cytoplasmic PR and no increase of nuclear PR after hormone administration.

Similar results were later published by Perrot-Applanat et al. (9), using antibodies to rabbit PR on paraffin sections of rabbit uterus. Numerous studies have also shown the exclusively nuclear localization of the estrogen receptor, even in absence of hormonal ligand (10,11). More recently, studies designed to test the impact of technical artifacts on our observations brought forth new experimental arguments in support of an "all nuclear" concept. It had been contended that when a piece of tissue is placed in a fixative solution, molecules originally in the cytoplasm may be displaced toward the nucleus. There are arguments strongly suggesting this is not the case for PR. On frozen sections of fresh, unfixed tissue, postfixed by immersion in a fixative solution, the PR immunostaining is nuclear, as on paraffin sections, although the possibility of artifactual translocation is minimized (Fig. 1C). Indeed, it was shown that when a frozen section is immersed in a buffer solution, similar to the kind used for tissue homogenization, what occurs is a loss of PR from the nucleus into the solution, and not the opposite movement from the cytoplasm toward the nucleus. It is only if the buffer solution contains a fixative (formaldehyde or else) that the loss of nuclear PR is limited or blocked, thus allowing the detection of PR in cell nuclei. In order to completely exclude any nuclear displacement during fixation by immersion, we resorted to an unusual technique of fixation. Frozen sections were fixed in vapors of a mixture of formaldehyde and acetic acid in conditions specially established for this system. At no point between the freezing of the tissue and the end of the fixation procedure were sections exposed to a liquid phase, thus preventing any artifactual nuclear translocation of PR to occur. In all cases, independently of the presence or absence of hormonal ligand, PR was always revealed in cell nuclei, following the same pattern of stained cells as in regular frozen sections and paraffin sections (Fig. 1D). It appears, therefore, highly probable that PR is originally nuclear even in its hormone-free form, with the exception of the molecules being synthesized.

The lack of large amounts of PR in the cytoplasm is more difficult to demonstrate. A complete loss of cytoplasmic PR may occur in the case of frozen sections fixed by immersion as the cytoplasm is directly exposed to the aqueous phase of the fixative solution. A similar loss is impossible when frozen sections are fixed in vapors but this technique has not been sufficiently tested with other cytoplasmic antigens, to conclude only on the basis of a negative result. The fixation procedure may be inadequate to detect PR in the cytoplasm of the same cells in which PR is detected in the nuclei. In the case of paraffin sections, even though some loss of cytoplasmic material is possible, a complete loss of PR, below the threshold of detection, is improbable.

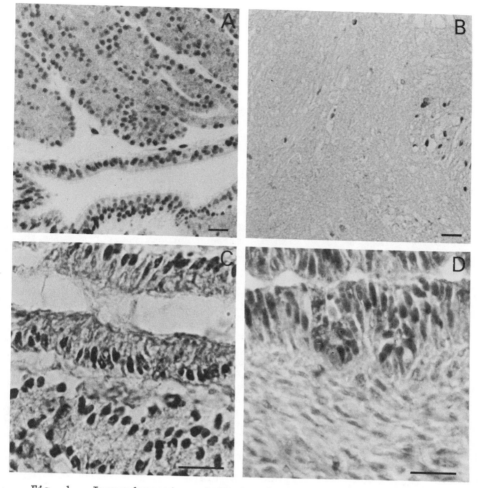

Fig. 1. Immunodetection of PR in the oviduct of young sexually immature chicken. (A) On a paraffin section PR is
revealed exclusively in cell nuclei of luminal and glandular
epithelia, and stroma; a great majority of the nuclei appear
immunostained. (B) Paraffin section of the centrifugation
pellet obtained after tissue homogenization for the preparation of a cytosolic extract from the same oviduct as shown in
A. After immunostaining very few cell nuclei appear as still
containing PR. The PR positive nuclei are usually in areas
where tissue organization (strips of epithelium or bundles of
smooth muscle fibers) is still recognizable. Most nuclei
which contained PR in the intact tissue (see A) have lost
their receptors during cytosol preparation and appear now PR
negative in the sedimentation pellet. (C) On a frozen section
fixed by immersion in a formaldehyde-glutaraldehyde solution,
the immunostaining appears identical to that on a paraffin
section: most nuclei are stained in all tissues although no
artifactual translocation from cytoplasm to the nucleus can
have occurred. (D) On a frozen section fixed in vapors of
formaldehyde and acetic acid, PR is revealed exclusively in
cell nuclei although any intracellular redistribution of PR is
excluded in these conditions. As this animal had no gland
differentiated, only nuclei of the luminal epithelium appear
positive. No counterstain; Bar: 20 μmeters.

Another argument supports the exclusively nuclear localization of PR and is not in keeping with a nuclear translocation process. When small explants of chick oviduct are incubated at 4°C with a radioactive synthetic progestagen (^{3}H-Organon 2058) and submitted to the special autoradiographic technique for steroid hormones, no cytoplasmic labeling is found while nuclear labeling appears progressively as the duration of incubation increases (12). At least some ^{3}H-Org 2058-PR complexes should be detected within the cytoplasm according to the nuclear translocation hypothesis since those present in the nucleus were formed in the cytoplasm and the translocation is a temperature dependent process. This lack of cytoplasmic labeling added to the constant failure to find any evidence of cytoplasmic PR with antibodies lead to the conclusion that there is no PR stored in the cytoplasm and, consequently, the hormone-receptor complexes form directly in the nucleus.

Another question one can address with this methodology is the intracellular localization of the heat shock protein of molecular weight 90 kDa (hsp 90). It is associated with all steroid hormone receptors under their hormone-free, untransformed form (13). Its role in the mechanism of action of the receptors is still not completely established (see details in the chapter by E. E. Baulieu). Hsp 90 is revealed in both the cytoplasm and nuclei with a predominance in either one or the other compartment depending on the type of fixation and the tissue (7). On paraffin sections the hsp 90 immunostaining is stronger in nuclei than in cytoplasm of glandular cells in oviduct after glutaraldehyde fixation. After fixation of the same tissue in acidified alcohol, the immunostaining is more evenly distributed between the two cellular compartments. Such a discrepancy is due to the difficult fixation of glandular cells and, consequently, to the only partial retention of hsp 90 inside the cells under certain fixation conditions. Hsp 90 is a cytosolic protein found in large amount in the supernatant of tissue homogenates and similar losses or intracellular displacements cannot be excluded in our technical conditions. It is, however, improbable that such artifacts account for the presence of hsp 90 in cell nuclei since on frozen sections it is also revealed in the nucleus, and as explained above for PR, an artifactual nuclear translocation of cytoplasmic material is highly improbable in the case of frozen sections. All the observations, therefore, indicate the presence of hsp 90 in the cytoplasm and the nucleus of PR containing cells and confirm the possible association of hsp 90 and PR. The cytoplasmic hsp 90 is obviously not associated to PR, but rather related to the still ill-defined functions of this protein.

If PR is exclusively nuclear, even under its untransformed form, why is it recovered in the cytosolic fraction after tissue homogenization? The two following experiments are an attempt to answer this question. In intact chick oviduct, PR was detected in the cell nuclei. When a chick oviduct is homogenized to prepare a cytosol, the centrifugation pellet, observed after histological fixation and processing, appears to contain cellular debris, organelles, nuclei, and also pieces of tissues still displaying a tissular structure. The immunostaining of the sections shows nuclei deprived of reaction with anti PR antibodies while in intact chick oviduct PR was detected in almost all cell nuclei (Fig. 1A and 1B). Only when pieces of still organized tissue are visible (strips of luminal epithelium, or bundles of smooth muscles), the nuclei are immunostained. When the nucleus has been well preserved from the drastic conditions of homogenization by its natural cytoplasmic environment, PR is still detectable in the nucleus. When the cell nuclei were exposed to abnormal ionic strength after cellular disruption, PR immunoreactivity is totally absent. This experiment, which suggests a leak of PR from the nucleus during the cytosol preparation, is confirmed by another carried out with frozen sections. When an unfixed frozen section is immersed in a buffer solution for 1 to 60 min, then fixed and immunostained, the staining rapidly decreases as the time of immersion prior to fixation increases. On such frozen sections, as in a tissue homogenate, nuclei are exposed directly to the buffer solution. The loss of immunostaining illustrates the progressive leak of PR from the nuclei, and this phenomenon reproduces on a histological slide what takes place during tissue homogenization.

All the results demonstrate that PR is a nuclear protein and hormone-receptor complexes form in the nucleus. Going one step further, recent reports at electron microscopy level, show an intranuclear translocation from eu- to heterochromatin following the formation of the complexes (14). Such studies open the way to new investigations on the cell biology of the receptor at ultrastructural level. An important question remaining unsolved is the mechanism by which hsp 90 associates with and dissociates from the hormone binding subunit of PR, and the physiological role of this process.

INTRACELLULAR LOCALIZATION OF THE GLUCOCORTICOID RECEPTOR

Contrary to PR, which was found exclusively in the cell nuclei, GR was initially shown to be cytoplasmic and nuclear. The initial work on cultured cells (15,16) and further in vivo studies with adrenalectomized rats all showed an increase in nuclear GR after hormone administration (17,18) interpreted as an evidence for nuclear translocation. This discrepancy between two receptors which are very similar by many other aspects, prompted us to reexamine the intracellular distribution of GR with the same techniques as used for PR, with particular attention to possible experimental artifacts.

In liver of adrenalectomized rats, processed for paraffin histology under the same conditions as the chick oviduct for PR, GR immunostaining was detected in cytoplasm and nuclei. The cytoplasmic staining was usually weak and displayed some irregularity between cells (Fig. 2A). The nuclei were also weakly and irregularly stained. After administering the animals with dexamethasone, the nuclear staining increased while the cyto-plasmic staining did not appear significantly modified (Fig. 2B). This observation agrees with that already published for the rat liver (17).

The presence of GR in cell nuclei of rat liver more than one week after adrenalectomy, and the increase in nuclear immunostaining after giving the hormone, was confirmed on frozen sections fixed by immersion (Fig. 2C and 2D). Based on our own experiments of antibody dilution, one can estimate the increase in nuclear GR after dexamethasone treatment to at least 40 times. The nuclear immunostaining was more regular than on paraffin sections of liver, from the same animal. In contrast to paraffin sections, the cytoplasm of frozen sections appear devoid of GR. However, the lack of cytoplasmic is meaningless since cells are cut open and cytosolic proteins are free to diffuse into the buffer solution in which the frozen section is immersed.

A vapor fixation technique also used for PR (Fig. 1D) was tried to avoid any contact of the cells with a liquid phase until after the end of the fixation process, thus preventing intra- and extracellular displace-ments. The results were completely different from those obtained with PR. GR was detected in the cytoplasm, and the nuclei appeared free of immuno-staining or only weakly stained (Fig. 3). The cytoplasmic staining was not visibly modified after hormone administration. The meaning of the results obtained after vapor fixation of liver sections is debatable since, in the case of GR, this technique lacks reproducibility. While some liver blocks constantly show a cytoplasmic staining, others are

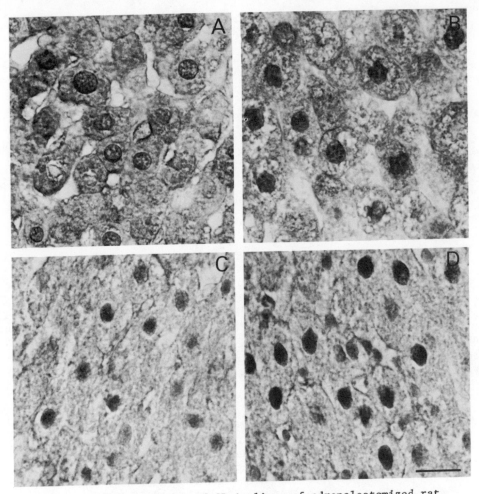

Fig. 2. Immunodetection of GR in liver of adrenalectomized rat.
(A) On a paraffin section from a control animal the cytoplasm is
weakly stained, and cell nuclei display a staining irregular in
intensity from negative to medium level although this animal was
adrenalectomized 12 days earlier. (B) After dexamethasone
treatment, under identical technical conditions, the GR immunostaining increases in cell nuclei and is not modified in the
cytoplasm. (C) On a frozen section fixed by immersion in
formaldehyde-glutaraldehyde solution, GR is revealed in cell
nuclei with a weak to medium intensity level. The cytoplasmic
staining is not specific. (D) After dexamethasone treatment GR
immunostaining is greatly increased in most cell nuclei. No
counterstain; Bar: 20 µmeters.

deprived of any staining under these technical conditions. The fact that
GR is reproducibly detectable in the nuclei after fixation by immersion of
the same blocks of liver makes the failure of the vapor fixation technique
still less comprehensible. Despite this lack of reproducibility, the
cytoplasmic staining meets the criteria for a specific immunostaining, in
particular it is abolished by presaturation of the antibody by purified
GR. Still more intriguing is the lack of nuclear staining on sections
which, processed differently, show the presence of nuclear GR. Since the
same technique of vapor fixation shows the presence of nuclear PR in the
chick oviduct, one must admit it is adequate at least for some nuclear

antigens. The cause for the failure to detect nuclear GR in liver sections remains unknown. Because of these uncertainties, the results obtained with this vapor fixation technique are only a confirmation, under conditions precluding any intracellular displacement, of the presence of GR in cytoplasm as already shown on paraffin sections.

Another monoclonal antibody to GR also used in the present study (I-GR 49/4 from Dr. M. Beato) produced exactly the same observations as above described.

All these results are in complete agreement with those reported by J. A. Gustafsson and collaborators using the same antibody to localize GR in cultured cells (19) and brain sections (18). These authors reported that the results are clearly in favor of a mechanism of nuclear translocation which appears to cope with the increase of nuclear GR immunostaining after hormone administration. This conclusion distinguishes GR from PR and ER, and also vitamin D receptor which is always recovered in the nucleus (20). There are, however, at least two observations that do not fit the nuclear translocation concept. One is the presence of GR in nuclei of adrenalectomized rat liver in absence of hormone treatment (Fig. 2A) and the other is the lack of decrease of the cytoplasmic GR after hormonal treatment (Fig. 2A and 2B). Because the observations are only partially in agreement with the translocation hypothesis and also because a difference between receptors is difficult to accept without a strong evidence, we propose an explanation of the results on GR which is an alternative to the nuclear translocation.

Hormone-free GR would be a cytosolic protein with very low affinity for nuclear structures and thus easily extracted from the nuclei. In a

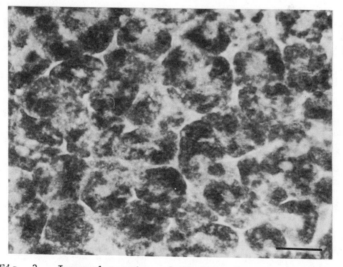

Fig. 3. Immunodetection of GR in a frozen section of adrenalectomized rat liver after fixation in vapors of formaldehyde-acetic acid. Under conditions which preclude any artifactual redistribution during fixation GR is revealed in cytoplasm and occasionally also in cell nuclei. After dexamethasone treatment the same intracellular distribution of GR is observed (not shown). The failure of this technique to reveal a strong nuclear staining remains obscure. No counterstain; Bar: 20 μmeters.

recent study (unpublished results of the authors), we observed the rapid decrease of the GR immunostaining on frozen sections when they are immersed in a buffer solution prior to fixation. Interestingly, the free GR is lost more rapidly (after 5 min of immersion no GR is detectable) while the hormone-bound GR remains longer (still present after 60 min of immersion). This observation clearly illustrates the strong tendency of the hormone-free GR to leak very rapidly out of the nucleus when exposed to the buffer solution. A similar leak may occur during the first minutes or seconds of the fixation procedure when the hormone-free GR molecules are exposed to the buffer solution but not yet all immobilized by the fixative (formaldehyde and glutaraldehyde). On the contrary, the hormone-complexed GR already bound to nuclear structures is better retained in the nucleus during the fixation process and little loss occurs, resulting in a strong immunostaining. A lesser loss in nuclear GR after hormone administration is then interpreted as an increase in nuclear GR, a false evidence of nuclear translocation. The question comes immediately of how to explain the discrepancy between PR and GR. One must assume that the hormone-free PR is less easily lost because of tighter binding to nucleus than free GR. In effect, preliminary observations show that the hormone-free PR behaves more like the hormone-bound GR by its ability to be retained longer in nuclei of cells exposed to buffer solution.

There are to date two experimental arguments to support the alternative hypothesis to the nuclear translocation of GR that we develop here. One is the decrease in nuclear staining after immersion and the other is the irregularity in intensity of nuclear staining in absence of hormone. This is particularly visible on paraffin sections of liver which show side by side nuclei with all levels of immunostaining between negative and strong (although not so strong as after hormone administration) (Fig. 2A). This difference implies that some cells must have an abundant nuclear GR even though the animals had been adrenalectomized at least one week earlier. One may therefore extrapolate that all cells had originally the same high level of nuclear GR, and that local conditions produce differential losses between cells. The result is an irregular intensity of the nuclear staining always lower than after hormone administration. Another argument is provided by the experiments of enucleation in which GR is recovered in the nucleoplasm fraction even when cells are grown in absence of hormone (21). The nearly total recovery of GR in nuclei of cells depleted in ATP by dinitrophenol treatment also accords well with the nuclear localization of hormone-free GR (22). Finally, the low level and the constancy of the cytoplasmic immunostaining even after hormonal treatment appears in contradiction with the nuclear translocation process.

DISCUSSION

The different observations made in the same experimental conditions on PR and GR point to the necessity to further study the movements of receptor molecules inside the cells. Our alternative hypothesis to the nuclear translocation of GR accounts for the apparent increase of nuclear GR, and does not take into account the presence of GR in the cytoplasm. In the nuclei GR and PR would act similarly with only a difference in affinity of the free receptor for nuclear structures. In the cytoplasmic compartment the difference is not easily reducible to technical artifacts: there is no evidence for cytoplasmic PR, while GR is constantly found in that cellular compartment. The constant level of cytoplasmic GR before and after hormone treatment does not agree with a nuclear translocation process, particularly since the increase in nuclear GR appears very high. If the cytoplasmic GR is a real entity and not receptor artifactually lost from the nucleus, what role does it play in cell physiology? The report of a specific binding of GR to transfer RNA may provide an explanation

(23). The possibility of a mutant molecule lacking affinity for nuclear structures appears more attractive. A mutant GR, the β-receptor described by Hollenberg et al. (24) does not bind the hormone but it is not known if it also lacks affinity for nuclear structures. In cultured lymphoma cells, other mutant GR forms have been described and one of them has a reduced affinity for DNA (25). Whether receptor molecules other than the α-form are present in rat liver cells and neurons, in sufficient amount to be detected, remains to be documented. The low affinity of normal hormone-free GR for nuclear structures may also account for the presence of GR in the cytoplasm. If free GR is weakly bound to the nucleus, the equilibrium maintains a low but detectable concentration of receptor molecules in the cytoplasm. This is similar to the interpretation proposed by Sheridan and Martin to explain the intracellular movements of PR and ER (26).

The question of the existence of mutant molecules not only for GR, but also PR and ER is directly linked to the use of antibodies in the distinction between hormone sensitive and insensitive tumors. It will be critical to validate the immunoassays in comparison to other assays before antibodies become of routine use in pathology laboratories (27-29). Another important step in that direction is the quantification of the immunostaining. The attempts by Agnati et al. (30) to automatize the reading of immunostained GR on brain sections illustrate the great potential of quantitative studies and their application in fundamental and clinical research.

The studies at electronmicroscopic level is another aspect of the immunocytochemical analysis which deserves more attention in the future. A few reports have already been published which illustrate the feasibility, and also pitfalls, of this approach (14,31). More than in regular histological techniques, at submicroscopical level the questions of intracellular movements are essential. Most of the present article discusses possible undetected displacements of receptors inside and outside the cells. Similar experimental artifacts become more critical and have to be strictly taken into account and controlled in studies on the ultra-structural localization of steroid hormone receptors.

ACKNOWLEDGMENTS

The authors particularly thank J. M. Renoir, P. Tuohimaa, J. A. Gustafsson and M. Beato for gifts of antibodies, and F. Delahaye for her skillful and patient technical help. H. Deschaumes, C. Secco, F. Boussac and J. C. Lambert have assisted in the preparation of the manuscript.

REFERENCES

1. Nenci I, Dandliker WB, Meyers CY, Marchetti E, Marzola A, Fabris G. Estrogen receptor cytochemistry by fluorescent estrogen. J Histochem Cytochem 1980; 28:1081-8.
2. Sin Hang Lee. Validity of a histochemical estrogen receptor assay. J Histochem Cytochem 1984; 32:305-10.
3. Mercer WD, Edwards DP, Chamness GC, McGuire W. Failure of estradiol immunofluorescence in MCF-7 breast cancer cells to detect estrogen receptors. Cancer Res 1981; 41:4644-52.
4. Jensen EV, Suzuki T, Kawashima T, Stumpf WE, Jungblut PW, DeSombre ER. A two-step mechanism for the interaction of estradiol with rat uterus. Proc Natl Acad Sci USA 1968; 53:632-8.
5. Gorski J, Toft D, Shyamala G, Smith D, Notides A. Hormone receptors: studies on the interaction of estrogen with the uterus. Recent Prog Horm Res 1968; 24:45-80.

6. Gasc JM, Ennis BW, Baulieu EE, Stumpf WE. Recepteur de la progesterone dans l'oviducte de poulet: double revelation par immuno-histochimie avec des anticorps antirecepteur et par autoradiographie a l'aide d'un progestagene tritie. C R Acad Sci [II] (Paris) 1983; 297:477–82.

7. Gasc JM, Renoir JM, Radanyi C, Joab I, Tuohimaa P, Baulieu EE. Progesterone receptor in the chick oviduct: an immunohistochemical study with antibodies to distinct receptor components. J Cell Biol 1984; 99:1193–201.

8. Gasc JM, Baulieu EE. Immunohistochemical studies with antibodies to the chicken oviduct progesterone receptor. In: Pertschuk LP, Sin Hang Lee, eds. Localization of putative steroid receptors. Experimental systems; vol I. Boca Raton: CRC Press; 1985:125–41.

9. Perrot-Applanat M, Logeat F, Groyer-Picard MT, Milgrom E. Immuno-histochemical study of mammalian progesterone receptor using monoclonal antibodies. Endocrinology 1985; 116:1473–84.

10. King WJ, Greene GL. Monoclonal antibodies localize oestrogen receptor in the nuclei of target cells. Nature 1984; 307:745–7.

11. Press MF, Nousek-Goebl N, King WJ, Herbst AL, Greene GL. Immuno-histochemical assessment of estrogen receptor distribution in the human endometrium throughout the menstrual cycle. Lab Invest 1984; 51:495–503.

12. Ennis BW, Stumpf WE, Gasc JM, Baulieu EE. Nuclear localization of progesterone receptor before and after exposure to progestin at low and high temperatures: autoradiographic and immunohistochemical studies of chick oviduct. Endocrinology 1986; 119:2066–75.

13. Joab I, Radanyi C, Renoir JM, et al. Common non-hormone binding component in non-transformed chick oviduct receptors of four steroid hormones. Nature 1984; 308:850–3.

14. Perrot-Applanat M, Groyer-Picard MT, Logeat F, Milgrom E. Ultra-structural localization of the progesterone receptor by an immunogold method: effect of hormone administration. J Cell Biol 1986; 102: 1191–9.

15. Govindan MV. Immunofluorescence microscopy of the intracellular translocation of glucocorticoid-receptor complexes in rat hepatoma (HTC) cells. Exp Cell Res 1980; 127:293–7.

16. Papamichail M, Tsokos G, Tsawdaroglou N, Sekeris CE. Immunocytochemical demonstration of glucocorticoid receptors in different cell types and their translocation from the cytoplasm to the cell nucleus in the presence of dexamethasone. Exp Cell Res 1980; 125:490–3.

17. Antakly T, Eisen H. Immunocytochemical localization of glucocorticoid receptor in target cells. Endocrinology 1984; 115:1984–9.

18. Fuxe K, Wikstrom AC, Okret S, et al. Mapping of glucocorticoid receptor immunoreactive neurons in the rat tel- and diencephalon using a monoclonal antibody against rat liver glucocorticoid receptor. Endocrinology 1985; 117:1803–12.

19. Wikstrom AC, Bakke O, Okret S, Bronnegard M, Gustafsson JA. Intracellular localization of the glucocorticoid receptor: evidence for cytoplasmic and nuclear localization. Endocrinology 1987; 120:1232–42.

20. Walters MR, Hunziker W, Norman AW. Unoccupied 1,25-dihydroxyvitamin D3 receptors. Nuclear/cytosol ratio depends on ionic strength. J Biol Chem 1980; 255:6799–805.

21. Welshons WV, Krummel BM, Gorski J. Nuclear localization of unoc-cupied receptors for glucocorticoids, estrogens, and progesterone in GH3 cells. Endocrinology 1985; 117:2140–7.

22. Mendel DB, Bodwell JE, Munck A. Glucocorticoid receptors lacking hormone-binding activity are bound in nuclei of ATP-depleted cells. Nature 1986; 324:478–80.

23. Ali M, Vedeckis W. Interaction of RNA with transformed glucocor-

ticoid receptor. Identification of the RNA as transfer RNA. J Biol Chem 1987; 262:6778–84.

24. Hollenberg SM, Weinberger C, Ong ES, et al. Primary structure and expression of a functional human glucocorticoid receptor cDNA. Nature 1985; 318:635–41.

25. Danielsen M, Northrop JP, Ringold GM. The mouse glucocorticoid receptor: mapping of functional domains by cloning, sequencing and expression of wild-type and mutant receptor proteins. EMBO J 1986; 5:2513–22.

26. Sheridan PJ, Buchanan JM, Anselmo VC, Martin M. Unbound progesterone receptors are in equilibrium between the nucleus and cytoplasm in cells of the rat uterus. Endocrinology 1981; 108:1533–7.

27. King WJ, DeSombre ER, Jensen EV, Greene GL. Comparison of immuno-cytochemical and steroid-binding assays for estrogen receptor in human breast tumors. Cancer Res 1985; 45:293–304.

28. Pertschuk LP, Eisenberg KB, Carter AC, Feldman JG. Immunohistologic localization of estrogen receptors in breast cancer with monoclonal antibodies. Cancer 1985; 55:1513–8.

29. Perrot-Applanat M, Groyer-Picard MT, Lorenzo F, et al. Immunocyto-chemical study with monoclonal antibodies to progesterone receptor in human breast tumors. Cancer Res 1987; 47:2652–61.

30. Agnati LF, Fuxe K, Yu ZY, et al. Morphometrical analysis of the distribution of corticotropin releasing factor, glucocorticoid receptor and phenylethanolamine-N-methyltransferase immunoreactive structures in the paraventricular hypothalamic nucleus of the rat. Neurosci Lett 1985; 54:147–52.

31. Isola J, Pelto-Huikko M, Ylikomi T, Tuohimaa P. Immunoelectron microscopic localization of progesterone receptor in the chick oviduct. J Steroid Biochem 1987; 26:19–23.

4

IMMUNOCYTOCHEMISTRY OF ESTROGEN AND PROGESTIN RECEPTORS

IN THE PRIMATE REPRODUCTIVE TRACT

Robert M. Brenner, Maryanne C. McClellan,*
Neal B. West

Oregon Regional Primate Research Center
Beaverton, OR 97006, and *Reed College,
Portland, OR 97202

The central focus of our research program, since its inception, has been on steroid receptors as components of regulatory mechanisms that control tissue structure and function in the reproductive tract in female primates. Our approach has been to correlate fluctuations in the levels of receptors with the morphological and physiological effects of the gonadal steroids. Our long-term goal is to deepen our understanding of how steroids bring about the various transformations that occur in the primate reproductive tract during the individual's life history. Our current research depends heavily on immunocytochemical techniques that have come to maturity in our laboratory over the last few years (1-3). Our findings to date support the hypothesis (4) that there are significant stromal-epithelial interactions involved in steroid hormone action in the adult reproductive tract. Our findings also support the view that in vivo, the bulk of the estrogen receptor (ER) and progestin receptor (PR) are located in target cell nuclei, even in the absence of ligand (5-7).

In what follows, we will review the data that supports these conclusions. In particular, we will point out several specific hormonal conditions during which the epithelial cells in a target organ are dramatically influenced by a steroid, even though the only cells in that organ that possess the appropriate steroid receptor are in the stroma, not the epithelium. One example is the striking lack of nuclear staining for ER and PR in the endothelial cells that form the innermost lining of the small blood vessels of the reproductive system, while the smooth muscle cells in the walls and the perivascular stroma of these vessels contain both receptors. This suggests that the effects of steroids on blood vessel permeability (8) may not be directly mediated by steroid receptors in endothelial cells, but by steroid receptors in adjacent stromal cells. How these and other analogous observations will ultimately fit into our understanding of steroid hormone-mediated differentiation and function in the primate reproductive tract remains to be determined.

In addition, we and others have published studies on progesterone-induced suppression of the ER (9-12). Most of these observations were based on bulk biochemical assays which do not discriminate between the different cell types within the tissues. We now have information on how the cellular compartments of the oviduct, uterus, and cervix differ in their susceptibility to the suppressive effects of progesterone. The evidence suggests that progesterone antagonism develops at different rates within the different tissue compartments. Here we review our most recent studies (13) of the rate of change in the pattern of immunocytochemical staining for both ER and PR in the stromal, epithelial and smooth muscle components of the reproductive tract during progesterone antagonism. Most of our published work to date concerns the ER; our unpublished work on PR will be presented in preliminary form.

METHODS

Animals

We used rhesus (Macaca mulatta), cynomolgus (Macaca fascicularis) and pigtail (Macaca nemestrina) monkeys in these studies. All animal handling procedures were approved by the Institutional Animal Care and Use Committee of the Oregon Regional Primate Research Center according to guidelines established by the NIH. Some animals were laparotomized under Fluothane/ nitrous oxide anesthesia at different times during the menstrual cycle and the reproductive tract was removed for study. In other experiments, animals were ovariectomized and subsequently treated by subcutaneous implantation of Silastic capsules filled with crystalline steroids (14). The reproductive tract was then removed as above after various periods of hormone treatment.

Tissue Handling

Within 15 min of surgery, the uterus was separated from the cervix and oviducts. The uterus was first cut along the fundal-cervical axis into two halves, and these segments were halved again along the same axis. Thin cross-sectional slices of the whole uterine wall were cut at the point where the endometrium was the thickest. These slices were used for immunocytochemistry and morphology, and the remainder of the endometrium and myometrium were homogenized for receptor assays. The oviducts were trimmed of fat and connective tissue, and divided into fimbriae, ampulla and isthmus regions. The cervix was cross-sectioned with razor blades. Samples of all tissue slices were fixed in a fixative containing glutaraldehyde and formaldehyde (15) and embedded in araldite or glycolmethacrylate for morphological study.

Immunocytochemistry

The immunocytochemical technique was generally the same as described by McClellan et al. (14) for indirect immunocytochemistry with the avidin-biotin complex (ABC) method. Thin tissue slices (approximately 1-2 mm in thickness) were placed into drops of Tissue Tek II O.C.T. compound (Miles Laboratories, Naperville, IL) on small pieces of aluminum foil and plunged into liquefied propane cooled with liquid N_2. Frozen samples were stored up to 6 months over liquid N_2 (approximately -150 to -190°C). Blocks of frozen tissue were mounted on cryostat chucks with O.C.T. in a freezing chamber at -70°C, transferred to a Hacker/Bright cryostat, sectioned at 4-6 μm and thaw-mounted onto glass slides coated with 1% gelatin. In our early studies, the frozen sections were stored at -30°C until prepared for immunocytochemistry. Recently we have placed the frozen sections in anhydrous acetone at -80°C for 2 days before fixing the sections. This freeze-substitution step improves the morphology of the tissues and helps preserve the fragile cilia of the oviductal epithelium and other delicate structures.

The frozen (or freeze-substituted) tissue sections were fixed at 0-4°C in 0.2% picric acid-2% paraformaldehyde in 0.1M phosphate buffer pH

7.3 with 0.02% glutaraldehyde for 2 to 3 min, followed by the same picric acid-paraformaldehyde mixture without glutaraldehyde for 10 min, and then 85% ethanol for 4 min. The glutaraldehyde step is eliminated when freeze-substituted tissues are processed. The slides were rinsed with phosphate buffered saline (PBS), pH 7.6, placed in 0.05% sodium borohydride for 4 min, and then rinsed with PBS containing gelatin (1% w/v).

For ER, tissue sections were incubated with a combination of 2 monoclonal rat IgG_{2a} anti-ER antibodies (H222, courtesy Abbott Laboratories, and D75, courtesy Dr. Geoffrey Greene, University of Chicago; each at a concentration of 3.5 µg/ml) overnight in a moist chamber at 0-4°C after a 30-min incubation with normal rabbit serum. Sections were then rinsed with PBS, blocked with normal rabbit serum, incubated with biotinylated-antirat IgG (prepared in rabbit) for 30 min at 20°C, rinsed again and transferred to a solution containing avidin-biotin-peroxidase complex (Vector) prepared according to the directions included with the kit, and then reacted with diaminobenzidine and H_2O_2. Controls for nonspecific staining were obtained for each tissue by using a rat IgG_{2a} monoclonal antibody (AT) that was prepared against a different antigen (namely, antigen B of Timothy grass pollen; courtesy Dr. Arthur Malley, ORPRC) as a substitute for the anti-ER antibodies. Sections of nontarget tissue such as duodenum, colon, skeletal muscle or esophagus were also used as method controls.

For PR, a monoclonal rat IgG_{2a} anti-PR antibody (B39, 0.5 µg/ml; courtesy of Dr. Geoffrey Greene, University of Chicago) was used exactly as described above. Immunocytochemically stained tissue sections were counterstained with hematoxylin (Gill's 3X) after postfixation with OsO_4 (0.1%).

All slides to be compared for staining intensity (for example, all slides of oviducts from spayed, estrogen-treated and sequential progestin-treated animals) were processed in the same immunocytochemical run. At least two observers judged the slides for staining intensity as well as number of stained cells, and then ranked the results as strong (+++), moderate (++), weak (+) or absent (0), and also commented on the cellular distribution of staining (e.g., nuclear, cytoplasmic, stromal, epithelial, etc.). Photographs to document the distribution of stain and the differences in staining intensity were taken with planapochromatic lenses on a Zeiss light microscope with the aid of an automatic exposure meter, which resulted in negatives of closely matched density and contrast. Prints of closely matched density and contrast were prepared with a Durst enlarger and Schneider-Componon lenses.

Steroid-Binding Assays

Nuclear and cytosolic E_2 receptors were analyzed with previously published procedures (16). Briefly, the tissues were homogenized in Tris-EDTA buffer and centrifuged to prepare nuclear and cytosolic fractions. The nuclei were washed and an exchange assay performed at 37°C for 1 h. We used the tritiated synthetic estrogen Moxestrol (R2858) as the radioligand. Cytosols were incubated for 3 h at 0°C to measure unoccupied ER. Nonspecific binding was subtracted from all data by including one hundredfold radioinert R2858 in parallel tubes.

DISTRIBUTION OF THE ESTROGEN RECEPTOR IN THE ESTROGENIZED STATE

To examine ER distribution in the estrogenized state, we sampled either intact females during the follicular phase or spayed animals treated with E_2 for 2 weeks. The specificity of the anti-ER monoclonal antibodies used has been well established (17). Moreover, we and others (1,5) have shown that all specific staining was in the nuclei, not the cytoplasm of the positively stained cells.

In the uterus of estrogenized monkeys, nuclear staining was evident in the glandular epithelium and the stromal fibroblasts of the endometrium (Fig. 1a) and in the smooth muscle cells of the myometrium (Fig. 1b). Cytoplasmic staining was pale and was not significantly altered when control antibodies (AT) were used instead of antiestrophilins. Nuclear staining was always absent when control antibodies were used, but pale cytoplasmic staining was present (Fig. 1, c and d).

In control nontarget tissues, such as the duodenum, there was no nuclear staining with antiestrophilins (Fig. 2a). There was moderate cytoplasmic staining in this tissue which was not abolished when AT was used as the first antibody (Fig. 2b). All control nontarget tissues behaved similarly. The endothelial lining cells of blood and lymph

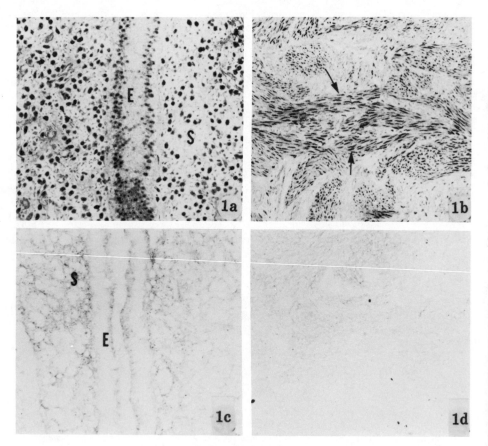

Fig. 1. Immunocytochemistry of endometrium (a and c) and myometrium (b and d) from a monkey treated with E_2 for 14 days. Note the intense staining of glandular, stromal, and myometrial nuclei in a and b which were stained with the antiestrophilins. Only nonspecific staining of the cytoplasm and extracellular matrix is evident in c and d, for which AT was used as the first antibody. Magnification: a and c, X300; b and d, X150; E, epithelium; S, stromal. Reprinted with permission from Endocrinology (1).

50

vessels in the uterus were unstained, but the perivascular stromal cells and the smooth muscles in the wall of the larger arteries were usually stained.

The oviduct, cervix, and vagina all contained cells that exhibited specific nuclear staining when immunostained with the antiestrophilins.

Both epithelial and stromal nuclei were stained in fimbriae of the oviduct (Fig. 3a). Within the oviductal epithelium, however, nuclear staining was detectable only in the secretory, not the ciliated, cells. Smooth muscle nuclei of the myosalpinx were positive, but all cell types

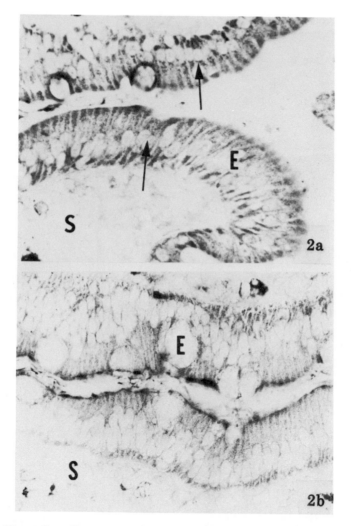

Fig. 2. Immunocytochemistry of frozen sections of duodenum from an E_2-treated monkey. Sections were incubated with anti-ER antibodies (a) or with a control antibody AT (b). Duodenal nuclei (arrows) did not exhibit a positive reaction regardless of whether the antiestrophilins (a) or AT (b) were used as the first antibody. E, epithelium or mucosa; S, stroma of lamina propria. Magnification, X400. Reprinted with permission from Endocrinology (1).

in oviductal blood vessels were negative. In the cervix, stromal and secretory cells were positive (Fig. 3b). The macaque cervix has many fewer ciliated cells than the oviduct, but the cervical ciliated cells were also negative for ER. In the vagina, stromal nuclei were intensely stained, but only the nuclei of the epithelial cells of the basal layers were positive (Fig. 3c). Cytoplasmic staining in the vagina was comparable to that found in histotypically similar nontarget tissues, such as the esophagus. This nonspecific cytoplasmic staining was also evident when the antiestrophilins were replaced by AT.

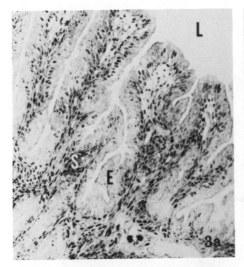

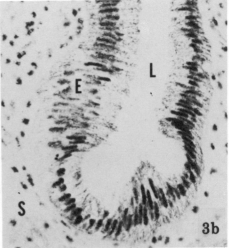

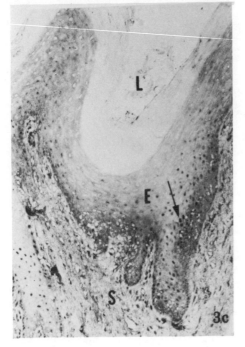

Fig. 3. Immunohistochemically stained cryostat sections of oviduct (a), cervix (b), and vagina (c) also displayed a positive nuclear reaction when incubated with a mixture of antibodies D75 and H222. Both epithelial (E) and stromal (S) nuclei were reactive in all target organs. In the stratified squamous epithelium of the vagina, only the nuclei in the basal layers (arrow) were intensely stained. L, lumen. Magnification: a, X150; b, X400; c, X150. Reprinted with permission from Endocrinology (1).

THE ESTROGEN RECEPTOR DURING ESTROGEN-PROGESTIN TREATMENTS

We (13) compared ER levels determined by steroid-binding assays with the intensity of nuclear staining revealed by immunocytochemistry during both long-term and short-term estrogen-progestin treatments. For the long-term studies, 36 sexually mature cynomolgus macaques were ovariectomized and held for 6 weeks. Some were untreated, others were treated with a 2 cm estradiol (E_2) implant for 2 weeks, and the remainder were treated with E_2 for 2 weeks, and then a 6 cm progestin implant was added for 2 additional weeks (sequential P). Reproductive tracts were removed from spayed (n=8), 14-day E_2 stimulated (n=15) and sequential progestin-treated (n=13) animals. For the short-term studies, the reproductive tracts of spayed pigtail macaques were removed after 14 days of E_2 treatment (n=3) and then on 1 (n=5), 3 (n=5), 12 (n=1), 18 (n=1), and 24 (n=1) h after the insertion of a progestin implant.

Long-Term Estradiol and Progesterone Treatments

Receptor binding assays. The results are summarized in Figure 4. The endometrium, oviduct, cervix and myometrium from spayed, untreated animals had low levels of nuclear but substantial amounts of cytosolic ER. After 14 days of E_2 treatment, there was a significant increase in cytosolic and nuclear ER obtained from the endometrium, oviduct and cervix; the myometrium showed no significant change. After sequential progestin, the endometrium and the oviduct had significantly lower nuclear and cytosolic ER, the cervix had decreased cytosolic levels, and the myometrium showed no significant change in ER. In the endometrium and oviducts of animals treated sequentially with progestin, cytosolic ER values were lower than in the same tissues of untreated spayed animals (t-test, P<0.01). However, nuclear ER levels in endometria of sequential progestin-treated animals were higher than in the endometria of untreated spayed animals (t-test; P<0.05).

Immunocytochemistry. Changes in the endometrium and oviduct will be illustrated here; the photomicrographs of the cervical and myometrial changes can be reviewed in reference 13.

In spayed macaques, nuclear staining for ER was evident in the epithelial and stromal cells of the endometrium (Fig. 5a), oviduct (Fig. 6a), and cervix and smooth muscle cells of the myometrium. All cytoplasmic or extracellular staining was nonspecific, just as was seen in estrogenized animals. After 14 days of E_2, there was a dramatic increase both in the intensity of staining and in the number of ER positive epithelial and stromal cells in endometrium (Fig. 5b), oviduct (Fig. 6b), and cervix as well as a modest increase in these parameters in the smooth muscle cells of the myometrium. Sequential progestin treatment abolished staining in epithelial and stromal cells in endometrium (Fig. 5c) and oviduct (Fig. 6c), and greatly reduced it in stromal cells in the cervix. ER staining was only slightly reduced in cervical epithelial cells and smooth muscle cells of the myometrium after long-term progestin treatment.

Short-Term Progestin Treatment of Estrogenized Animals

Receptor binding assays. The results are summarized in Figure 7. Nuclear ER was significantly reduced after 1 and 3 h of progestin treatment in both endometrium and oviduct. Cytosolic ER was decreased in endometrium by 3 h but not until 12-24 h in oviduct. In the cervix, nuclear and cytosolic ER were not lowered until 12-24 h of progestin treatment. Myometrial ER was unchanged at all times of treatment.

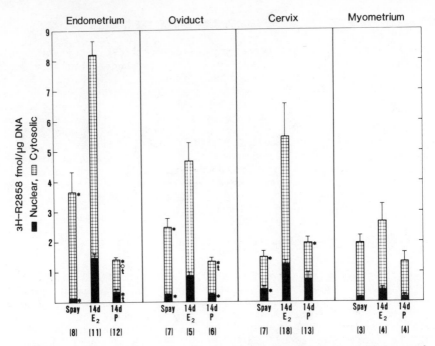

Fig. 4. ER levels measured by R2858 binding in nuclear and cytosolic fractions of reproductive tract tissues obtained from spayed 14-day E_2-treated and sequential progestin-treated macaques. The number of animals in each group is shown in parentheses. Fractions marked with asterisks are significantly different (by ANOVA–Duncans, $P<0.05$) from the same fractions of the 14-day E_2 treatment group. The cytosolic fraction of the sequential progestin group is marked with an open circle to indicate that it is significantly lower (by ANOVA–Duncans, $P<0.05$) than the same fraction in the spayed group. t indicates those cytosolic fractions in the sequential progestin groups that are significantly different by unpaired t test ($P<0.05$) from those in the corresponding fractions of spayed macaques. P, progestin. Reprinted with permission from Endocrinology (13).

<u>Immunocytochemistry</u>. In endometrium, nuclear staining was intense after 14 days of E_2 (Fig. 8a), unchanged after 1 h (Fig. 8b), noticeably reduced by 3 h (Fig. 8c) and greatly reduced by 12–24 h (Fig. 8d). In the oviduct, the initial level of nuclear staining intensity (Fig. 9a) was not unequivocally reduced until 12–24 h (Fig. 9d). In the cervix, reduction in nuclear staining intensity was not evident until 12–24 h, and this was more noticeable in stromal than epithelial cells. There was no noticeable decrease in nuclear staining intensity in the myometrium.

To summarize the above, our binding assays showed that in spayed animals most of the receptor was cytosolic but our immunocytochemistry indicated that all of the specific staining was nuclear. This supports the view that in the absence of E_2, the unoccupied, nontransformed form of ER can be easily stripped away from the nucleus during homogenization and becomes detectable in the cytosolic fraction. After 14 days of E_2 treatment, more ER is found in the nuclear fraction, presumably because the binding of E_2 results in an activated receptor with more affinity for nuclear components. More cytosolic ER is also found because E_2 treatment leads to synthesis and accumulation of excess unoccupied receptor. There

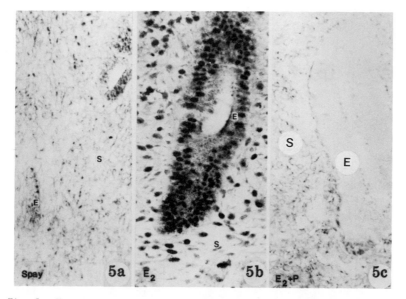

Fig. 5. Upper functionalis of the endometrium. The spayed group (a) had light nuclear staining in cells of both the glandular epithelium (E) and stroma (S). After 14 days of E_2 treatment (b), the cells had hypertrophied, and more intense nuclear staining was found in both epithelial (E) and stromal (S) cells. Sequential progestin treatment for 14 days (c) virtually abolished staining in cells of both epithelium (E) and stroma (S). Magnification, X450. Reprinted with permission from Endocrinology (13).

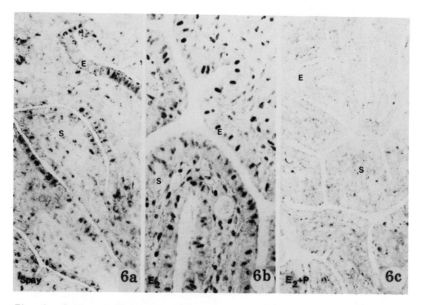

Fig. 6. Oviductal fimbriae. The spayed group (a) had a moderate level of nuclear staining in epithelial (E) and stromal (S) cells. After 14 days of E_2 treatment (b), strong nuclear staining was evident in a larger number of stromal (S) and epithelial (E) cells. Although not evident at this magnification, only nuclei of the secretory epithelial cells are stained; the nuclei of the ciliated cells are unstained. After 14 days of sequential progestin treatment (c), staining is virtually abolished in stromal and epithelial cells. Magnification, X450.

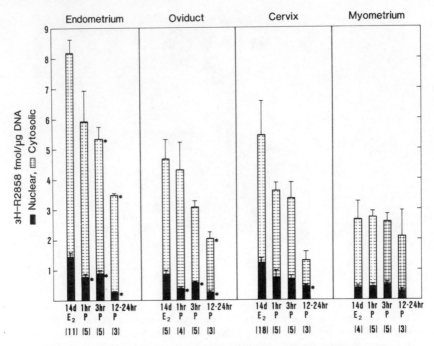

Fig. 7. ER levels in reproductive tract tissues obtained after 0, 1, 3 or 12-24 h of sequential progestin treatment of macaques that had been estrogenized for 14 days. The number of animals in each group is shown in parentheses. The asterisks indicate the nuclear or cytosolic fractions that contain significantly less ER (by ANOVA-Duncans, P<0.05) than the corresponding fractions of the 0 h, 14-day, E_2-treated group. P, progestin. Reprinted with permission from Endocrinology (13).

was an overall increase in nuclear staining after 2 weeks of E_2 treatment, presumably because there were more ER molecules, both occupied and unoccupied, in the nuclei of a larger number of cells.

Sequential progestin treatment for 2 weeks lowers cytosolic and nuclear ER in the oviduct and endometrium significantly below the amount present in these tissues in E_2-treated animals and lowers the cytosolic, but not the nuclear, levels significantly below the levels found in the oviduct and endometrium of spayed animals. After such sequential progestin treatment, nuclear staining was undetectable, well below the amount seen in spayed animals. If the nuclear ER was the major receptor fraction detected by the antibody, then the progestin-suppressed tissues should have had as much nuclear staining as the spayed animals because the latter had equivalent amounts of biochemically detectable nuclear ER. Because progestin treatment of estrogenized animals suppressed cytosolic, but not nuclear, ER to levels below those in spayed animals, it follows that the progestin-induced reduction in nuclear staining is mainly due to the progestin-induced suppression of cytosolic, not nuclear, ER. The results of our short-term progestin treatments led to similar conclusions. For example, in oviduct and endometrium, concentrations of nuclear ER determined by exchange assay were significantly decreased as early as 1 h after the beginning of sequential progestin treatment in both tissues, but there was no unequivocal decline in ER staining after 1 h of progestin treatment in either of them. There were substantial declines in nuclear staining intensity found after 3 h in endometrium and 12-24 h in oviduct, and these were paralleled by significant decreases in cytosolic and total ER deter-

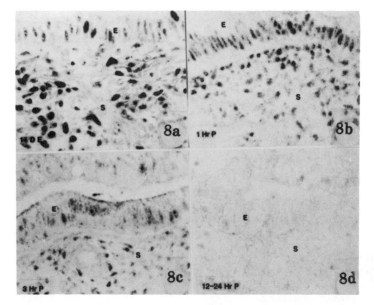

Fig. 8. Upper functionalis of endometrium. There was intense
nuclear staining in all stromal (S) and epithelial (E) cells in the
14-day E_2-treated animals (a). There was no obvious decline in
staining after 1 h of sequential E_2 plus progestin treatment (b),
but by 3 h of progestin treatment (c), there was a noticeable
decrease in nuclear staining of both epithelial (E) and stromal (S)
cells. By 12-24 h of progestin treatment (d), ER staining was
virtually abolished. Magnification, X775. Reprinted with permission from Endocrinology (13).

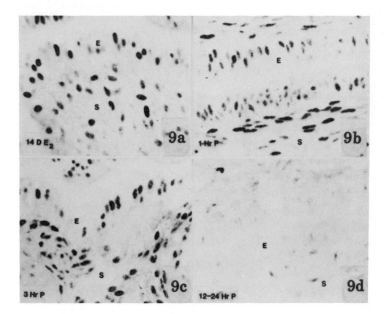

Fig. 9. Oviductal fimbriae. Intense nuclear staining was seen in
the 14-day E_2-treated group (a). No change was evident after 1 h
(b) or 3 h (c) of sequential progestin treatment, but after 12-24 h
of progestin treatment (d), staining for ER was greatly reduced in
both stromal and epithelial cells. Magnification, X775. Reprinted
with permission from Endocrinology (13).

mined biochemically in both tissues. In summary, the data suggest that the bulk of the cytosolic receptor is in the nucleus when cells are frozen. We assume that the ER, like other nuclear proteins, is synthesized in the rough endoplasmic reticulum and shipped so rapidly to specific nuclear sites that its concentration in the cytoplasm always remains low.

THE ARTIFICIAL LUTEAL-FOLLICULAR TRANSITION

Because approximately two-thirds of the endometrium is lost and regenerated every menstrual cycle, the macaque uterus is uniquely suited for the study of the mechanisms of estrogen-dependent cellular growth and differentiation in adult organisms. After menses and repair, there is a period of hypertrophy and hyperplasia that results from the action of E_2 in the absence of progestin (18,19). As noted above, we have studied the suppressive effects of progestin on ER in hormone-treated spayed animals. A similar suppression occurs during the luteal phase of the natural menstrual cycle (20). In the early follicular phase, as serum progestin levels decline, the progestin suppression is relieved and ER levels rise, but it was not known whether ER was renewed at the same rate in the different uterine cell types.

To study this question, we (14) created artificial menstrual cycles in spayed macaques through the use of E_2 and progestin-filled Silastic capsules, and sampled the endometrium during the transition period between the end of one cycle and the beginning of the next (the luteal-follicular transition). We measured ER levels with binding assays and used immunocytochemistry with monoclonal antiestrophilins to evaluate changes in the distribution of ER among the various uterine cell types.

Twenty-seven spayed cynomolgus macaques were implanted subcutaneously with 2 cm E_2-filled Silastic capsules, and these were left in place throughout the experiment. After 14 days of E_2 treatment, a 6 cm progestin-filled Silastic capsule was implanted, left in place for 14 days and then removed. Animals were brought to surgery 0, 0.5, 1, 2, 3, 4, 5, 7, or 14 days later and their reproductive tracts were removed. When menstruating tissues were sampled for biochemical assays, the sloughing surface tissues were washed away and only the intact endometrium was used.

Binding Assays of ER

The ER concentrations measured on day 0 were low, similar to amounts present during the late luteal phase of the natural cycle (20). No changes were detected during the first 2 days of progestin withdrawal, but receptor concentrations approximately doubled by day 3 of progestin withdrawal (Table 1). This day was equivalent to day 1 of a normal menstrual cycle as menstruation was externally detected in most animals on this day. Total ER concentrations increased in a linear fashion (Fig. 10) through day 7 with no further increase on day 14 of progestin withdrawal.

Morphological Changes

Endometria from day 0-0.5 (Fig. 11a) specimens were characteristic of the late luteal phase of the natural cycle (21). No distinct morphological changes were evident until 1-2 days of progestin withdrawal when there was the typical premenstrual increase in the number of leukocytes in the outer zones (Fig. 11b). In the inner zones (III and IV), there were numerous dead and dying glandular epithelial cells undergoing apoptosis and pyknosis, and an increased number of macrophages filled with cellular debris and nuclear fragments. During this period, there was a great

Table 1. Effects of progesterone withdrawal on estrogen receptor levels in macaque endometrium.

	14d E_2 + P	12,24 + 48 h P withdrawal	3 + 4 d P withdrawal	5,7 + 14d P withdrawal
Number of animals	9	9	6	9
Serum E_2 pg/ml	129 ± 12	132 ± 13	129 ± 24	110 ± 12
Serum progestin ng/ml	6.78 ± 0.80	0.41 ± 0.04[a]	0.19 ± 0.02[a]	0.22 ± 0.03
Cytosol receptor fmol/mg DNA	941 ± 73[a]	1287 ± 158[b]	2156 ± 255[a,b]	5878 ± 619[a,b]
Nuclear receptor fmol/mg DNA	389 ± 160[a]	198 ± 75[b,c]	606 ± 172[b]	1447 ± 314[a,c]
Total receptor fmol/mg DNA	1330 ± 201[a]	1483 ± 205[b]	2762 ± 190[a,b]	7325 ± 829[a,b]

All data mean ± SEM.
Groups having the same lower-case letter for each parameter are significantly different (P<0.05 or less). P, progesterone. Reprinted with permission from Endocrinology (14).

decrease in interstitial edema. This resulted in compaction of the stroma, increased crowding of the stromal fibroblasts and development of close associations between the basal lamina of the endometrial glands and the subepithelial stromal cells. By the third and fourth days of progestin withdrawal, typical menstrual hemorrhage and sloughing of the outer zones had occurred and the stroma had become further compacted (Fig. 11c). From day 3-5, intimate associations of periglandular stromal cells and glandular epithelial cells were apparent (Fig. 11d); there was minimal extracellular matrix and marked stromal hypertrophy. By day 5, epithelial cells had migrated from the mouths of the glands and formed a new luminal surface. On day 5, epithelial mitoses in the glands had increased (Fig. 11e), except in the basalis and the flattened surface epithelial cells. By day 7, the surface was healed and zones I and II had reformed. In the newly formed zone II, numerous mitotic figures were evident in the glandular epithelium, the extracellular matrix had increased in amount, and the stromal fibroblasts were spaced further apart and had lost their intimate association with the basal lamina of the glands (Fig. 11f). By day 14 of progestin withdrawal, there was an increase in overall endometrial thickness and a further loosening of the stroma in all zones, including the basalis.

Immunocytochemistry of the Endometrium

On day 0, nuclear staining for ER was detectable only in zone IV of the basalis, where a few glandular epithelial cells were positive, and in the walls of some spiral arteries, in which some stromal fibroblasts and smooth muscle cells were stained. All other stromal and glandular epithelial cells were negative (Fig. 12a). On days 0.5-1 of progestin withdrawal, additional stromal, but not glandular epithelial cells became positively stained (Fig. 12b). Staining of the glandular epithelium of zone IV of the basalis decreased during this time. On days 2 (Fig. 12c) and 4 (Fig. 12d), stromal cells were still the only cell type stained.

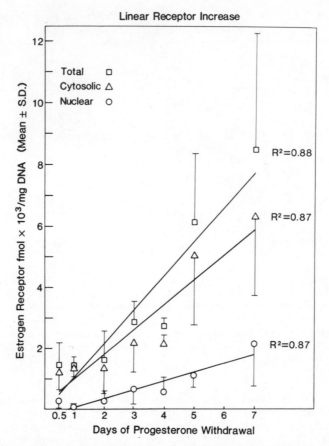

Fig. 10. Concentrations of nuclear, cytosolic, and
total ER in partially purified subcellular fractions
of endometria from cynomolgus macaques after 0.5
through 7 days of progestin withdrawal. Values in
femtomoles per mg DNA are means ± SD. Regression
analysis demonstrated a distinct linear trend for
all three values. Reprinted with permission from
Endocrinology (14).

The first epithelial staining occurred on day 5 (in 1 out of 3 animals),
in the glands of the lower, surviving portions of the functionalis and the
upper regions of the basalis (Fig. 12e). Only by day 7 was the glandular
epithelium positively stained throughout the endometrium in all animals
(Fig. 12f). On day 14 there was no apparent change in the number of
stained cells, though the intensity of nuclear staining in both glandular
epithelial and stromal cells had lessened. During days 3-4 of progestin
withdrawal, in the upper regions of the endometria that were undergoing a
combination of sloughing and repair, most of the stromal and epithelial
cells were negative. At no time was there any evidence of receptor
staining in endothelial cells lining blood vessels of either the endometrium or myometrium. In sections treated with AT in place of D75 and
H222, the nuclei of stromal and epithelial cells were never stained.

These results show that bulk endometrial ER concentrations increase
linearly during an artificially induced proliferative phase in the primate
endometrium. The immunocytochemical results reveal that up to and including the time when epithelial growth is initiated, most of the ER is

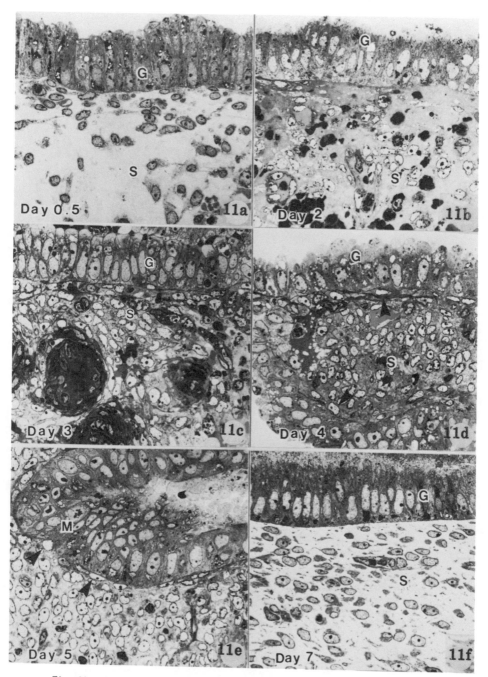

Fig. 11. Araldite-embedded specimens of zones II through III of the endometrium on days 0-7 of progestin withdrawal. a: Day 0. Enlarged stromal
cells scattered throughout an abundant extracellular matrix. G, glandular
epithelium; S, stroma. b: Day 2. Leukocytes become more numerous within
the stroma matrix. c: Day 3. Extracellular matrix diminishes and stromal cells become densely crowded. d: Day 4. Numerous stromal cells
(arrows) are very closely opposed to the epithelial cells of the glands.
e: Day 5. Mitotic figures (M) become prevalent. f: Day 7. Extracellular matrix increases and stromal cells become more separated. Glycogen
develops in basal regions of the glandular epithelium. Magnification,
X700. Reprinted with permission from Endocrinology (14).

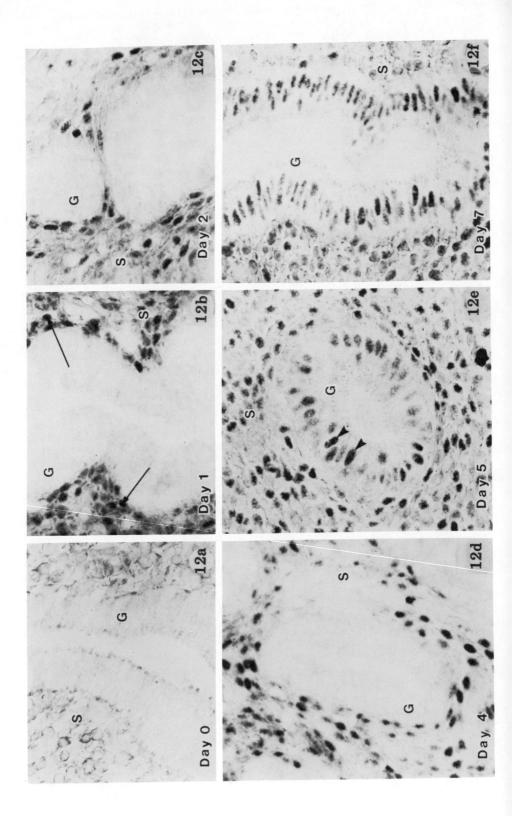

specifically localized in the stromal fibroblasts. Many epithelial cells were ER-negative at 5 days of progestin withdrawal when the mitotic activity in the glands had become maximal. Compaction of the stroma resulted in close associations between stromal fibroblasts and epithelial cells. Such a stromal-epithelial association has been shown to influence the proliferation of normal and neoplastic mammary epithelium (22,23).

During the menstrual sloughing process (days 3-5 of progestin withdrawal), ER staining is negative in the sloughing cells themselves and in the glands and stroma that reorganize to form the upper regions of the endometrium (zone I and upper part of zone II). ER staining is initially negative in the epithelial cells that migrate out from the mouths of the glands to form the new luminal epithelial surface. Clearly, the epithelial and stromal cells that participate in early endometrial surface repair do not require estrogen receptors to carry out such repair. Ferenczy (24) has suggested that menstrual repair is estrogen independent and our observations support that view. Such estrogen-independent "wound healing" of the endometrial surface repair must also occur in ovariectomized animals, which often menstruate for 2-3 days after ovariectomy.

The evidence for an inductive role for stromal cells on epithelial differentiation in sex steroid target tissues during fetal and neonatal life has been reviewed (4). The data clearly indicate that stromal-epithelial interactions play a vital role in steroid hormone action. Cunha (25) has also suggested that the stroma continues to regulate the epithelial hormonal response in the adult. In cyclic tissues, such as uterus, oviduct, vagina and cervix, the state of differentiation of the epithelium fluctuates on a regular basis with changes in prevailing hormonal environment. The appearance of steroid receptors in stromal but not epithelial cells at the onset of hormone action would be consistent with a regulatory role for the stroma.

To further clarify the relationship between estrogen-receptor interaction and cell proliferation, combined autoradiographic/immunocytochemical studies of endometrial slices incubated in vitro with H^3-thymidine are being done. Preliminary results indicate that the majority of epithelial cells that incorporate thymidine on days 4.5-5 lack immunocytochemically detectable ER. These data indicate that the effects of E_2 on epithelial mitosis in the endometrium during the early proliferative stage may be mediated indirectly through estrogen-induced growth factors in stromal cells.

Fig. 12 (opposite page). Frozen sections of the upper functionalis (zones II and III) of endometria from macaques treated with E_2 plus progestin, (a) or after 1 (b), 2 (c), 4 (d), 5 (e), or 7 (f) days of progestin withdrawal. No glandular epithelial (G) nuclear staining was observed on days 0-4 of progestin withdrawal (a-d). Stromal (S) nuclear staining (arrow) was evident as early as 1 day after removing progestin (b) and persisted in all samples, including 14 days of E_2. The earliest evidence of nuclear ER in glandular epithelial cells was on day 5 of progestin withdrawal when 1 of 3 animals exhibited immunostaining for ER (e; arrowhead). By day 7, all endometria sampled exhibited nuclear ER staining in both stromal and epithelial cells (f). Magnification, X575. Reprinted with permission from Endocrinology (14).

THE ESTROGEN RECEPTOR DURING THE NATURAL MENSTRUAL CYCLE

In addition to the above studies with hormone-treated animals, we have begun collecting the reproductive tracts of naturally cycling animals. So far, we have only examined the tracts of a few animals at representative intervals during the cycle. A complete set of photomicrographs of these tissues will be published separately.

Endometrium

At the very beginning of the cycle, the pattern of ER staining is exactly as described above for the hormonally induced luteal-follicular transition (see Figure 12 for examples). There is minimal staining on the first day of menstruation except in the glandular epithelium of the basalis. The first cells to develop ER staining are the stromal cells in the inner zones, and the number of positive ER stromal cells increases steadily through the period of menses and repair. Glandular epithelial cells do not become ER positive throughout the endometrium until repair of the endometrial surface is well underway. The same intense packing of the stromal cells with close stromal-epithelial apposition is evident throughout the early follicular phase (see Figure 11 for examples). By midcycle, the majority of stromal fibroblasts and glandular epithelial cells are positively stained for ER. Vascular endothelium and nonfibroblast stromal cells are unstained. After ovulation there is a decline in the intensity of both stromal and epithelial staining that is evident first in the outer zones (I and II) and later in zone III. The stromal cells in zone IV are also suppressed, but the glandular epithelium of zone IV (the basalis) retains its ER staining. The stromal cells around the spiral arteries and some of the smooth muscle cells in these vessels also retain their ER staining throughout the luteal phase. In the myometrium, ER staining is intense during the follicular phase and only slightly diminished during the luteal phase.

The Oviduct

During the early follicular phase, ER becomes detectable in many, but not all, stromal and epithelial cells. All smooth muscle cells of the myosalpinx appear ER-positive. By mid-cycle when the epithelium has fully differentiated into ciliated and secretory cells (21), ER staining is clearly present only in the secretory epithelial cells, stromal cells and smooth muscle cells. Ciliated cells lack detectable levels of ER. At this time, the oviduct has the appearance shown in Figures 3a and 6b. After ovulation, when serum progestin levels rise above 1 ng/ml, ER staining is suppressed in all stromal and secretory cells, similar to the appearance shown in Figure 6c. ER staining in smooth muscle cells is less suppressed than in the other cell types during the luteal phase. During the luteal-follicular transition to the next menstrual cycle, stromal cells appear to develop positive ER staining more rapidly than the epithelial cells, as in the endometrium. However, this phenomenon is less marked in the oviduct than the endometrium; oviductal epithelial cells develop ER more rapidly than endometrial ones.

THE PROGESTERONE RECEPTOR DURING DIFFERENT HORMONAL STATES

In a preliminary report (2) we have described our findings with the anti-PR antibody B39. As with the anti-ER antibodies, all cytoplasmic staining with B39 appears nonspecific, as the same degree of cytoplasmic staining occurs with AT and other nonimmune rat IgG_{2a} antibodies in all target cells. B39 also lightly stains the cytoplasm, but not the nuclei, of intestinal epithelial and other nontarget cells. However, B39 is an extremely high affinity antibody that is effective at a lower concentration and shows much less nonspecific cytoplasmic and pericellular staining than any of the anti-ER antibodies we have used.

Endometrium

We have examined the endometria of rhesus monkeys that were spayed, estrogenized and sequentially progestin treated with the regimens described above. Intact, cycling animals have also been studied. In spayed animals PR was usually absent, though a few animals had considerable amounts of PR detectable in glandular epithelial cells. Estrogen treatment for 14 days led to great increases in the number of PR-positive stromal and epithelial cells in all zones in all animals. The functionalis of an estrogenized animal is shown in Figure 13. After 2 additional weeks of sequential progestin treatment, PR had been suppressed in the glandular epithelial cells of the functionalis (Fig. 14), was retained in the glandular epithelial cells of the basalis (Fig. 15) and remained easily detectable in the stromal cells of all of the endometrial zones (Fig. 14 and 15).

In the natural menstrual cycle, during the luteal-follicular transition the pattern of PR staining is identical to that of ER. Stromal cells become intensely positive for PR while epithelial cells remain PR-negative. Most glandular epithelial cells do not become PR-positive until after menses and repair are complete. After ovulation there is a reduction in PR staining that is evident in the glandular epithelium, first in the outer zones and later in the inner zones. As was the case with ER staining, the deepest region of the basalis (zone IV) retains its PR staining longer than the other zones. However, at the very beginning of the next cycle, this zone loses its PR staining. Throughout the thickness of the endometrium, stromal cells showed only a slight reduction in the intensity of PR staining during the luteal phase. Luteal progestin appears to suppress PR staining much more in glandular epithelium than in the stroma. Perivascular stroma and smooth muscle cells remain PR-

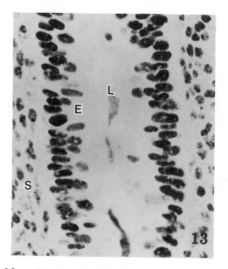

Fig. 13. PR in the functionalis (zones II-III) of an estrogenized rhesus monkey. PR staining is intense in the glandular epithelium and the stroma. E = epithelium; S = stroma; L = lumen of gland. Magnification, X600.

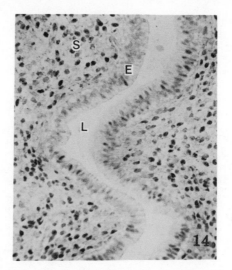

Fig. 14. PR in functionalis (zones II-III)
of a sequentially progestin-treated rhesus
monkey, equivalent to the late luteal phase
of the cycle compared to the estrogenized
state. PR staining is greatly reduced in
the glandular epithelium but remains intense
in the stroma. E, S, L as above. Magnification, X350.

positive during the luteal phase, though vascular endothelium is PR
negative at all times. In the myometrium, the intensity of the PR
staining does not change during the cycle. The retention of PR in most
stromal cells, and its loss in most glandular epithelial cells during the
luteal phase, suggests that the effects of luteal progestin on the
glandular epithelium may be indirectly mediated by stromal cells. As with

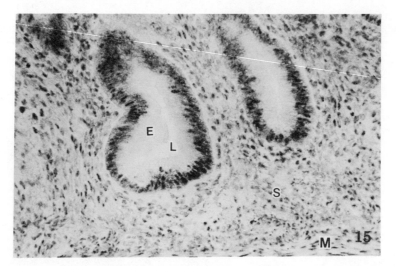

Fig. 15. PR in the basalis-myometrial region (zone IV) of the
endometrium of the same sequentially progestin treated as in
Figure 14. PR staining is retained in both the stroma and the
glandular epithelium of the basalis region. E, S, L as above.
Magnification, X350.

E_2, the effects of progestin on the endometrial vascular endothelium may be mediated indirectly by perivascular stromal and smooth muscle cells. Luteal progestin can act directly on myometrial smooth muscle cells as these cells retain PR staining at all times.

The Oviduct

In spayed animals, most cells lack PR staining, though stromal cells have barely detectable levels. After estrogenization, when the epithelium differentiates into ciliated and secretory cells, PR is present in the stromal, secretory and smooth muscle cells but, like ER, is absent from the ciliated cells (Fig. 16). After long-term progestin treatment of estrogenized animals, the oviduct atrophies and the epithelium deciliates and stops secreting due to progestin antagonism (26). PR becomes non-detectable in the secretory cells but, most importantly, remains in the stromal cells (Fig. 17). Consequently, the only cells remaining in the mucosa that could mediate the continuing antagonistic effects of progestin on the epithelium are the stromal cells. Because the oviductal epithelium will remain atrophied as long as progestin treatment continues, it follows that the suppressive effects of progestin on the epithelium must be mediated indirectly through the stromal cells.

In the follicular phase of the natural cycle, PR is present in the smooth muscle cells, the stroma and the secretory epithelial cells but not the ciliated ones. After ovulation, PR is suppressed dramatically in the secretory epithelial cells but only minimally in the stroma, just as described above for progestin-treated spayed animals. The long-term antagonistic effects of progestin on the oviductal epithelium appear to be mediated by PR in stromal cells in naturally cycling as well as hormonally treated animals.

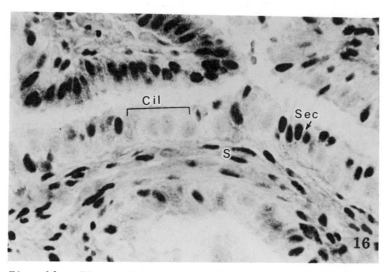

Fig. 16. PR in the oviduct of an estrogenized rhesus monkey. Intense staining is evident in stromal (S) and secretory epithelial (SEC) cells, but not in the ciliated epithelial (CIL) cells. Magnification, X600.

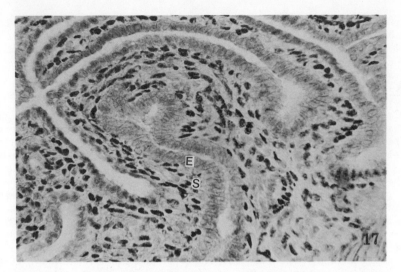

Fig. 17. PR in the oviduct of a sequentially progestin-
treated rhesus monkey. PR staining is only evident in the
stroma (S), not the epithelium (E). Magnification, X400.

SUMMARY

The above data suggest that the major portion of ER that contributes
to immunocytochemical staining of target cell nuclei is that portion
detectable in the cytosol after tissue homogenization. In untreated,
spayed animals, most of the receptor was recovered in the cytosol, yet the
specific immunostaining was nuclear. This important case strongly
suggests that the staining seen in the nucleus represents most of the ER
in the cell. With various hormonal treatments, the changes in the degree
of nuclear staining revealed by immunocytochemistry always paralleled the
changes in cytosolic and total ER, but not always the amount found in the
nuclear fraction by binding assays. Because immunocytochemistry of frozen
sections most likely reveals antigens in their native locations, these
findings support the view that the so-called cytosolic ER resides in the
nucleus in living cells, and that the techniques of homogenization and
centrifugation artifactually separate the total cellular ER into nuclear
and cytosolic fractions (6).

Another major conclusion that we have drawn from the above research
is that some of the important actions of both E_2 and progestin on the
epithelial components of the sex steroid target organs may be mediated in
paracrine fashion through factors secreted by neighboring stromal cells.
This is evident from studies of the endometrium during the luteal-
follicular transition, when stromal cells develop their ER several days
before the glandular epithelial cells, yet the latter cells undergo
estrogen-dependent mitosis. It is also evident in the progestin-
suppressed oviduct, where ciliated cells that lack PR are suppressed by
the action of progestin, and the only PR-positive cells that persist
throughout the period of progestin antagonism are in the stroma. We
suggest that new research on the paracrine action of regulatory factors
secreted by stromal cells under steroid hormone influence is needed to
gain more insight into the mechanism by which steroid hormones regulate
the cyclic changes of the adult female reproductive tract.

ACKNOWLEDGMENTS

We thank Dr. Geoffrey Greene of the Ben May Laboratories of the University of Chicago, and Chris Nolan of Abbott Laboratories for the monoclonal antibodies. We also thank Bev Cole and Kunie Mah for their technical assistance, Kay S. Carlisle for photographic work and Angela Adler for secretarial help.

REFERENCES

1. McClellan MC, West NB, Tacha DE, Greene GL, Brenner RM. Immunocytochemical localization of estrogen receptors in the macaque reproductive tract with monoclonal antiestrophilins. Endocrinology 1984; 114:2002-14.
2. Brenner RM, West NB. Immunocytochemistry of the progestin receptor in the reproductive tract of female macaques [Abstract]. Program and Abstracts of the 69th Annual Meeting of The Endocrine Society, Indianapolis, IN, 1987:79.
3. Bentley JP, Brenner RM, Linstedt AD, et al. Increased hyaluronate and collagen biosynthesis and fibroblast estrogen receptors in macaque sex skin. J Invest Dermatol 1986; 87:668-73.
4. Cunha GR, Chung LWK, Shannon JM, Taguchi O, Fujii H. Hormone-induced morphogenesis and growth: role of mesenchymal-epithelial interactions. Recent Prog Horm Res 1983; 39:559-98.
5. King WJ, Greene GL. Monoclonal antibodies localize oestrogen receptor in the nuclei of target cells. Nature 1984; 307:745-7.
6. Welshons WV, Lieberman ME, Gorski J. Nuclear localization of unoccupied oestrogen receptors. Nature 1984; 307:747-9.
7. Gravanis A, Gurpide E. Enucleation of human endometrial cells: nucleo-cytoplasmic distribution of DNA polymerase alpha and estrogen receptor. J Steroid Biochem 1986; 24:469-74.
8. Resnik R. The endocrine regulation of uterine blood flow in the nonpregnant uterus: a review. Am J Obstet Gynecol 1981; 140:151.
9. Brenner RM, West NB. Hormonal regulation of the reproductive tract in female mammals. Annu Rev Physiol 1975; 37:273-302.
10. Brenner RM, West NB, Norman RL, Sandow BA, Verhage HG. Progesterone suppression of the estradiol receptor in the reproductive tract of macaques, cats and hamsters. Adv Exp Med Biol 1979; 117:173-96.
11. Katzenellenbogen BS. Dynamics of steroid hormone receptor action. Annu Rev Physiol 1980; 42:17-36.
12. Leavitt WW, MacDonald RG, Okulicz WC. Hormonal regulation of estrogen and progesterone receptor systems. In: Litwack G, ed. Biochemical actions of hormones; vol X. New York: Academic Press, 1983: 323-56.
13. West NB, McClellan MC, Sternfeld MD, Brenner RM. Immunocytochemistry versus binding assays of the estrogen receptor in the reproductive tract of spayed and hormone treated macaques. Endocrinology 1987; 121:1789-800.
14. McClellan M, West NB, Brenner RM. Immunocytochemical localization of estrogen receptors in the macaque endometrium during the luteal-follicular transition. Endocrinology 1986; 119:2467-75.
15. Sandow BA, West NB, Norman RL, Brenner RM. Hormonal control of apoptosis in hamster uterine luminal epithelium. Am J Anat 1979; 156:15-36.
16. West NB, Brenner RM. Progesterone-mediated suppression of estradiol receptors in cynomolgus macaque cervix, endometrium and oviduct during sequential estradiol-progesterone treatment. J Steroid Biochem 1985; 22:29-37.
17. Greene GL, Press MF. Structure and dynamics of the estrogen receptor. J Steroid Biochem 1986; 24:1-7.

18. Bartelmez GW. Cyclic changes in the endometrium of the rhesus monkey (<u>Macaca mulatta</u>). Contrib Embryol 1951; 34:99–144.

19. Ferenczy A, Bertrand G, Gelfand MM. Studies on the cytodynamics of human endometrial regeneration III. <u>In vitro</u> short-term incubation historadioautography. Am J Obstet Gynecol 1979; 134:297–304.

20. West NB, Brenner RM. Estrogen receptor levels in the oviducts and endometria of cynomolgus macaques during the menstrual cycle. Biol Reprod 1983; 29:1303–12.

21. Brenner RM, Carlisle KS, Hess DL, Sandow BA, West NB. Morphology of the oviducts and endometria of cynomolgus macaques during the menstrual cycle. Biol Reprod 1983; 29:1289–302.

22. Enami J, Enami S, Koga M. Growth of normal and neoplastic mouse mammary epithelial cells in primary culture: stimulation by conditioned medium from mouse mammary fibroblasts. Gann 1983; 74:845–53.

23. McGrath CM. Augmentation of the response of normal mammary epithelial cells to estradiol by mammary stroma. Cancer Res 1984; 43:1355–60.

24. Ferenczy A. Studies on the cytodynamics of experimental endometrial regeneration in the rabbit. Historadioautography and ultrastructure. Am J Obstet Gynecol 1977; 128:536–45.

25. Cunha GR, Bigsby RM, Cooke PS, Sugimura Y. Stromal-epithelial interactions in adult organs. Cell Differ 1985; 17:137–48.

26. Brenner RM, Resko JA, West NB. Cyclic changes in oviductal morphology and residual cytoplasmic estradiol binding capacity induced by sequential estradiol-progesterone treatment of spayed rhesus monkeys. Endocrinology 1974; 95:1094–104.

5

STRUCTURE, FUNCTIONAL DOMAINS AND SUBCELLULAR
DISTRIBUTION OF GLUCOCORTICOID RECEPTOR

Jan Carlstedt-Duke, Ann-Charlotte Wikstrom, and
Jan-Ake Gustafsson

Department of Medical Nutrition, Karolinska Institutet
Huddinge University Hospital F69, S-141 86 Huddinge,
Sweden

INTRODUCTION

Much interest has been focused on the steroid hormone receptor proteins during recent years. These proteins are transcriptional regulatory factors and have proven to be of central interest for research on gene regulation in eukaryotic cells. It was hypothesized early that the steroid hormones exerted their biological effects via the genome with the help of soluble receptor proteins (1), and this model, with minor modifications, holds true today, even with the more detailed information available. Our interest has focused on the glucocorticoid receptor protein (GR) and its mechanism of action. We have worked predominantly with the rat liver GR, although some work on the mouse and human GR has also been carried out at our laboratory. There are only minor differences between species. The structure and function of GR will be discussed in this chapter.

INTRACELLULAR LOCALIZATION OF GR

According to the original dogma proposed (1), GR was a cytoplasmic protein that underwent a nuclear translocation first after the binding of the steroid to the protein (Fig. 1A). After translocation, the receptor complex interacted with the genome resulting in both transcriptional stimulation and inhibition of specific genes. This model was based on the occurrence and distribution of GR in crude cytosolic and nuclear preparations, assuming that these preparations represent the cytoplasm and nucleus in vivo, respectively. However, studies on the subcellular localization of estrogen receptors (ER) and progestin receptors (PR), using either immunocytochemical staining techniques (2-5) or cellular enucleation followed by biochemical measurement of ER content (6) or GR and PR content (7), have indicated a strictly nuclear location of ER and PR. It was assumed that the presence of ER and PR in cytosol preparations was a result of a redistribution of receptor from the nucleus, to which it was loosely associated. It is first after the binding of steroid to the receptor that the complex becomes tightly associated with the chromatin in the nucleus. This form of receptor remains associated with the nucleus throughout the preparation of subcellular fractions and is released from the nucleus first after incubation at high ionic strength. Thus, the unique nuclear localization of ER and PR proposed maintains the two-step model of steroid-binding followed by DNA-binding, although both steps would then occur within the nucleus without any intervening translocation (Fig. 1B).

In view of the results obtained with ER and PR, it was considered of interest to reassess the cellular localization of GR. Antibodies against GR have been raised by several groups and several immunocytochemical and immunohistochemical studies of GR have been published (8-15). Using a monoclonal antibody raised against rat liver GR (16), an immunocytochemical analysis of the intracellular localization was performed, including the use of several fixation and permeabilization procedures (17). With all fixation methods tested, it was possible to obtain specific GR staining. Further studies were carried out using fixation with para-formaldehyde. Solubilization with Triton X-100 or saponin at various concentrations was evaluated by using antibodies against core-nucleosome proteins and tubulin, cellular constituents with well-defined localization. Three different systems were used for these studies: rat Rueber hepatoma H-4-II-E and human uterus carcinoma NHIK 3025 cell lines as well as cultured rat hepatocytes. Specific GR staining was obtained using the peroxidase antiperoxidase technique or with second antibodies labeled with fluorescein isothiocyanate.

Permeabilization of the cells was shown to be a factor of importance for the intracellular localization of GR (17). If the cells were fixed but not permeabilized, an intense staining for GR was seen in some areas of the cytoplasm with a general weaker cytoplasmic staining. No nuclear GR staining was seen. Mild permeabilization with 0.05% Triton resulted in a more intense general staining of the cytoplasm, and nuclear staining was detectable in some cells. Permeabilization with 0.5% Triton resulted in a more extensive staining of the nuclei, at the same time as the cytoplasmic staining was reduced. Double staining with antibodies against GR and core nucleosomes or tubulin showed that the intensity of GR staining within the different cellular compartments paralleled the accessibility of the different compartments to antibodies, depending on the solubilization. Thus, a mild permeabilization enabled an intensive staining of tubulin in all cells whereas there was only staining of core nucleosomes in a small fraction of the cells. GR staining in these cells was very similar to the tubulin staining, with intensive cytoplasmic staining in a fibrillar pattern. Only those cells that demonstrated staining of core nucleosomes following mild permeabilization stained for GR in the nucleus. Thus, the occurrence of nuclear GR staining in these cells is dependent on the accessibility of the nucleus to the antibodies. Extensive permeabiliza-

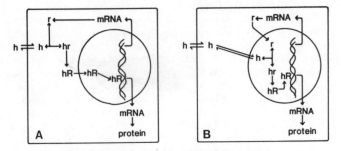

Fig. 1. Mechanism of action of steroid hormone receptors. (A) The cytoplasmic-nuclear transloca-tion model. (B) The nuclear localization model. Abbreviations: h, hormone; r, receptor protein; hr, nonactivated hormone-receptor complex; hR, activated hormone-receptor complex.

tion results in a concomitant intensive staining of all nuclei for both core nucleosomes as well as GR. The nucleoli remained unstained with both antibodies. However, extensive permeabilization also resulted in the loss of the cytoplasmic GR staining. Experiments on MCF-7 cells with parallel staining for GR and ER showed the same pattern of cytoplasmic and nuclear GR staining, dependent on the permeabilization, whereas ER staining was seen exclusively within the nucleus (17), in accordance with previous results published (2-4). Thus, the intracellular localization of GR appears to be both cytoplasmic and nuclear, in contrast to the localization of ER and PR.

Previous studies have reported a dexamethasone-dependent nuclear translocation of GR in the rat brain (10,13) or cultured cells (8,9), based on the intensification of the nuclear GR staining following the addition of dexamethasone. When H-4-II-E cells were grown in medium supplemented with serum treated with dextran-coated charcoal and dialyzed, dexamethasone addition to the medium resulted in an intensification of the nuclear GR staining. This effect was seen within 30 min incubation with 25 nM dexamethasone and may represent nuclear translocation (Fig. 1A).

STRUCTURE OF THE ACTIVATED GR

The two-step model for the mechanism of action of steroid receptors described above entails first the binding of steroid followed by the interaction of the complex with the genome, whether or not the nonliganded receptor is localized in the cytoplasm or the nucleus (Fig. 1). Thus, prior to the binding of the steroid, the receptor is incapable of binding to DNA whereas the steroid-receptor complex acquires this capability. The transition from the non-DNA-binding state to the DNA-binding state has been called activation (which is the term used here) or transformation. In vitro, a variety of conditions favor the activation process of the steroid-receptor complex such as increased temperature, increased ionic strength, dilution or gel filtration (18). It is believed that the activation process represents a conformational change of the receptor protein. Activation is paralleled by the dissociation of a dimer of the heat-shock protein hsp 90 from the receptor (19). The purification scheme established at this laboratory to purify active preparations of GR centers around the activation process.

Purification of GR

Rat liver GR from 8 adrenalectomized animals is purified following the incubation of the cytosol with ^{3}H-triamcinolone acetonide at 0°C and rapid passage through phosphocellulose (20). The flow-through volume from the phosphocellulose column is diluted and incubated at 25°C which results in activation of over 90% of the GR (21). This is then subjected to DNA-cellulose chromatography and the activated GR eluted with 27.5 mM MgCl$_2$. A final purification by chromatography on DEAE-Sepharose eluted with a linear NaCl gradient results in the recovery of about 50 µg GR. This preparation consists of two predominant proteins according to SDS-poly-acrylamide electrophoresis (SDS-PAGE) with apparent MW 94,000 and 72,000. The MW 94,000 protein binds the ^{3}H-steroid and reacts specifically with antibodies raised against GR. The MW 72,000 protein binds neither steroid nor anti-GR antibodies and appears to bear no relation to GR at all.

The peak of radioactivity obtained after DEAE-Sepharose was pooled and can be stored at -80°C in the presence of 20 mM DTT and 200 µg insulin/ml as carrier, without losing appreciable activity for months. This preparation has been used for the studies on purified GR and the interaction with DNA described below.

Limited Proteolysis of GR

Both crude cytosolic and purified GR are highly susceptible to limited proteolysis with a variety of enzymes (22-25). Proteolysis of crude cytosolic GR gives rise to two specific fragments with Stokes radii of about 3 and 2 nm (22). The 3 nm GR fragment was found to retain both the DNA- and steroid-binding sites whereas the 2 nm fragment only contained the steroid-binding site (23). This led to the postulation of at least two functional domains, one containing the steroid-binding site and one containing the DNA-binding site. It was later shown that a third domain, containing the determinants recognized by our antibodies, could be demonstrated (24).

Limited proteolysis of purified GR (25) also resulted in the demonstration of two major GR fragments with apparent MW 39,000 and 27,000 according to SDS-PAGE, corresponding to the crude cytosolic fragments with Stokes radii of 3 and 2 nm, respectively. Digestion of the MW 39,000 fragment with trypsin gave rise to the MW 27,000 fragment (26). Thus, the smaller fragment can be found entirely within the larger fragment. The MW 39,000 fragment binds both steroid and DNA whereas the MW 27,000 fragment binds only steroid. In addition to these two major fragments, several intermediary minor GR fragments were also seen with apparent MW 91,000, 79,000, 69,000, 60,000 and 51,000. These appear to be intermediary minor GR fragments since very mild proteolytic digestion gives rise to the larger fragments, which are not recovered after more extensive digestion. All the fragments can be shown to bind steroid and the larger fragments also bind the anti-GR antibodies raised at this laboratory (25).

The purified preparations of GR contain two major proteins, the MW 94,000 GR and an MW 72,000 protein. As described above, the MW 94,000 GR is highly susceptible to proteolytic digestion resulting in specific fragments. Analysis by SDS-PAGE shows that the MW 72,000 protein appears to be unaffected by either trypsin or chymotrypsin at the concentrations required to digest GR (25). Furthermore, the MW 72,000 protein binds neither steroid nor anti-GR antibodies and thus appears to be completely unrelated to GR.

Mutant Forms of GR and Corticosteroid Resistance

The development of resistance towards glucocorticoids is of clinical relevance following long-term high-dose therapy with glucocorticoids such as during the treatment of acute lymphoblastic leukemia or lung fibrosis. Some of these patients develop a resistance towards glucocorticoids in the pathological organ or tissue whereas normal tissue is still sensitive to the steroids giving rise to the side effects associated with glucocorticoid therapy. Mouse lymphoma cells have been shown to be a working model system for the development of glucocorticoid resistance.

The most common mechanism by which corticosteroid resistance arises is a mutation resulting in the apparent lack of functional GR or in a nonsteroid-binding form of GR (27-29), and this form of mutation has been called r^-. Other mutations of GR giving rise to resistance have also been described (29,30). The nt^- form binds steroid but the complex does not then interact with purified nuclei or DNA. Both the r^- and nt^- mutant GR forms have apparently the same size as wt GR (31-33). However, a third mutant form, the nt^1 form, was found to be much smaller than the wt GR (27-34). The nt^1 form binds steroid with normal affinity and the complex has even higher affinity for nonspecific DNA than the wt form (27,35). The nt^1 form has a similar size to the chymotryptic fragment of GR containing the steroid- and DNA-binding sites (31,32,36,37). Analysis with anti-GR antibodies showed that the rest of the receptor could not be found in the cells (37). This mutant GR form is of great interest with regard to the function of different parts of the protein as described below.

A general resistance towards glucocorticoids has been associated with a different form of GR (38). In this condition, the receptor was found to be relatively labile at increased temperatures above 37°C. The cause of this thermo-lability is unclear but the condition appears to be familial. A similar form of the androgen receptor has also been associated with androgen resistance (39,40).

DOMAIN STRUCTURE OF GR

Analysis of the GR function and the fragments obtained following limited proteolysis, as described above, resulted in the definition of three functional domains within the protein (24). Digestion with chymotrypsin gave rise to a fragment containing both the DNA- and steroid-binding domains whereas digestion with trypsin gave rise to a fragment corresponding to the steroid-binding domain (Fig. 2). Thus, the steroid-binding domain corresponds to the MW 27,000 fragment on SDS-PAGE and the DNA-binding domain corresponds to the rest of the MW 39,000 fragment. The third domain contains the determinants for the anti-GR antibodies raised at our department (24).

The primary structures of rat (41), human (42), and mouse (43) GR have been deduced from the cDNA sequences. Eight segments of the deduced

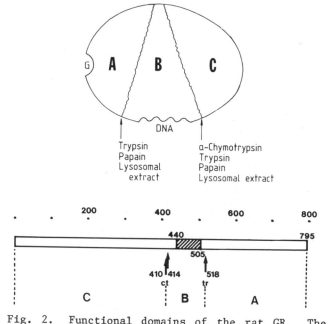

Fig. 2. Functional domains of the rat GR. The upper figure represents the result of limited proteolysis of crude cytosolic GR. The lower figure represents the localization of the domain borders in comparison with the primary structure of rGR (41). The hatched region is the highly conserved Cys-, Lys-, Arg-rich segment. The numbers represent amino acid residues based on the deduced primary structure.

rat GR primary structure have been confirmed by protein sequence analysis of peptides derived from purified GR (26). These segments range from close to the N-terminus (residue 28) to close to the C-terminus (residue 790), thus inferring that the cDNA clone described (41) represents the intact receptor protein. The deduced GR primary structure has been a prerequisite for the studies described below. All further discussion will be related to the primary structure of rat GR (rGR).

Steroid-binding Domain

The functional steroid-binding domain is defined by the tryptic cleavage site giving rise to the MW 27,000 GR fragment (Fig. 2). This fragment of purified GR was isolated by SDS-PAGE and sequenced from the N-terminus (26). The sequence obtained identified cleavage by trypsin after Lys-517. Assuming the steroid-binding domain continues to the C-terminus, the calculated molecular weight of this domain is 31,600 Da. Since deletion of the five C-terminal residues reduced the affinity of the receptor for steroid by thirtyfold (44), it is reasonable to assume that the steroid-binding domain stretches from residues 518 to 795 (the C-terminus).

Further analysis of the steroid-receptor interaction was carried out by photoaffinity-labeling with ^{3}H-triamcinolone acetonide and affinity-labeling with ^{3}H-dexamethasone mesylate (45). The affinity-labeled receptor complex was digested with trypsin, chymotrypsin or cyanogen bromide and the resultant peptide mixtures subjected to radiosequence analysis (Table 1). The radiosequence data in combination with the known specificity of proteolytic cleavage as well as the primary structure of rGR (41) identified three amino acid residues affinity-labeled by the steroid. Photoaffinity-labeling via the 3-keto-Δ^4 structure of ^{3}H-triamcinolone acetonide resulted in covalent binding of the steroid to Met-622 and Cys-754. Affinity-labeling via the side chain structure of ^{3}H-dexamethasone 21-mesylate resulted in covalent binding to Cys-656. Thus, the steroid-binding domain folds with Met-622 and Cys-754 in close proximity and at about 1.5 nm distance from Cys-656. All three residues lie within hydrophobic segments of the domain (45) and presumably the steroid-binding site is formed by a hydrophobic pocket.

The localization of the steroid-binding domain to the C-terminal region of GR described above agrees well with GR mutational data published. Deletion of a small number of residues at the C-terminus destroys the steroid-binding capacity (44). Deletion from the N-terminus to residue 497 has a small effect on steroid binding (sixfold lower affinity) whereas further deletion to residue 547 greatly reduces (300-fold) the steroid-binding capacity (44). Insertion at various sites between 568 and 714 interfered with steroid-binding (46). Interestingly, an insertion at residue 702 (46) had no effect on steroid-binding.

Cloning of two mutant forms of mouse GR (43) has identified two point mutations affecting the binding of steroid. A mutation at residue 558 (Glu → Gly) completely destroys the steroid-binding capacity whereas a mutation at residue 782 (Tyr → Asn) results in a three- to fourfold reduced affinity for steroid. Thus, the published data is not contradictory with the localization of the steroid-binding domain to residues 518-795.

DNA-binding Domain

The functional DNA-binding domain is defined by the chymotrypsin-cleavage site giving rise to the MW 39,000 fragment. Sequence analysis of this fragment showed a mixture of N-terminal sequences which enabled the identification of two cleavage sites after residues Phe-409 and Tyr-413

Table 1. Radiosequence analysis of GR affinity-labeled with ^{3}H-triamcinolone acetonide (TA) or ^{3}H-dexamethasone mesylate. The numbers refer to the cycle from which peaks of radioactivity were recovered.

Proteolytic cleavage	TA	MA
Cyanogen bromide	3, 11	_a
Trypsin without succinylation	16, 19	5
Trypsin with prior succinylation	19, 22	ND[b]
Chymotrypsin	ND[b]	4

[a] CNBr cleaved the covalent linkage of the steroid to GR.
[b] Not determined.

(26). Thus, the functional DNA-binding domain corresponds to residues 410/414-517 (Fig. 2), with a size of ≈11,400 Da. This region contains the highly conserved Cys-, Lys-, Arg-rich segment that is found in all steroid receptors and is believed to be the DNA-binding site. Insertion in proximity of the conserved Cys-residues destroys all DNA-binding whereas insertion within the intervening sequence destroys the transcriptional activating properties without affecting binding to nonspecific DNA (47). The repetitive Cys-structure is common to several DNA-binding proteins and it has been suggested that, in analogy to TFIIIA, the Cys_2 residues bind Zn^{2+} (48,49). However, attempts to label GR with $^{65}Zn^{2+}$, in vivo and in vitro under a variety of conditions, have not been successful (Stromstedt and Carlstedt-Duke, unpublished observations). Furthermore, 10 mM EDTA or 100 mM DTT does not have any effect on the specific interaction of purified GR with DNA, and neither does the addition of $ZnCl_2$. Thus, there is no conclusive evidence that GR is a metalloprotein.

Mutational studies on GR have identified approximately the same region as responsible for transcriptional activation as well as DNA-binding (44,46,47,50,51). Deletion mutation from the C-terminus results in steroid-independent constitutive transcriptional activation (44,50,51), and it is sufficient with a fragment of GR corresponding to residues 440-528 to give this constitutive activity. An insertion at residue 424 has no effect on transcriptional activity whereas an insertion at residue 441 completely destroys the activity (46,47). Thus, both insertional and deletion mutation indicate a border for the DNA-binding domain slightly C-terminal to the chymotryptic sites identified.

Mutations at the other border of this domain have even more dramatic effects. Insertion at residue 507-510 completely destroys the steroid-dependent transcriptional activation without affecting steroid-binding (46,47). Insertion at residue 515 or 532 reduces the steroid-dependent transcriptional activation to 10% (47) whereas an insertion at residue 534 has no effect (46). In fact, the sequence 510-518 is very rich in Lys and Arg and would be almost completely digested by trypsin. Thus, the tryptic cleavage site identified at residue 517 represents the C-terminal end of this region. The C-terminal sequence of the DNA-binding domain following cleavage with trypsin has not been identified. Thus, at the protein level, the DNA-binding domain appears to correspond to residues 414-517. Mutational data may indicate that the domain is slightly smaller than this.

One single point-mutation within this region has also been identified. The nt$^-$ mutant GR form was found to contain a mutation at residue 496 (Arg → His) that resulted in a GR form incapable of binding to purified nuclei (43).

N-terminal Domain

The remaining part of GR, the N-terminal half, consists of at least one functional domain (24). This part of the protein is immunodominant and it is this part of the receptor that is most divergent between the different steroid receptors. Deletion of the whole of this domain results in steroid-dependent transcriptional activation that is reduced to 10% compared to intact GR (50). In fact, this deletion mutant is equivalent to the nt^1 mutant form of GR in corticosteroid-resistant cells, as described above. However, it is unknown whether the nt^1 mutant contains any point-mutations in addition to the truncation. Insertion at residue 141 or 235 resulted in only 2-3% steroid-dependent activity (46) whereas deletion of residues 98-282 resulted in 10% steroid-dependent activity (47). Thus, this domain appears to play an important role in transcriptional activation, possibly by interaction with other transcriptional factors, and the region responsible has been called the τ_1-region (46).

Analysis of the specific interaction of GR or the chymotryptic MW 39,000 fragment with DNA, using the mouse mammary tumor virus (MTV) promoter region and DNase I footprinting, shows that the DNA-binding for these two preparations is similar (Stromstedt and Carlstedt-Duke, unpublished observations). The footprints for intact GR and the chymotryptic fragment are identical. Also, the apparent affinity of the receptor and its fragment for the footprints is similar at 1 mM $MgCl_2$. Therefore, binding to DNA does not appear to be sufficient for transcriptional activation. Other factors or interactions are involved and this is probably the role of the N-terminal domain.

OLIGOMERIC STRUCTURE OF ACTIVATED GR

Prior to activation, the steroid-receptor complex is associated with a dimer of hsp 90 (19) and dissociation of this complex is an integral part of the activation process.

Specific binding regions for GR have been detected within a variety of glucocorticoid-dependent genes. One of the best characterized genes is the MTV gene which contains at least five regions that specifically bind GR (52). The binding region upstream of the promoter contains five GR-binding sites as judged by DNase I footprinting. Analysis of the GR-DNA interaction by electron microscopy showed a distribution of the purified GR complexes along the DNA corresponding to the distribution of the footprints (52). However, the size of the GR was much larger than that expected for a protein of 94,000 Da in size and it was suggested that the activated DNA-binding GR species could be an oligomer of the 94,000 Da species (52).

The stoichiometry of the GR-DNA interaction was investigated using double isotope-labeling with ^{3}H-GR and ^{32}P-DNA of known specific activity (21). Freshly prepared purified GR was incubated with a mixture of ^{32}P-DNA consisting of a 185 bp fragment containing three of the five binding sites (footprints) from the MTV promoter region and a 2.3 kbp nonspecific vector DNA fragment. The GR, DNA and GR-DNA complexes were separated by glycerol gradient centrifugation and analyzed for ^{3}H and ^{32}P (Fig. 3). By incubating GR with various concentrations of DNA and quantitating the radioactivity in the various peaks, it was possible to estimate the number of GR molecules bound per binding site (footprint) (Fig. 4). At saturating concentrations of DNA, the ratio of GR:footprint was 0.8-0.9. This was confirmed by quantitative footprinting (21). Thus, one molecule of MW 94,000 GR appears to bind at each individual binding site and the activated GR seems to be monomeric in nature.

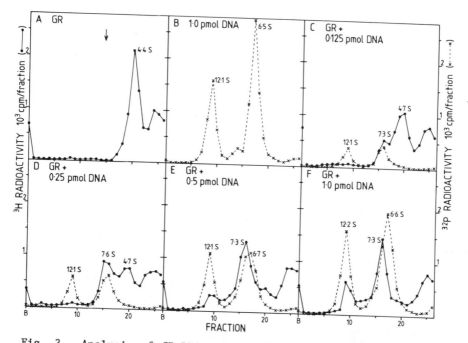

Fig. 3. Analysis of GR-DNA stoichiometry by glycerol gradient centrifugation. Two pmol ^{3}H-GR was incubated with 0-1.0 pmol ^{32}P-DNA of known specific activity. Free GR sediments at 4.4 S, the 185 bp MTV fragment containing three footprints at 6.5 S, the specific GR-DNA complex at 7.3 S, and the 2.3 kbp vector DNA fragment as well as the nonspecific GR-DNA complex at 12.1 S. The arrow shows the position of the internal standard ^{14}C-aldolase (7.9 S). From reference 21.

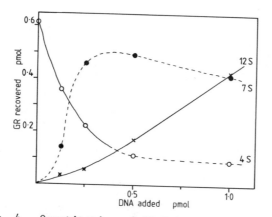

Fig. 4. Quantitation of GR following analysis of GR-DNA interaction by glycerol gradient centrifugation (Fig. 3). The 4 S peak represents free GR and the background in this area is shown by the dotted line. The 7 S peak represents the specific GR-DNA complex whereas the 12 S peak represents the nonspecific GR-DNA complex. From reference 21.

Analysis of the protein distribution following the glycerol gradient centrifugation showed that the MW 72,000 protein was partially separated from the MW 94,000 GR. However, after the binding of the GR to DNA, the MW 72,000 protein cosedimented with the specific GR-DNA complex in apparently equimolar amounts to the MW 94,000 GR as judged by SDS-PAGE. Thus, the interaction between the two proteins appears to be stabilized by the binding of GR to DNA. The physiological role of this interaction is still unclear and it may simply represent an artifact arising during tissue preparation for the purification procedure.

SUMMARY

The activated GR complex appears to consist of a single monomeric protein with apparent MW 94,000. This protein consists of at least three functional domains that can be defined by limited proteolysis. Using purified preparations of rat GR, the steroid-binding domain has been localized at the C-terminal corresponding to residues 518-795. Probing of the steroid-receptor interaction by affinity-labeling has identified three residues widespread within this domain that bind steroid. The domain folds to form a hydrophobic pocket which is the steroid-binding site. Within this pocket, Met-622 and Cys-754 are in close proximity and interact with the 3-keto-Δ^4 structure of the steroid (Fig. 5). Cys-656 also lies within this pocket and interacts with the side chain structure of the steroid. It must therefore lie at about 1.5 nm distance from the other two residues identified. The DNA-binding domain corresponds to residues 414-517 which corresponds well with the functional domain defined on the basis of mutational data. Within this domain lies the Cys-, Lys-, Arg-rich region that is highly conserved between the different steroid receptors. The N-terminal domain appears to be of importance for maximal transcriptional activation but does not play any major role in the specific GR-DNA interaction. The receptor appears to be localized in both the cytoplasm and nucleus. Following the addition of dexamethasone, there is an intensification of GR staining in the nucleus which may be indicative of nuclear translocation and interaction with the genome in vivo.

The use of modification of amino acid residues within GR in connection with functional studies is a powerful tool and a valuable complement to mutational studies. Further probing of steroid-GR and GR-DNA interaction is at present under progress and should prove to be an important step in the understanding of receptor function.

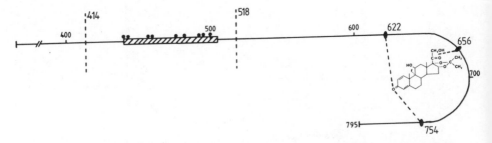

Fig. 5. Summary of GR structure based on limited proteolysis and sequence analysis as well as affinity-labeling and radiosequence analysis. The domain borders are represented by dashed lines. The affinity-labeled amino acid residues identified and their interaction with triamcinolone acetonide are shown. The hatched region represents the Cys-, Lys-, Arg-rich segment and the dots, the nine conserved Cys residues.

ACKNOWLEDGMENTS

The studies from this department described in this report were supported by grants from the Swedish Medical Research Council (grant 2819), the Swedish National Board for Technical Development and Pharmacia, Uppsala, Sweden. Ann-Charlotte Wikstrom is the recipient of a fellowship from the Swedish Medical Research Council.

REFERENCES

1. Baxter JD, Tomkins GH. Specific cytoplasmic glucocorticoid hormone receptors in hepatoma tissue culture cells. Proc Natl Acad Sci USA 1971; 68:932-7.
2. King WJ, Greene GL. Monoclonal antibodies localize oestrogen receptor in the nucleus of target cells. Nature 1984; 307:745-7.
3. King WJ, DeSombre ER, Jensen EV, Greene GL. Comparison of immunocytochemical and steroid-binding assays for estrogen receptor in human breast tumors. Cancer Res 1985; 45:293-304.
4. Press MF, Nousek-Goebl NA, Greene GL. Immunoelectron microscopic localization of estrogen receptor with monoclonal estrophilin antibodies. J Histochem Cytochem 1985; 33:915-24.
5. Perrot-Applanat M, Logeat F, Groyer-Picard MT, Milgrom E. Immunocytochemical study of mammalian progesterone receptor using monoclonal antibodies. Endocrinology 1985; 116:1473-84.
6. Welshons WV, Lieberman ME, Gorski J. Nuclear localization of unoccupied oestrogen receptors. Nature 1984; 307:747-9.
7. Welshons WV, Krummel BM, Gorski J. Nuclear localization of unoccupied receptors for glucocorticoids, estrogens and progesterone in GH_3 cells. Endocrinology 1985; 117:2140-7.
8. Govindan MV. Immunofluorescence microscopy of the intracellular translocation of glucocorticoid-receptor complexes in rat hepatoma (HTC) cells. Exp Cell Res 1980; 127:293-7.
9. Papamichail M, Tsokos G, Tsawdaroglou N, Sekeris CE. Immunocytochemical demonstration of glucocorticoid receptors in different cell types and their translocation from the cytoplasm to the cell nucleus in the presence of dexamethasone. Exp Cell Res 1980; 125:490-3.
10. Gustafsson J-A, Carlstedt-Duke J, Fuxe K, Carlstrom K, Okret S, Wrange O. Studies on the glucocorticoid receptor. In: Fuxe F, Wetterberg L, Gustafsson J-A, eds. Steroid hormone regulation of the brain. Oxford: Pergamon Press, 1981:31-9.
11. Bernard PA, Joh TH. Characterization and immunocytochemical demonstration of glucocorticoid receptor using antisera specific to transformed receptor. Arch Biochem Biophys 1984; 229:466-76.
12. Antakly T, Eisen HJ. Immunocytochemical localization of glucocorticoid receptor in target cells. Endocrinology 1984; 115:1984-9.
13. Fuxe K, Wikstrom A-C, Okret S, et al. Mapping of glucocorticoid receptor immunoreactive neurons in the rat tel- and diencephalon using a monoclonal antibody against rat liver glucocorticoid receptor. Endocrinology 1985; 117:1803-12.
14. Agnati LF, Fuxe K, Yu ZY, et al. Morphometrical analysis of the distribution of corticotropin releasing factor, glucocorticoid receptor and phenylethanolamine-n-methyltransferase immunoreactive neurons in the paraventricular hypothalamic nucleus of the rat. Neurosci Lett 1985; 54:147-52.
15. Fuxe K, Harfstrand A, Agnati LF, et al. Immunocytochemical studies on the localization of glucocorticoid receptor immunoreactive nerve cells in the lower brain stem and spinal cord of the male rat using a monoclonal antibody against rat liver glucocorticoid receptor. Neurosci Lett 1985; 60:1-6.
16. Okret S, Wikstrom A-C, Wrange O, Andersson B, Gustafsson J-A.

Monoclonal antibodies against the rat liver glucocorticoid receptor.
Proc Natl Acad Sci USA 1984; 81:1609-13.

17. Wikstrom A-C, Bakke O, Okret S, Bronnegard M, Gustafsson J-A.
Intracellular localization of the glucocorticoid receptor: evidence
for cytoplasmic and nuclear localization. Endocrinology 1987;
120:1232-42.

18. Schmidt TJ, Barnett CA, Litwack G. Activation of the glucocorticoid-
receptor complex. J Cell Biochem 1982; 20:15-27.

19. Denis M, Wikstrom A-C, Gustafsson J-A. The molybdate-stabilized
non-activated glucocorticoid receptor contains a dimer of M_r 90,000
non-hormone binding protein. J Biol Chem 1987; 262 (in press).

20. Wrange O, Carlstedt-Duke J, Gustafsson J-A. Purification of the
glucocorticoid receptor from rat liver cytosol. J Biol Chem 1979;
254:9284-90.

21. Wrange O, Carlstedt-Duke J, Gustafsson J-A. Stoichiometric analysis
of the specific interaction of the glucocorticoid receptor with DNA.
J Biol Chem 1986; 261:11770-8.

22. Carlstedt-Duke J, Gustafsson J-A, Wrange O. Formation and characteristics of hepatic dexamethasone-receptor complexes of different
molecular weight. Biochim Biophys Acta 1977; 497:507-24.

23. Wrange O, Gustafsson J-A. Separation of the hormone- and DNA-binding
sites of the hepatic glucocorticoid receptor by means of proteolysis.
J Biol Chem 1978; 253:856-65.

24. Carlstedt-Duke J, Okret S, Wrange O, Gustafsson J-A. Immunochemical
analysis of the glucocorticoid receptor: identification of a third
domain separate from the steroid-binding and DNA-binding domains.
Proc Natl Acad Sci USA 1982; 79:4260-4.

25. Wrange O, Okret S, Radojcic M, Carlstedt-Duke J, Gustafsson J-A.
Characterization of the purified activated glucocorticoid receptor
from rat liver cytosol. J Biol Chem 1984; 259:4534-41.

26. Carlstedt-Duke J, Stromstedt P-E, Wrange O, Bergman T, Gustafsson
J-A, Jornvall H. Domain structure of the glucocorticoid receptor
protein. Proc Natl Acad Sci USA 1987; 84:4437-40.

27. Yamamoto KR, Stampfer MR, Tomkins GM. Receptors from glucocor-
ticoid-sensitive lymphoma cells and two classes of insensitive
clones: physical and DNA-binding properties. Proc Natl Acad Sci USA
1974; 71:3901-5.

28. Sibley CH, Yamamoto KR. Mouse lymphoma cells: mechanism of resistance to glucocorticoids. In: Baxter JD, Rousseau GG, eds. Glucocorticoid hormone action. Heidelberg: Springer-Verlag, 1979:357-76.

29. Northrop JP, Gametchu B, Harrison RW, Ringold GM. Characterization
of wild type and mutant glucocorticoid receptors from rat hepatoma
and mouse lymphoma cells. J Biol Chem 1985; 260:6398-403.

30. Gehring U, Tomkins GM. A new mechanism for steroid unresponsiveness:
loss of nuclear binding activity of a steroid hormone receptor. Cell
1974; 3:301-6.

31. Dellweg H-G, Hotz A, Mugele K, Gehring U. Active domains in wild-
type and mutant glucocorticoid receptors. EMBO J 1982; 1:285-9.

32. Gehring U, Holz A. Photoaffinity labeling and partial proteolysis of
wild-type and variant glucocorticoid receptors. Biochemistry 1983;
22:4013-8.

33. Westphal HM, Mugele K, Beato M, Gehring U. Immunochemical characterization of wild-type and variant glucocorticoid receptors by monoclonal antibodies. EMBO J 1984; 3:1493-8.

34. Stevens J, Stevens Y-W. Physicochemical differences between glucocorticoid-binding components from the corticoid-sensitive and -resistant
strains of mouse lymphoma P1798. Cancer Res 1979; 39:4011-21.

35. Stevens J, Stevens Y-W, Rhodes J, Steiner G. Differences in nuclear
glucocorticoid binding between corticoid-sensitive and corticoid-
resistant lymphocytes of mouse lymphoma P1798 and stabilization of
nuclear hormone receptor complexes with carbobenzoxy-L-phenylalanine.
J Natl Cancer Inst 1978; 61:1477-85.

36. Stevens J, Stevens Y-W. Influence of limited proteolysis on the physicochemical and DNA-binding properties of glucocorticoid receptors from corticoid-sensitive and -resistant mouse lymphoma P1798. Cancer Res 1981; 41:125-33.

37. Okret S, Stevens Y-W, Carlstedt-Duke J, Wrange O, Gustafsson J-A, Stevens J. Absence in glucocorticoid-resistant mouse lymphoma P1798 of a glucocorticoid receptor domain responsible for biological effects. Cancer Res 1983; 43:3127-31.

38. Bronnegard M, Werner S, Gustafsson J-A. Primary cortisol resistance associated with a thermolabile glucocorticoid receptor in a patient with fatigue as the only symptom. J Clin Invest 1986; 78:1270-8.

39. Griffin JE, Durrant JL. Qualitative receptor defects in families with androgen resistance: failure of stabilization of the fibroblast cytosol androgen receptor. J Clin Endocrinol Metab 1982; 55:465-74.

40. Kovacs WJ, Griffin JE, Weaver DD, Carlson BR, Wilson JD. A mutation that causes lability of the androgen receptor under conditions that normally promote transformation to the DNA-binding state. J Clin Invest 1984; 73:1095-104.

41. Miesfeld R, Rusconi S, Godowski PJ, et al. Genetic complementation of a glucocorticoid receptor deficiency by expression of cloned receptor cDNA. Cell 1986; 46:389-99.

42. Hollenberg SM, Weinberger C, Ong ES, et al. Primary structure and expression of a functional human glucocorticoid receptor cDNA. Nature 1985; 318:635-41.

43. Danielsen M, Norhrop JP, Ringold GM. The mouse glucocorticoid receptor: mapping of functional domains by cloning, sequencing and expression of wild-type and mutant receptor proteins. EMBO J 1986; 5:2513-22.

44. Rusconi S, Yamamoto KR. Functional dissection of the hormone and DNA binding activities of the glucocorticoid receptor. EMBO J 1987; 6:1309-15.

45. Carlstedt-Duke J, Stromstedt P-E, Persson B, Cederlund E, Gustafsson J-A, Jornvall H. Identification of hormone-interacting amino acid residues within the steroid-binding domain of the glucocorticoid receptor in relation to other hormone receptors. EMBO J (submitted for publication).

46. Giguere V, Hollenberg SM, Rosenfeld MG, Evans RM. Functional domains of the human glucocorticoid receptor. Cell 1986; 46:645-52.

47. Hollenberg SM, Giguere V, Segui P, Evans RM. Colocalization of DNA-binding and transcriptional activation functions in the human glucocorticoid receptor. Cell 1987; 49:39-46.

48. Berg JM. Potential metal-binding domains in nucleic acid binding proteins. Science 1986; 232:485-7.

49. Miller J, McLachlan AD, Klug A. Repetitive Zinc-binding domains in the protein transcription factor IIIA from Xenopus oocytes. EMBO J 1985; 4:1609-14.

50. Miesfeld R, Godowski PJ, Maler BA, Yamamoto KR. Glucocorticoid receptor mutants that define a small region sufficient for enhancer activation. Science 1987; 236:423-7.

51. Godowski PJ, Rusconi S, Miesfeld R, Yamamoto KR. Glucocorticoid receptor mutants that are constitutive activators of transcriptional enhancement. Nature 1987; 325:365-8.

52. Payvar F, DeFranco D, Firestone GL, et al. Sequence-specific binding of glucocorticoid receptor to MTV DNA at sites within and upstream of the transcribed region. Cell 1983; 35:381-92.

6

HORMONE-DEPENDENT PHOSPHORYLATION OF THE
AVIAN PROGESTERONE RECEPTOR

William P. Sullivan, David F. Smith, and David O. Toft

Department of Biochemistry and Molecular Biology
Mayo Medical School, Rochester, MN 55905

Considerable effort has been devoted to the isolation and characterization of the avian progesterone receptor. Methods have been
developed for purification of the A and B receptor forms (1-5) and both
immunological (2-4,6) and cDNA (7-9) probes for these proteins have
recently become available to provide new opportunities for further characterization of the receptor proteins.

While these advances are very encouraging, at the present time many
structural and functional properties of the progesterone receptor are
poorly understood. Soon after its purification, the progesterone receptor
was shown to be a phosphoprotein (10,11), and studies over the past
several years indicate that most, if not all, steroid receptors are
phosphorylated (12-16). However, the significance of this phosphorylation
to receptor structure or function has remained unclear. In this report we
will summarize our recent efforts to describe more clearly the significance of receptor phosphorylation in progesterone action.

METHODS

Immature chicks stimulated with daily injections of diethylstilbestrol (5 mg) were used. In some experiments, chicks were treated with
R5020 or progesterone by sc injection of hormone in 200 µl sesame oil.
The oviducts were homogenized in 4 volumes of 50 mM Tris, 10 mM Na_2MoO_4,
10 mM thioglycerol, pH 7.4 (homogenization buffer) using a Polytron PT-20
homogenizer. Where indicated, the following protease inhibitors were
included during homogenization: leupeptin, 0.1 mM; bacitracin, 100 µg/ml;
aprotinin, 77 µg/ml; pepstatin, 1.5 µM; and phenylmethylsulfonyl fluoride,
0.5 mM. After centrifugation at 800 x g for 5 min, the supernatant was
centrifuged for 30 min at 100,000 x g. The low speed pellet containing
nuclear material was washed with 4 ml homogenization buffer, and any
residual receptors extracted by incubation for 1 h on ice in buffer
containing 10 mM Tris, 1.5 mM EDTA, 0.4 M KCl, pH 8. The insoluble
material was pelleted at 4000 x g for 30 min. Saturated ammonium sulfate
adjusted to pH 7.4 was added to an equal volume of high speed supernatant
(cytosol) and to the soluble nuclear extract. After 30 min incubation at
4°C on a rocker platform, the precipitate was pelleted by centrifugation
at 400 x g for 30 min. The precipitate was redissolved in 300 µl of
distilled water and mixed with 300 µl 2x sample buffer (0.25 M Tris, 2%
(w:v) SDS, 20% (v:v) glycerol, 0.05% (w:v) bromphenol blue pH 6.8) con-

taining 10% (v:v) mercaptoethanol. After 15 min incubation at room
temperature with intermittent vortexing, the samples were heated for 2 min
in a boiling waterbath.

Western Blotting Procedure

Proteins were resolved by electrophoresis on discontinuous polyacrylamide gels according to the method of Laemmli (17). The resolving
gel was 7.5% acrylamide. Following electrophoresis, the proteins were
transferred to nitrocellulose using a TE Series Transphor Electrophoresis
Unit with Transphor Power-Lid, Model TE50 (Hoefer Scientific Instruments,
San Francisco, CA) set at 1 Amp for 2 h. The transfer buffer was 20 mM
sodium phosphate, 20% (v:v) methanol, 0.2% (w:v) sodium dodecyl sulfate,
pH 6.5. The nitrocellulose sheet was blocked with 20 mM Tris, 150 mM
NaCl, 0.5% (v:v) polyoxyethelenesorbitan monolaurate (Tween-20), 1.0%
(w:v) bovine serum albumin, pH 7.4 (Western buffer) for 30 min at 37°C.
The sheet was then incubated overnight in Western buffer containing the
indicated monoclonal antibody at 10 μg/ml. The nitrocellulose was washed
three times with Western buffer. Then alkaline phosphatase conjugated
anti-mouse IgG (Southern Biotechnology Associates, Birmingham, AL),
diluted 1:500 in Western buffer, was added for 4 h at room temperature.
The nitrocellulose was washed as above and the alkaline phosphatase
complexes were detected by the method of Blake et al. (18) modified as
follows: nitrocellulose sheets were rinsed for 2 min with substrate
buffer (100 mM Tris, 100 mM NaCl, 50 mM $MgCl_2$, pH 9.5). Nitro blue
tetrazolium (Sigma, St. Louis, MO) was added to substrate buffer to a
final concentration of 330 μg/ml from a stock solution of nitro blue
tetrazolium (75 mg/ml) in 70% dimethylformamide stored at -20°C. The
reaction was initiated by addition of 3 bromo - 4 chloro -5-indolyl
phosphate (BCIP) to a final concentration of 166 μg/ml substrate buffer.
BCIP was added from 2 mg/ml stock prepared just before use. In some cases
the intensity of stained bands was quantitated by densitometry. The
stained nitrocellulose sheet was first photographed to prepare a positive
transparency. This was then scanned using a Helena Cliniscan with the
gain set manually to allow comparison between lanes. Peaks of interest
were selected and quantified in arbitrary integral units.

Antibodies

Monoclonal antibodies have been prepared against avian progesterone
receptor isolated from oviduct cytosol by steroid affinity chromatography.
Their characterization has been described elsewhere (6). In summary αPR
11, 13, 16, and 22 recognize both the A and B forms of the progesterone
receptor while αPR6 is specific for the B form.

Hormone Dependent Phosphorylation

Dulbecco's Minimal Essential Medium without phosphate (Irvine Scientific, Santa Ana, CA) was reconstituted according to manufacturer's
protocol and supplemented with 10 μM NaH_2PO_4.

A diethylstilbestrol stimulated chick was killed and the oviduct
removed to medium. It was divided into four 400 mg pieces. In each case,
the tissue was minced to pieces approximately 2 mm^2. The mince was washed
with several changes of medium by sedimentation at unit gravity. The
tissue was suspended in 4 ml of medium; approximately 1 mCi of ortho [^{32}P]
phosphate (NEN) was added and the mixture incubated at 37°C with agita-
tion. After 20 min, progesterone dissolved in medium was added at varying
times to the incubations to a final concentration of 1 x 10^{-7} M. The time
points for progesterone exposure were 40, 20, and 5 min. The fourth
incubation received medium without progesterone. After 60 min the medium

was removed, the tissue was washed with 10 ml each ice cold saline, ice cold homogenization buffer (50 mM K_2HPO_4, 10 mM Na_2MoO4, 10 mM EDTA, 50 mM NaF, 10 mM thioglycerol pH 7.0) and resuspended in 1.6 ml (4 volumes) of homogenization buffer. The tissue was homogenized with a glass/glass homogenizer. The homogenate was centrifuged at 800 x g for 5 min and the resulting supernatant was centrifuged at 100,000 x g for 30 min. Monoclonal antibody αPR13 (20 µg) was added to each sample. After 2 h on ice, 50 µl (packed gel) of antimouse IgG agarose (Sigma) was added to each tube and incubation continued for 1 h with intermittent vortexing. The resin was pelleted by centrifugation, washed 3 times with 4 ml of homogenization buffer, followed by 2 wash steps with 4 ml of homogenization buffer with 0.4 M KCl. The resin was transferred to clean tubes in 4 ml of 50 mM K_2HPO_4 pH 7.0. After pelleting, the resin was mixed with an equal volume of 2 x sample buffer and boiled for 2 min. The supernatant containing approximately one-half of the immuno-precipitated material was subjected to electrophoresis. Following electrophoresis, the gel was incubated in a solution of 25% methanol, 10% acetic acid for 1 h. After equilibration in distilled water, the gel was dried under vacuum. The ^{32}P-labeled proteins were visualized by exposure of film (Kodak X-Omat AR5) in a cassette with lighting plus intensifier screens (Dupont) at -70°C.

Two-Dimensional Mapping

Receptor proteins were labeled with ^{32}P and purified as described above. The proteins were resolved on 7.5% polyacrylamide gels and transferred to nitrocellulose. The protein bands of interest were identified by fluorography and excised. Unreacted sites on the nitrocellulose were blocked by incubation in PBS (8.1 mM Na_2HPO_4, 1.5 mM KH_2PO_4, 2.7 mM KCl, 137 mM NaCl, pH 7.2) containing 0.1% Tween 20 (polyoxyethylene sorbotan monolaurate) for 30 min at 37°C. The nitrocellulose pieces were rinsed with 50 mM ammonium bicarbonate buffer pH 7.8 and placed in tubes containing 400 µl of the buffer and either 25 µg of V8 protease from staphylococcus aureus (Sigma) or 10 µg of TPCK treated trypsin (Sigma). Two 10 µg additions of trypsin were added at 2-h intervals. Incubations were continued overnight at either 37°C (V8) or 22°C (trypsin). After incubations, the supernatant from the nitrocellulose pieces was collected and lyophilized and dissolved in 10 µl of electrophoresis buffer consisting of formic acid:acetic acid:water (5:15:80). Digests were analyzed by two-dimensional mapping by spotting on a 20 x 20 cm cellulose plate as described previously (30). The electrophoresis was performed in the stated buffer system at 500 V for 60-90 min. Thin layer chromatography in the second dimension was carried out in a solvent system containing 1-butanol:pyridine:acetic acid:water (32.5:25:5:20) for 3-4 h. After drying the cellulose sheet, the ^{32}P-labeled peptides were identified by autoradiography.

RESULTS

Antibody Probes for the Progesterone Receptor

Our studies were enhanced considerably by the availability of monoclonal antibodies to the progesterone receptor (6). Because of this, we will first describe some important applications of these antibodies to receptor characterization. These have been used as a means of receptor measurement which is independent of hormone binding activity. Antibodies have also been used as a rapid method for receptor isolation. Figure 1 illustrates the use of five different antibodies for detection of the progesterone receptor by Western blotting. As described previously (6), four antibodies called PR 11, 13, 16, and 22 recognize the A (80 kDa) and B (110 kDa) receptor forms equally. However, one antibody, PR6, is

specific for the B receptor (lane 2). In the example in Figure 1, PR6
also reacts with a band just above the A receptor. The appearance of this
band is variable and we believe that it is a breakdown product of receptor
B (19). Liver cytosol is not believed to contain progesterone receptor
and no specific immune reactivity was observed with liver cytosol.
However, an antibody against the 90 kDa heat shock protein, hsp 90, does
show a reaction band in both oviduct and liver samples (lane D7). While
hsp 90 has been shown to associate with the progesterone receptor and
other steroid receptors (20-22), it is a protein that is prevalent in most
eukaryotic cells.

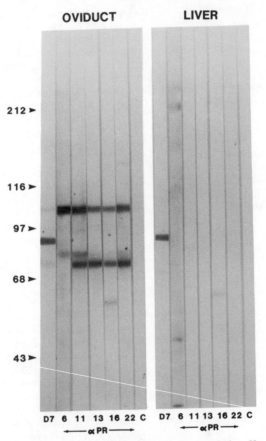

Fig. 1. Antibody interactions demonstrated by Western blotting. Cytosol fractions from chick oviduct and liver were
fractionated by ammonium sulfate precipitation (45% of saturation). The precipitated proteins were resolved by SDS-polyacrylamide gel electrophoresis and electrophoretically
transferred to nitrocellulose. Strips of nitrocellulose were
incubated with 40 µg of the indicated antibodies or with
Western buffer alone. After incubation with alkaline phosphatase-conjugated antimouse IgG, the antibody complexes were
stained with a phosphatase-sensitive dye. Lane 1, D7, anti-
hsp 90 antibody D7a; lanes 2-6, anti-receptor antibodies,
αPR6, αPR11, αPR13, αPR16 and αPR22; lane 7, c, no primary
antibody. The molecular weight standards (BioRad) were myosin
(212,000), β-galactosidase (116,000) phosphorylase b (97,000),
bovine serum albumin (68,000), and ovalbumin (43,000).
Reprinted with permission from reference 31.

The equivalent reaction of four antibodies with receptor forms A and B indicate that these are closely related antigens. Similar conclusions have been made using polyclonal antisera to the avian progesterone receptor (2-4) and it now seems likely that the two receptors are coded by the same gene (7-9). However, there has been controversy as to the significance of the smaller A receptor, both in the chicken and in mammalian systems (2-4,23,24). This may be a significant form of receptor within the cell or a proteolytic product formed after cell disruption.

To test these possibilities, Western blotting was used to measure the proportion of A and B receptor that existed immediately after homogenization or after preparation of supernatant fractions (Fig. 2). In another sample the homogenate was incubated on ice for 1.5 h before processing. In each case, comparisons were made between samples prepared in the presence or absence of protease inhibitors. The results of Figure 2 show that under all conditions used, approximately equal proportions of A and B receptor were observed and neither form is very susceptible to protease damage. In additional studies (19), the A and B receptors were shown to be quite stable even when the cytosol was incubated at 37°C, a condition which destroys steroid binding activity. However, receptor breakdown was observed when the tissue was homogenized more harshly or when it had been stored frozen (19). These results indicate that A and B receptors are quite stable and are very likely to represent receptor forms in the cell. However, the biological significance of the two receptor forms remains unknown.

Effects of Progesterone Treatment

Western blotting provides a rapid and convenient method for receptor analysis in crude extracts. We used this procedure to see if progesterone treatment had any effect on the quantity or electrophoretic properties of progesterone receptor. In the experiment shown in Figure 3, chickens were treated with the synthetic progestin, R5020, for up to 20 h. At the times indicated, oviduct cytosol and nuclear extracts were prepared, subjected to SDS gel electrophoresis, and the receptor analyzed by Western blotting.

There were two very noticeable changes in the receptor patterns after hormone treatment. First, while the level of nuclear receptor, particularly receptor A, increased during the first hour of treatment, the level declined dramatically at later times as did the receptor in the cytosol fraction. Thus, there appears to be extensive loss or down-regulation of the receptor after R5020 administration. Very similar results were obtained when the natural hormone, progesterone, was used (19).

A second observation was a change in the mobility of the A receptor form to a slower migrating species termed A'. This appeared in both the cytosol and the nuclear fractions and it was the major receptor form in the nuclear fraction at all times after hormone treatment. Additional studies have shown that the A' receptor is also observed after administration of progesterone and that this effect is dose-dependent (19). The A' receptor is generated within 15 min, the earliest time studied, and it reacts with all four antibodies that recognize the A receptor, but not with the B-specific antibody, PR6. Thus, it is clearly derived from the A receptor.

Receptor Phosphorylation

One possible explanation for the mobility shift from A to A' is an increased phosphorylation of receptor after hormone treatment. Similar mobility shifts have been observed for progesterone receptor from the rabbit (15) and human (25-26), and for vitamin D receptor (16). In these cases there is evidence for a phosphorylation event following hormone treatment and phosphorylation has been shown to alter or retard the electrophoretic mobility of some other proteins on SDS gels (27-29).

The avian progesterone receptor has been shown to be phosphorylated on serine residues (10,11). However, these earlier studies were performed with receptor from oviducts that were not treated with a progestin. To test for additional hormone-dependent phosphorylation, the incorporation of ^{32}P-labeled orthophosphate into the receptor was measured using a protocol similar to that of Milgrom and co-workers in their studies with the rabbit progesterone receptor (15). Oviduct minces were incubated in culture medium with [^{32}P] orthophosphate for 1 h. During this incubation, progesterone was added for 0, 5, 20, or 40 min. Tissue cytosols were then prepared and the receptor was isolated by immune adsorption with antibody

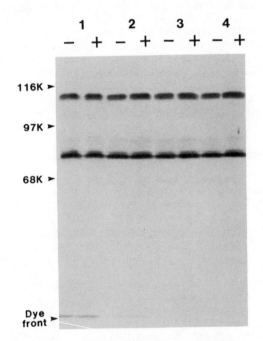

Fig. 2. Effect of protease inhibitors on receptor stability. Chick oviduct tissue was homogenized without (-) or with (+) a mixture of protease inhibitors as described in Methods. Samples were removed, adjusted to 2% (w:v) SDS, and 5% (v:v) mercapto-ethanol and boiled for 2 min immediately after homogenization (1), low speed centrifugation (2) or high speed centrifugation (3). Alternatively, each homogenate was incubated on ice for 1.5 h before processing to cytosol (4). Loads equivalent to 1.6 µl of homogenate or supernatants were applied to gels. Western blotting was done with αPR13 which reacts with both the 110 kDa B receptor (upper band) and the 80 kDa A receptor (lower band). The molecular weight markers indicated by arrows are β-galacto-sidase, 116K; phosphorylase b, 97K; and bovine serum albumin, 68K.

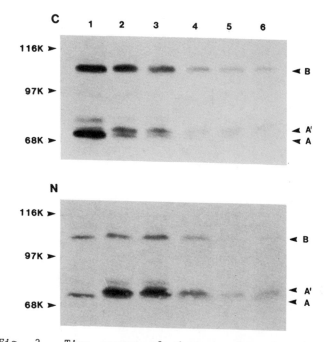

Fig. 3. Time course of changes after in vivo administration of R-5020. Chicks were injected sc with either sesame oil alone (lane 1) or with 2 mg of R-5020 in oil (lanes 2-6) at the following times: 30 min (lane 2), 60 min (lane 3), 2 h (lane 4), 4 h (lanes 1 and 5) or 20 h (lane 6). At the end of the time course, chicks were killed and their oviducts removed. Cytosolic (C) and nuclear (N) extracts were prepared from each as described in Methods. Western blotting was done with αPR13 as the primary antibody.

PR13 and antimouse IgG linked to agarose. It was then eluted from the resin and analyzed by gel electrophoresis and autoradiography (19). This procedure provides highly purified receptor preparations where the ^{32}P-labeled receptor forms are the major phosphoproteins and can be readily observed after electrophoresis. As shown in Figure 4, incorporation of ^{32}P into the A and B receptor forms is readily apparent without hormone treatment (lane one). However, the extent of incorporation is increased quite dramatically by the addition of progesterone. This is noticeable with only 5 min of treatment and appears to be near a maximum by 20 min. These results are very similar to those obtained for progesterone receptor in the rabbit uterus (15). Thus, receptor phosphorylation does occur very early after progesterone treatment and may be related to the mobility effects observed on SDS gels. The bands of radioactivity shown in Figure 4 are quite broad and do not allow one to resolve A and A' receptor forms. However, when similar experiments were performed and analyzed by Western blots, generation of the A' receptor was clearly evident after hormone treatment.

Two additional phosphoproteins can be seen in Figure 4. The band migrating below the 68 kDa standard has not been identified. It is not observed consistently and is likely to be a protein contaminant unrelated to the receptor. The 90 kDa protein that is clearly observed in lane 1 above receptor A is the heat shock protein, hsp 90. This was identified by Western blotting similar samples with antibodies specific for this protein. Hsp 90 is a phosphoprotein and its association with nontransformed receptor was established in earlier studies (20–22). Thus, it was isolated along with the receptor in the experiment of Figure 4. However, the amount of hsp 90 recovered with the receptor decreases with time of hormone treatment. This has recently been confirmed by Western blotting analysis rather than ^{32}P measurement. This suggests that hormone treatment alters the receptor, or hsp 90, in a way which weakens the interaction between these two proteins.

We have recently used peptide mapping analysis in an attempt to more clearly describe the sites of phosphorylation on the progesterone recep-

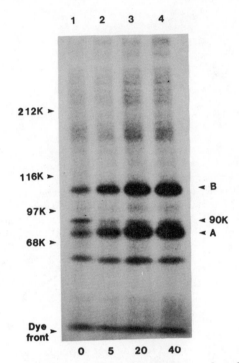

Fig. 4. Time course of receptor phosphorylation following progesterone treatment. Oviduct tissue minces were incubated for $\frac{1}{2}$ h at 41°C in culture medium containing [^{32}P] orthophosphate. Progesterone (50 nm) was added to individual incubation flasks for 5, 20, or 40 min before incubation was terminated. Cytosol samples were prepared in 50 mM potassium phosphate, 10 mM Na_2MoO_4, 10 mM thioglycerol, 10 mM EDTA, and 50 mM NaF, pH 7, and incubated with antibody αPR13 for 2 h on ice, and the immune complexes were then purified by adsorption to antimouse IgG covalently linked to agarose. Protein was eluted from the resin into SDS sample buffer and resolved by gel electrophoresis. An autoradiogram of the gel is illustrated. Lane 1, no progesterone treatment; lanes 2–4, treatment with progesterone for 5, 20, or 40 min. Receptors A and B are indicated by arrows.

tor. In our earlier studies to describe phosphorylation of the nontransformed receptor (without hormone treatment), we found that multiple
phosphopeptides were observed after trypsin digestion (30). This is also
the case when receptor is analyzed after treatment with progesterone.
Figure 5 illustrates two-dimensional mapping of the phosphopeptides
generated by digestion of receptor A and A' with trypsin (panel A) or with
V8 (panel B). In both cases, four major phosphopeptides were observed.
In repeated experiments, the pattern with V8 protease is very consistent.
However, the tightly grouped trypsin phosphopeptides shown at the top of
panel A show some variation ranging between two to four peptides. The
patterns observed with receptor B are almost identical to those shown for
A and A' providing additional evidence that a similar process is occurring
with both receptor forms. Additional studies are needed, but the present
results indicate that receptor phosphorylation occurs at multiple sites.
Studies are in progress to identify the regions, and eventually, the
actual sites on the receptor where phosphorylation occurs.

DISCUSSION

The results presented here indicate that receptor phosphorylation is,
indeed, a very early event following hormone binding. The stimulation of
receptor phosphorylation offers a likely explanation for the mobility
shift from receptor A to A', but this is still uncertain and other possible modifications of the receptor should also be considered. While the
extent of ^{32}P incorporation into the A and B receptor forms appears to be
about equal, there is little change in the electrophoretic mobility of the
B receptor after hormone treatment. The mechanism by which phosphorylation alters protein mobility in SDS gels is not clear (27-29) and it is
certainly possible that some phosphorylation can occur at sites that do
not influence the electrophoretic mobility. Another factor that may
contribute to this is the fact that the progesterone receptor migrates on
SDS gels with an apparent molecular weight that is much larger than that
calculated from the cDNA sequence (9). The margin of difference here
appears to be greater for the B receptor than for the A receptor and it
has been suggested that the retarded mobility of the B receptor is due to
the high content of glutamic acid near its amino terminus.

The significance of phosphorylation to receptor function remains
unknown, although several suggestions have been made (12-16). The most
obvious possibilities would be for the modulation of steroid binding or
the interaction of receptors with DNA or chromatin proteins. Phosphorylation could also modify the turnover of the receptor and, thus, influence
the down-regulation following hormone treatment. The apparent loss of
interaction between the receptor and hsp 90 that is indicated in our
studies could relate to receptor phosphorylation. The significance of
this interaction is unknown, but it is possible that hsp 90 maintains the
receptor in an inactive form. A phosphorylation event may then promote a
release and activation of the receptor protein. It should now be possible
to test these and other possibilities.

The analysis of progesterone receptor phosphorylation by peptide
mapping indicates that there are multiple sites of phosphorylation. Thus,
it is possible that phosphorylation influences more than one aspect of
receptor structure or function. It will be important to identify the
actual phosphorylation sites and to measure the extent to which these are
modified during the course of hormone action.

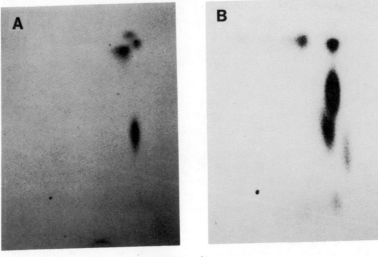

Fig. 5. Phosphopeptide mapping of ^{32}P-labeled progesterone receptor. Progesterone receptor was ^{32}P-labeled in tissue minces incubated with 10^{-7}M progesterone for 30 min and purified by immune isolation (see Methods). After transfer from an SDS gel to nitrocellulose, the receptor A bands were cut out, digested with trypsin (panel A) or with V8 protease (panel B), and the phosphopeptides were resolved on thin layer sheets. Electrophoresis was done in the first dimension from left to right toward the anode followed by chromatography in the second dimension from bottom to top. The figure represents autoradiograms of the cellulose thin layer sheets.

REFERENCES

1. Puri RK, Grandics P, Dougherty JJ, et al. Purification of "nontransformed" avian progesterone receptor and preliminary characterization. J Biol Chem 1982; 257:10831-7.

2. Renoir JM, Mester J, Buchou T, et al. Purification by affinity chromatography and immunological characterization of a 110kDa component of the chick oviduct progesterone receptor. Biochem J 1984; 217:685-92.

3. Gronemeyer H, Govindan MV, Chambon P. Immunological similarity between the chick oviduct progesterone receptor forms A and B. J Biol Chem 1985; 6916-25.

4. Birnbaumer M, Hinrichs-Rosello MV, Cook RG, et al. Chemical and antigenic properties of pure 108,000 molecular weight chick progesterone receptor. Mol Endocrinol 1987; 1:249-59.

5. Simpson RJ, Grego B, Govindan, et al. Peptide sequencing of the chick oviduct progesterone receptor form B. Mol Cell Endocrinol 1987; 52:177-84.

6. Sullivan WP, Beito TG, Proper J, et al. Preparation of monoclonal antibodies to the avian progesterone receptor. Endocrinology 1986; 119:1549-57.

7. Conneely OM, Sullivan WP, Toft DO, et al. Molecular cloning of the chicken progesterone receptor. Science 1986; 233:767-70,

8. Jeltsch JM, Krozowski Z, Quirin-Stricker C, et al. Cloning of the chicken progesterone receptor. Proc Natl Acad Sci USA 1986; 83: 5424-8

9. Conneely OM, Dobson ADW, Tsai M-J, et al. Sequence and expression of a functional chicken progesterone receptor. Mol Endocrinol 1987; 1:517-25.

10. Dougherty JJ, Puri RK, Toft DO. Phosphorylation in vivo of chicken oviduct progesterone receptor. J Biol Chem 1982; 257:14226-30.

11. Dougherty JJ, Puri RK, Toft DO. Polypeptide components of two 8S forms of chicken oviduct progesterone receptor. J Biol Chem 1984; 259:8004-9.

12. Dougherty JJ, Puri RK, Toft DO. Phosphorylation of steroid receptors. Trends Pharm Sci 1985; 6:83-5.

13. Housley PR, Sanchez ER, Westphal HM, et al. The molybdate-stabilized L-cell glucocorticoid receptor isolated by affinity chromatography or with a monoclonal antibody is associated with a 90-92-kDa nonsteroid-binding phosphoprotein. J Biol Chem 1985; 260:13810-7.

14. Migliaccio A, Rotondi A, Auricchio F. Estradiol receptor: phosphorylation on tyrosine in uterus and interaction with antiphosphoty-rosine antibody. EMBO J 1986; 5:2867-72.

15. Logeat F, Le Cunff M, Pamphile R, et al. The nuclear bound form of the progesterone receptor is generated through a hormone-dependent phosphorylation. Biochem Biophys Res Commun 1985a; 131:421-7.

16. Pike JW, Sleator NM. Hormone-dependent phosphorylation of the $1,25$-dihydroxyvitamin D_3 receptor in mouse fibroblasts. Biochem Biophys Res Commun 1985; 131:378-85.

17. Laemmli UK. Cleavage of structural proteins during the assembly of the head of bacteriophage T4. Nature 1970; 227:680-5.

18. Blake MS, Johnston KH, Russel-Jones GJ, et al. A rapid, sensitive method for detection of alkaline phosphatase-conjugated anti-antibody on Western blots. Anal Biochem 1984; 136:175-9.

19. Sullivan WP, Smith DF, Beito TG, et al. Hormone-dependent processing of the avian progesterone receptor. J Cell Biochem (in press).

20. Schuh S, Yonemoto W, Brugge J, et al. A 90,000-dalton binding protein common to both steroid receptors and the Rous sarcoma virus transforming protein, $pp60^{v-src}$. J Biol Chem 1985; 260:14292-6.

21. Sanchez ER, Toft DO, Schlesinger MJ, et al. Evidence that the 90-kDa phosphoprotein associated with the untransformed L-cell glucocor-ticoid receptor is a murine heat shock protein. J Biol Chem 1985; 260:12398-401.

22. Catelli MG, Binart N, Jung-Testas I, et al. The common 90kDa protein component of non-transformed "8S" steroid receptors is a heat-shock protein. EMBO J 1985; 4:3131-5

23. Loosfelt H, Logeat F, Hai MTV, et al. The rabbit progesterone receptor. Evidence for a single steroid-binding subunit and char-acterization of receptor mRNA. J Biol Chem 1984; 259:14196-202.

24. Wei LL, Horwitz KB. The structure of progesterone receptors. Steroids 1985; 46:678-95.

25. Horwitz KB, Francis MD, Wei LL. Hormone-dependent covalent modifica-tion and processing of human progesterone receptors in the nucleus. DNA 1985; 4:451-60.

26. Wei LL, Sheridan PL, Krett NL, et al. Immunologic analysis of human breast cancer progesterone receptors. 2. Structure, phosphoryla-tion, and processing. Biochemistry 1987; 26:6262-72.

27. Sekimizu K, Kubo Y, Segawa K, et al. Difference in phosphorylation of two factors stimulating RNA polymerase II of Ehrlich ascites tumor cells. Biochemistry 1981; 20:2286-92.

28. Wegener AD, Jones LR. Phosphorylation-induced mobility shift in phospholamban in sodium dodecyl sulfate-polyacrylamide gels. J Biol Chem 1984; 259:1834-41.

29. Georges E, Mushynski WE. Chemical modification of charged amino acid moieties alters the electrophoretic mobilities of neurofilament subunits on SDS/polyacrylamide gels. Eur J Biochem 1987; 165:281-7.

30. Puri RK, Toft DO. Peptide mapping analysis of the avian progesterone

receptor. J Biol Chem 1986; 261:5651-7.

31. Toft DO, Sullivan WB, Smith DF, et al. Immuological analysis of the avian progesterone receptor. In: Spelsberg TC, Kumar R, eds. Steroid and sterol hormone action. Boston, MA: Martinus Nijhoff Publishing, 1987:25-39.

III. RECEPTOR MODIFICATIONS AND HORMONE REGULATION

7

HORMONE-DEPENDENT AND HORMONE-INDEPENDENT

CONFORMATIONAL TRANSITIONS OF THE ESTROGEN RECEPTOR

Jeffrey C. Hansen and Jack Gorski

Department of Biochemistry
University of Wisconsin
Madison, WI 53706

INTRODUCTION

From a chemical perspective, steroid hormones are simple molecules. Yet from a biological perspective, steroid hormones are complex molecules that are capable of coordinating and regulating a diverse number of biological processes. At the cellular level, the crucial links between the chemically simple and biologically complex nature of steroid hormones are specific receptor proteins that bind steroids with very high affinity, and are found exclusively in cells that respond to hormone. In effect, steroid hormone receptors are macromolecular information transducers in that they couple broad biological input, i.e., the cumulative information that leads to synthesis of a steroid molecule, to dramatic cellular response. Since cellular responses are strictly dependent on the interaction of hormone and receptor, it has been of considerable interest to biochemists and molecular biologists to define the molecular mechanisms involved in hormone-dependent modulation of steroid receptor activity. In addition, the emerging evidence that steroid receptors are also intimately involved in many diseases has provided additional impetus to understand better the mechanism of steroid receptor action in target cells.

The Temperature-Sensitive Structure of Steroid Receptors in Vitro

As might be expected, the structure of steroid receptors has been found to be quite dynamic in vitro (1-4). Central among these observations is that steroid receptors of all types undergo a temperature-dependent structural change in vitro that modulates receptor interactions with DNA-cellulose (5,6), isolated nuclei (7,8), and a 90 KD heat shock protein (9-11). These temperature-dependent changes in receptor structure have been termed receptor "transformation" (and in some cases "activation") and most commonly serve as the basis for molecular models of steroid receptor function (1-4,12).

Despite the long-standing belief in the in vivo relevance of receptor transformation, there are still a number of questions that remain unanswered. Most important, what are the consequences of hormone binding on receptor structure and the transformation process? We know that hormone binding is an absolute requirement in vivo, yet all studies of in vitro receptor transformation have been done with hormone-occupied receptor complexes. Thus, the processes associated with receptor transformation must be strictly hormone-dependent in order to be considered biologically relevant. In addition, what is the origin of the effects of temperature on receptor structure in vitro, i.e., why does moderate temperature (25-30°C) influence the structure of a protein that was recently isolated from the 37°C environment of the intact cell? In an attempt to determine the answers to these questions, we have characterized the behavior of both unoccupied and hormone-bound estrogen receptors in aqueous two-phase polymer systems.

Aqueous Two-Phase Partitioning of Steroid Receptors

Why aqueous two-phase partitioning? First and foremost, this technique can be used to study the physicochemical properties of unoccupied steroid receptors in vitro (13). This ability to directly characterize unoccupied receptors is necessary both to determine the molecular consequences of hormone binding, and to define the relationship between hormone binding and receptor transformation. In addition, aqueous two-phase partitioning provides an alternative type of structural information than the standard approaches (e.g., sedimentation, column chromatography, etc.) most commonly used to characterize the properties of steroid receptors. As predicted by theory and as has been demonstrated empirically by the continuously elegant work of Albertsson (14-16), the partitioning of macromolecules in aqueous two-phase systems is dependent on both the net molecular charge and the net hydrophobic/hydrophilic content on the molecule's surface. Thus in the case of steroid receptors, the partitioning technique will in principle provide information regarding the effect(s) of hormone binding and temperature on the chemical composition of the receptor's surface, even if these treatments do not change the size and shape of the protein. Furthermore, knowledge of the surface properties of native steroid receptors are increasingly useful in light of the recent determination of the steroid receptor amino acid primary sequences (17-20).

The feasibility of using aqueous two-phase partitioning to characterize steroid hormone receptors has been repeatedly demonstrated by the pioneering studies of Andreasen (21-27). Working with the glucocorticoid receptor, Andreasen used partitioning to perform detailed biochemical (21-23) and kinetic (25) studies of glucocorticoid receptor transformation, as well as to study the effects of in vitro proteolysis on receptor structure (26), and to characterize mutant glucocorticoid receptors from S49 lymphoma cells (24). Taken together, these studies indicate that partitioning in aqueous two-phase systems is a powerful and relevant means to characterize the information transducing properties of steroid hormone receptors.

HORMONE-DEPENDENT AND TEMPERATURE-DEPENDENT CHANGES IN ESTROGEN RECEPTOR PARTITIONING BEHAVIOR

Initially, we determined the partitioning behavior of three forms of the rat uterine estrogen receptor (ER): unoccupied, estrogen occupied at 0°C (nontransformed), and estrogen-occupied at 30°C (transformed). Receptors were partitioned to equilibrium in phase systems composed of 5.4% (w/w) each of dextran (MW 500,000) and PEG (MW 8,000) and the receptor concentration in each phase determined by hydroxylapatite assay. The data are expressed as the partition coefficient (K_{obs}), which is defined as the ratio of receptor concentrations in the upper and lower phases respectively:

$$K_{obs} = \frac{[ER]_{top}}{[ER]_{bottom}}$$

As shown in Figure 1, both estradiol binding and exposure of estradiol-receptor complexes to 30°C for 60 min dramatically alter the receptor partition coefficient. Significantly, binding of the nonsteroidal estrogen diethylstilbestrol causes the same partition change as estradiol binding (28), whereas binding of the competitive antagonist 4-OH-tamoxifen only partially induces the partition change observed with the estrogens (28, and Figure 1). Thus, the change in receptor structure that occurs upon hormone binding correlates with the biological activity of the ligand and not its steroidal or nonsteroidal structure. This immediately suggests that the hormone-dependent receptor transition plays an important role in receptor function. The observation that elevated temperature changes the partition coefficient of estradiol-receptor complexes indicates that estrogen receptor transformation can also be observed in aqueous two-phase polymer systems. From Figure 1, it can be seen clearly that both estrogen-receptor and antiestrogen-receptor complexes can be transformed by elevated temperature in vitro, although subtle differences in structure apparently exist in the final transformed states.

While these data are quite suggestive, it is necessary to determine the precise molecular changes in receptor structure that ultimately lead to altered partitioning behavior in order to understand the significance of the results contained in Figure 1. That is, since the experimentally derived partition coefficient is a composite of both the conformational and electrostatic properties of the receptor, and is sensitive to changes in receptor aggregation, there are many possible explanations of the data in Figure 1. For these reasons, we further characterized both the hormone-dependent and temperature-dependent changes in receptor partitioning in considerably more detail.

The Hormone-Dependent Estrogen Receptor Transition

In order to determine the molecular mechanism of the hormone-dependent receptor transition, we exploited the thermodynamic theory that

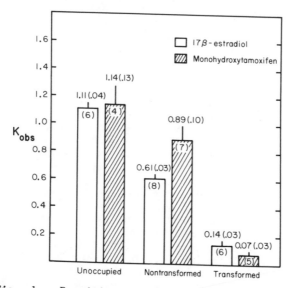

Fig. 1. Partition coefficients of unoccupied estrogen receptors, and nontransformed and transformed estrogen-receptor and antiestrogen-receptor complexes. Adapted from Hansen and Gorski (28).

dictates how molecules distribute in aqueous two-phase systems, and which is summarized by equation 2:

$$\ln K_{obs} = \ln K_o + \frac{ZF\Delta\Psi}{RT} = \Delta G^o_{tr}/2.303RT$$

Briefly, this relationship states that the value of the experimental partition coefficient is directly proportional to the change in the standard free energy of transfer that occurs during partitioning, and is a sum of two independent influences. The first component is the partition coefficient due to solute-solvent interactions (K_o), and is influenced by the degree of hydrophobicity and other conformational features. The second component is the electrostatic free energy change that results from the combination of net surface charge (Z) and an interfacial potential difference across the phase boundary ($\Delta\Psi$). Thus, the question we asked was which of these two terms is altered as a consequence of hormone binding? The data that resolves this question are shown in Figure 2. The electrostatic term can be manipulated in vitro by both salt and pH. Different salts create different values of $\Delta\Psi$ (29,30) and pH affects the net receptor charge (Z). Thus, at a pH where the receptor charge is significant (e.g., 7.4), the K_{obs} will be different in each salt; however, at the isoelectric point (pI) of the receptor (where Z = 0), the K_{obs} will be identical in all salts and will be equal to the value of K_o (16,31). Using such an approach, we observed that the pI (Fig. 2) and net charge (32) of both unoccupied and estrogen-occupied receptors were virtually identical, whereas the K_o term was dramatically lowered by estradiol binding. Thus, the hormone-dependent change in partition coefficients (Fig. 1) reflects a change in the conformation of the receptor surface that does not alter the net receptor charge. Besides having the same net charge, these results also indicate that the K_o value of both unoccupied and estrogen-bound receptors is unaffected by elevated ionic strength (0.3 M) and chaotropic salts (Li_2SO_4), together suggesting that these receptor forms are partitioning as stable monomers. Further support for this conclusion comes from the finding that the partition coefficients of both unoccupied and estrogen-bound receptors remain unchanged during >30-fold dilutions (to as low as 30 pM) (13). Further characterization of the hormone-dependent transition of the estrogen receptor monomer was performed using "affinity partitioning." With this approach receptors are partitioned in phase systems containing PEG-bound ligands such as palmitate (33-35) or triazine dyes (36-38). Using PEG-palmitate, we observed that hormone binding buries hydrophobic domain(s) originally present on the surface of the unoccupied receptor (28). In contrast, hormone binding dramatically increases the interaction of estrogen receptors with nucleotide analogs such as cibacron blue and procion green (39). Thus, the conformational change induced by hormone binding is linked to modulation of at least two different types of surface domains that may be important in receptor function.

Emerging evidence supports the concept that hormone-dependent conformational transitions are a general property of all steroid hormone receptors. Also using aqueous two-phase partitioning, Moudgil has recently reported that hormone binding alters the properties of both glucocorticoid (40) and progesterone (41) receptors. The recent demonstration by Green and Chambon (42) of induction of glucocorticoid gene expression upon estradiol binding to a chimeric receptor protein also suggests that direct structural rearrangement occurs upon hormone binding to estrogen and glucocorticoid receptors. Similarly, recent in vitro mutagenesis of glucocorticoid receptor genes (43,44) have led investigators to propose that the primary effect of hormone binding is to relieve steric hindrance at the transcription regulation domain of the protein. While it has not been established that the hormone-dependent

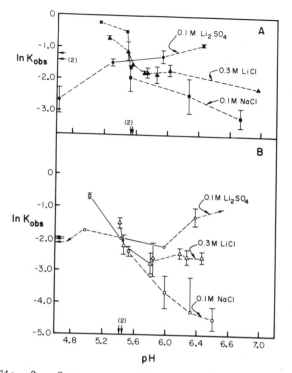

Fig. 2. Cross partitioning of unoccupied (A) and nontransformed (B) rat uterine estrogen receptors. Each estrogen receptor form was partitioned to equilibrium at the indicated pH and salt compositions. From the points of intersection on the y-axis, the K_o value of unoccupied and nontransformed ER is 0.25 ± 0.3 and 0.12 ± 0.2, respectively. From the points of intersection on the x-axis, the receptor pI is 5.55 ± .15 and 5.45 ± .15, respectively. Reproduced with permission from Hansen and Gorski (13), © 1985 American Chemical Society.

changes in steroid receptor structure observed with aqueous two-phase partitioning and molecular genetic analyses are in fact the same receptor transition, it is becoming increasingly clear that the structural effects of hormone binding per se can no longer be ignored.

The Temperature-Dependent Estrogen Receptor Transition

One of the most confusing aspects of steroid receptor transformation is its origin in vitro. It is most commonly believed that receptor transformation occurs only after hormone binding, at which point transformation can be "induced" by exposure of receptors to elevated temperature. In this two-step scenario, the in vivo role of hormone binding is to allow the events associated with receptor transformation to occur spontaneously in the 37°C environment of the cell. In order to address the question of the in vitro origin of estrogen receptor transformation, we have performed a detailed kinetic analysis of the effects of temperature on estrogen receptor partition coefficients.

As has been previously demonstrated by Andreasen (25), the phase partitioning technique is very well suited for studying macromolecular kinetics. In large part this is due to the fact that it only takes 5 sec of mixing to reach partitioning equilibrium (13), thus allowing for accurate determination of the fraction of transformed receptors over very short time intervals. The kinetics of the change in nontransformed estrogen receptor partition coefficients versus time at 30°C is shown in Figure 3. When plotted on a semilogarithmic plot, the transformation process is linear through >90% of the reaction. Similar studies over a fiftyfold range of estrogen receptor concentration yielded essentially identical results (32,45) and demonstrate rigorously that the temperature-dependent change in partition coefficients reflects a simple first-order process. This in turn indicates that the partition change is not due to 4S → 5S dimerization and does not involve associative interactions with other cytosolic components (both of which would be second-order processes —see reference 46). Incubation of temperature transformed receptors for even 18 h at 0°C did not change the partition coefficient from the value obtained after 60 min at 30°C, indicating that the process is irreversible with respect to temperature. Determination of the rate of partition change at 8 temperatures between 0-30°C indicates that the transformation process occurs significantly at 0-4°C. Thus, ER transformation is not induced by elevated temperature, but is simply accelerated by heating. Although the rate is dramatically affected, the same final extent of partition change occurs after 24 h at 0-4°C (and at all temperatures in between) as it does after 60 min at 30°C. Cumulatively, these kinetic data indicate that temperature-dependent change in ER partition coefficients represents an irreversible conformational change in the estrogen receptor monomer.

The ability of temperature to transform the estrogen receptor monomer has been documented previously using DNA-cellulose chromatography (47,48) and estradiol dissociation kinetics (49,50). Interestingly, it has recently been reported that the temperature-dependent change in the rate of estradiol dissociation is irreversible with respect to temperature, but can be reversed by addition of exogenous dithiothreitol at 20°C (51). These results support our conclusion that transformation of the estrogen receptor monomer in vitro is inherently an irreversible process.

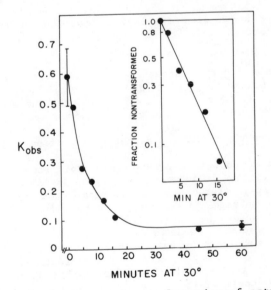

Fig. 3. Kinetics of transformation of estradiol-receptor complexes at 30°C. The inset is
a semilogarithmic plot of the same data.

Transformation of the Estrogen Receptor Monomer
Is Hormone-Independent in Vitro

As is the case with other studies of ER transformation, our kinetic experiments were performed with estradiol-receptor complexes (formed at 0°C prior to heating) and thus were lacking an important control experiment: does transformation occur to the unoccupied receptor? The results of experiments in which we heated the unoccupied estrogen receptor directly are illustrated in Figure 4. Quite to our surprise, exposure of unoccupied receptors to 30°C for 15 min significantly lowers the partition coefficient of this receptor form. Furthermore, binding of estradiol to the heated unoccupied receptor lowers the ER partition coefficient to a value that is indistinguishable from that of receptors that were heated after hormone binding. We have also determined that the temperature-dependent change in the unoccupied ER partition coefficient is a first-order process that occurs at the same rate as that of the estrogen occupied ("nontransformed") receptor (32,45). Thus, transformation of the estrogen receptor monomer in vitro is <u>hormone-independent</u>, which together with the earlier kinetic results indicates that the temperature-dependent ER transition is occurring irreversibly to unoccupied receptors in cytosol at 0°C. From these results, we further conclude that transformation of the estrogen receptor monomer occurs in vitro entirely as a consequence of tissue homogenization and subsequent extraction of receptors into cytosol.

In addition to changing the value of the partition coefficient, heating the unoccupied receptor at 30°C resulted in a loss of ER binding sites (receptor "inactivation"). The inactivation process was found to be second-order (32,45), consistent with enzymatic modification of the unoccupied receptor to a nonhormone binding form. Receptor inactivation also continued to occur well after the unoccupied ER partition change had reached completion, together indicating that temperature-dependent binding site inactivation is unrelated to ER transformation. Interestingly, inactivation of the steroid binding domain no longer occurs after binding of both estrogens and 4-OH-tamoxifen (28), indicating that even the partial conformational transition induced by 4-OH-tamoxifen binding is sufficient to disrupt surface features necessary for binding site inactivation (e.g., enzyme binding site, nucleotide binding site, etc.). It is also interesting that the structurally related processes of hormone binding and binding site inactivation are both independent of receptor

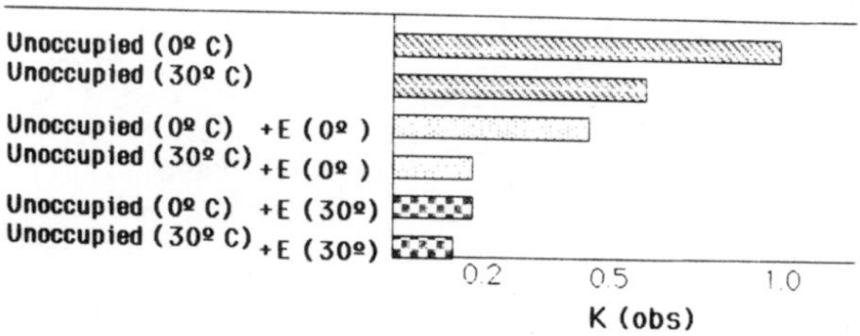

Fig. 4. Effect of temperature on unoccupied estrogen receptor properties. Unoccupied (0°C) refers to unoccupied ER that was kept at 0°C prior to addition of hormone. Unoccupied (30°C) refers to unoccupied ER that was exposed to 30°C for 15 min prior to partitioning. E_2 (0°C) refers to incubations with hormone at 0°C for 2.5 h. E_2 (30°C) refers to incubations with hormone where the last 15 min of the incubation occurred at 30°C. Adapted from Hansen and Gorski (28).

transformation, suggesting that the hormone-dependent and temperature-dependent receptor transitions occur in topologically distinct regions of the protein.

SUMMARY AND CONCLUSION: THE "ONE AND ONLY" STEP MODEL OF ESTROGEN ACTION

Partitioning of both unoccupied and hormone-bound estrogen receptors in aqueous two-phase polymer systems has demonstrated the existence of two conformational transitions that occur within the estrogen receptor monomer in vitro. The first structural change occurs upon estrogen binding, modulates a triazine dye binding domain and the hydrophobic content of the receptor surface and abolishes in vitro inactivation of the steroid binding site, but does not alter the net charge of the receptor. This receptor transition is only partially induced by antiestrogen binding. The temperature-dependent receptor transition (ER transformation) is a hormone-independent, irreversible structural change that apparently begins to occur immediately upon homogenization at 0-4°C and subsequent extraction of receptors into cytosol. In light of these findings, and in view of the results of recent molecular genetic studies that suggest that a simple hormone-dependent conformational change mediates the transcription-modulating activity of steroid receptors (42-44), the long presumed importance of steroid receptor transformation now seems suspect. Instead, the key event seems to be a hormone-induced structural transition that has been shown to influence at least four different structural and functional domains on the receptor surface. We believe, therefore, that in order to study the molecular details of steroid hormone action, it is necessary to focus on the effects of steroid and not on the effects of heating or other extraneous factors on the system. Until we have evidence to the contrary, the assumption should be that the receptor in the intact cell is responsive to only one environmental signal: the presence of estrogen.

REFERENCES

1. Jensen EV, DeSombre ER. Estrogen-receptor activation. Science 1973; 182:126.
2. Gorski J, Gannon F. Current models of steroid hormone action: a critique. Annu Rev Physiol 1976; 38:425-50.
3. Grody WW, Schrader WT, O'Malley BW. Activation, transformation, and subunit structure of steroid hormone receptors. Endocr Rev 1982; 3:141-62.
4. Andreasen PA. Aqueous two-phase partitioning for the study of steroid receptor activation. In: Litwack G, ed. Biochemical actions of hormones. New York: Academic Press, 1987:181-235.
5. Yamamoto K, Alberts BM. In vitro conversion of estradiol receptor protein to its nuclear form. Dependence on hormone and DNA. Proc Natl Acad Sci USA 1972; 69:2105-9.
6. Yamamoto KR. Characterization of the 4S and 5S forms of the estradiol receptor protein and their interaction with deoxyribonucleic acid. J Biol Chem 1974; 249:7068.
7. Jensen EV, Suzuki T, Kawashima T, Stumpf WE, Jungblut PW, DeSombre ER. A two-step mechanism for the interaction of estradiol with rat uterus. Proc Natl Acad Sci USA 1968; 59:632-8.
8. Atger M, Milgrom E. Mechanism and kinetics of the thermal activation of glucocorticoid hormone-receptor complex. J Biol Chem 1976; 251:4758-62.
9. Joab I, Radanyi C, Renoir M, et al. Common non-hormone binding component in non-transformed chick oviduct receptors of four steroid hormones. Nature 1984; 308:850-3.

10. Catelli MG, Binart N, Jung-Testas I, et al. The common 90-kd protein component of non-transformed '8S' steroid receptors is a heat-shock protein. EMBO J 1985; 4:3131-5.

11. Sanchez ER, Toft DO, Schlesinger MJ, Pratt WB. Evidence that the 90-kDa phosphoprotein associated with the untransformed L-cell glucocorticoid receptor is a murine heat shock protein. J Biol Chem 1985; 280:12398-401.

12. Sherman MR, Stevens J. Structure of mammalian steroid receptors: evolving concepts and methodological developments. Annu Rev Physiol 1984; 46:83-105.

13. Hansen JC, Gorski J. Conformational and electrostatic properties of unoccupied and liganded estrogen receptors determined by aqueous two-phase partitioning. Biochemistry 1985; 24:6078-85.

14. Albertsson PA. Partition between polymer phases. J Chromatogr 1978; 159:111-22.

15. Albertsson PA. Interaction between biomolecules studied by phase partition. Methods Biochem Anal 1983; 29:1-24.

16. Albertsson PA. Partition of cell particles and macromolecules. 3rd ed. New York: John Wiley & Sons, 1986.

17. Krust A, Green S, Argos P, et al. The chicken oestrogen receptor sequence: homology with v-erbA and the human oestrogen and glucocorticoid receptors. EMBO J 1986; 5:891-7.

18. Hollenberg SM, Weinberger C, Ong ES, et al. Primary structure and expression of a functional human glucocorticoid receptor cDNA. Nature 1985; 318:635-41.

19. Miesfeld R, Rusconi S, Godowski PJ, et al. Genetic complementation of a glucocorticoid receptor deficiency by expression of cloned receptor cDNA. Cell 1986; 46:389-99.

20. Jeltsch JM, Krozowski Z, Quirin-Stricker C, et al. Cloning of the chicken progesterone receptor. Proc Natl Acad Sci USA 1986; 83:5424-8.

21. Andreasen PA. Conversions of the glucocorticoid receptor complex of rat thymocyte cytosol, studied by partition in an aqueous dextran-polyethylene glycol two-phase system. Biochim Biophys Acta 1978; 540:484-99.

22. Andreasen PA, Mainwaring WIP. Aqueous two-phase partition studies of the glucocorticoid receptor. Activation and pH-dependent changes of rat liver glucocorticoid-receptor complex in partly purified preparations. Biochim Biophys Acta 1980; 631:334-49.

23. Andreasen PA. A specific adenine nucleotide effect on the rat liver glucocorticoid receptor, demonstrated by aqueous two-phase partitioning. Biochim Biophys Acta 1981; 676:205-12.

24. Andreasen PA, Gehring U. Activation and partial proteolysis of variant glucocorticoid receptors, studied by two-phase partitioning. Eur J Biochem 1981; 120:443-99.

25. Andreasen PA. Changes in net charge of glucocorticoid receptors by activation, and evidence for a biphasic activation kinetics. Mol Cell Endocrinol 1982; 28:563-86.

26. Andreasen PA. Aqueous two-phase partition studies of glucocorticoid receptors exposed to limited trypsinization. Mol Cell Endocrinol 1983; 30:229-39.

27. Andreasen PA, Junker K. Specific effects of monovalent cations and of adenine nucleotides on glucocorticoid receptor activation, as studied by aqueous two-phase partitioning. In: Moudgil VK, ed. Molecular mechanism of steroid hormone action. Berlin-New York: Walter de Gruyter & Co., 1985:199-224.

28. Hansen JC, Gorski J. Conformational transitions of the estrogen receptor monomer. J Biol Chem 1986; 261:13990-6.

29. Johansson G. Partition of proteins and micro-organisms in aqueous biphasic systems. Mol Cell Biochem 1974; 4:169-79.

30. Brooks DE, Sharp KA, Bamberger S, Tamblyn CH, Seaman GVF, Walter H.

Electrostatic and electrokinetic potentials in two polymer aqueous phase systems. J Colloid & Interface Sci 1984; 102:1-13.

31. Albertsson PA, Sasakawa S, Walker H. Cross partition and isoelectric points of proteins. Nature 1970; 228:1329-30.

32. Hansen JC. Characterization of the conformational transitions of the estrogen receptor monomer by partition in aqueous two-phase systems [Dissertation]. University of Wisconsin-Madison, 1986.

33. Axelsson C-G, Shanbhag VP. Histone-hydrocarbon interaction. Partition of histones in aqueous two-phase systems containing poly(ethylene glycol)-bound hydrocarbons. Eur J Biochem 1976; 71:419-23.

34. Pinaev G, Tartakovsky A, Shanbhag VP, Johansson G, Backman L. Hydrophobic surface properties of myosin in solution as studied by partition in aqueous two-phase systems: effects of ionic strength, pH and temperature. Mol Cell Biochem 1982; 48:65-9.

35. Johansson G, Shanbhag VP. Affinity partitioning of proteins in aqueous two-phase systems containing polymer-bound fatty acids. I. Effect of polyethylene glycol palmitate on the partition of human serum albumin and α-lactalbumin. J Chromatogr 1984; 284:63-72.

36. Kopperschlager G, Johansson G. Affinity partitioning with polymer-bound cibacron blue F3G-A for rapid, large-scale purification of phosphofructokinase from baker's yeast. Anal Biochem 1982; 124:117-24.

37. Kopperschlager G, Lorenz G, Usbeck E. Application of affinity partitioning in an aqueous two-phase system to the investigation of triazine dye-enzyme interactions. J Chromatogr 1983; 259:97-105.

38. Johansson G, Kopperschlager G, Albertsson P-A. Affinity partitioning of phosphofructokinase from baker's yeast using polymer-bound cibacron blue F3G-A. Eur J Biochem 1983; 131:589-94.

39. Miller CD, Hansen JC, Gorski J. Characterization of a potential (poly)nucleotide binding domain of the estrogen receptor by aqueous two-phase affinity partitioning [Abstract]. In: Endocrine Society program abstracts, 69th annual meeting, Indianapolis, June, 1987:62.

40. Moudgil VK, Vandenheede L, Hurd C, Eliezer N, Lombardo G. In vitro modulation of rat liver glucocorticoid receptor by urea. J Biol Chem 1987; 262:5180-7.

41. Moudgil VK, Hurd C. Transformation of calf uterine progesterone receptor: analysis of the process when receptor is bound to progesterone and RU38486. Biochemistry 1987; 26:4994-5001.

42. Green S, Chambon P. Oestradiol induction of a glucocorticoid-responsive gene by a chimaeric receptor. Nature 1987; 325:75-8.

43. Godowski PJ, Rusconi S, Miesfeld R, Yamamoto KR. Glucocorticoid receptor mutants that are constitutive activators of transcriptional enhancement. Nature 1987; 325:365-8.

44. Hollenberg SM, Giguere V, Segui P, Evans RM. Colocalization of DNA-binding and transcriptional activation functions in the human glucocorticoid receptor. Cell 1987: 49:39-46.

45. Hansen JC, Gorski J. A kinetic analysis of the temperature-dependent transition of the estrogen receptor monomer (submitted for publication).

46. Notides AC, Hamilton DE, Auer HE. A kinetic analysis of the estrogen receptor transformation. J Biol Chem 1975; 250:3945-50.

47. Bailly A, LeFevre B, Savouret J-F, Milgrom E. Activation and changes in sedimentation properties of receptors. J Biol Chem 1980; 255:2729-34.

48. Muller R, Traish AM, Wotiz HH. Estrogen receptor activation precedes transformation. J Biol Chem 1983; 258:9227-36.

49. Sakai D, Gorski J. Estrogen receptor transformation to a high-affinity state without subunit-subunit interactions. Biochemistry 1984; 23:3541-7.

50. Muller RE, Traish AM, Hirota T, Bercel E, Wotiz HH. Conversion of estrogen receptor from a state with low affinity for estradiol into a

state of higher affinity does not require 4S to 5S dimerization. Endocrinology 1985; 116:337-45.

51. Redeuilh G, Secco C, Mester J, Baulieu E-E. Transformation of the 8-9 S molybdate-stabilized estrogen receptor from low-affinity to high-affinity state without dissociation into subunits. J Biol Chem 1987; 262:5530-5.

8

HUMAN PROGESTERONE RECEPTORS A AND B:

TWO INDEPENDENT, FUNCTIONAL FORMS

Kathryn B. Horwitz

Departments of Medicine and Pathology
University of Colorado Health Sciences Center
Denver, CO 80262

The use of progesterone receptor (PR) measurements and progestins in the treatment of breast cancers (reviewed in reference 1) and the use of progesterone antagonists in contraception (2) has required an understanding of the actions of these hormones at a basic molecular level. To study the structure and function of human progesterone receptors (hPR), we have used T47D$_{\text{co}}$, a PR-rich human breast cancer cell line (3), and in situ photoaffinity labeling (4,5); we have also purified the PR from T47D cells and have made anti-PR monoclonal antibodies (6). This chapter describes some of our recent studies using these methods (7) to analyze the structure of hPR.

PHOTOAFFINITY LABELING AND THE ORIGIN OF THE A- AND B-PROTEINS

In situ photoaffinity labeling uses ultraviolet irradiation to covalently link the radioactive progestin R5020 (17,21-dimethyl-19-nor-pregn-4, 9-diene-3,20-dione; [17α-methyl-^{3}H]) to receptors in intact cells. Briefly, cells either attached to plastic, or harvested but still intact, are incubated with [^{3}H]R5020 for 2-4 h at 0°C to keep PR in the untransformed cytosolic state, or for 5-10 min at 37°C to transform PR to the tight nuclear binding state. The intact cells are then irradiated with UV for 2 min. The cells can be solubilized directly; or they can be homogenized and then receptors from various subcellular compartments including cytosols, nuclear extracts, microsomal pellets and residual nuclear pellets, can be solubilized and denatured. The denatured radioactive receptors are separated by SDS-polyacrylamide gel electrophoresis and visualized by fluorography. Alternately, after transfer to nitrocellulose, the proteins can be analyzed by combined immunoblotting and fluorography (7). In situ photolabeled untransformed hPR are composed of two major hormone binding species. The heavier B protein is a doublet or triplet of MW 117-120,000 daltons, and the smaller A protein is a singlet of MW 94,000 daltons.

These proteins are remarkably stable. Even incubation for 1 h at 37°C fails to degrade the B protein either to A or to any other fragments. We have previously shown that proteins A and B bind only progestins specifically (1), and that they are present in equimolar amounts (5). They can be demonstrated even if homogenization and centrifugation are eliminated, that is, by in situ photoaffinity labeling of intact cells, solubilization of the cells in buffer containing detergent plus protease inhibitors, denaturation, and immediate electrophoresis (1). The "doublet B—singlet A" is characteristic not only of activated and untransformed receptors, having low affinity for nuclei, but also of transformed receptors shortly after they have acquired tight chromatin binding capacity as a result of hormone treatment. Thus, equimolar amounts of B- and A-proteins are found whether receptors are soluble in cytosols or extracted from nuclei.

The argument has been made that A is formed in vitro as an artifactual proteolytic fragment of B; this argument is supported by several studies. First is the fact that despite repeated demonstrations of two progestin-binding proteins in chick oviduct and human breast cancer cells, two hormone-binding proteins are usually not demonstrated for the other steroid receptors (1). On occasions when two proteins are seen, the proteolysis explanation is invoked (8). Second are studies demonstrating structural similarity between chick or human A- and B-proteins by peptide mapping of photolabeled receptors (5,9,10), and by immunoreactivity (11). These are compelling findings but are also inconclusive, since they fail to reveal the approximately 25 kDa fragment that must be generated from B but not A if the proteolysis argument is true. Nor do the studies prove a proteolysis mechanism, since other explanations for the biosynthesis of partially homologous proteins are possible (see below). Third are immunoblot studies of rabbit uterine PR. These studies show that if homogenization is done quickly, little or no protein A is generated. Unfortunately, the antibody used for these experiments has not been fully characterized—receptor purification data are unpublished to our knowledge (12, 13), and the antibody used for the blotting studies failed to bind to 50% of native PR in salt-containing sucrose gradients (12), suggesting that it may have very different affinities for proteins A and B, and that it belongs to the class of B-specific antibodies commonly generated from partially purified PR (6). Thus, the protease hypothesis has not, in our opinion, been conclusively established. A cocktail of protease inhibitors is routinely added to homogenization buffers in our studies, but A-receptors levels are unaffected.

Our studies of breast cancer hPR suggest that protein B (MW 120,000) and protein A (MW 94,000) are integral intracellular proteins and that A is not generated by proteolysis: (a) Regardless of the site from which they are extracted (cytoplasmic or nuclear), proteins A and B are found in equimolar amounts (1,4). If a protease is degrading protein B, it must be present in cytosols as well as in nuclear extracts, it must be equally active in buffers of different ionic strengths and pH, and its activity must stop after degrading half of the B molecules. (b) Degradation of B to A cannot be demonstrated during in vitro incubations forcing the conclusion that the putative enzyme acts instantaneously on half of the B molecules when the cells are first broken. (c) Both receptor proteins are seen in cells photolabeled in situ then lysed directly in buffer containing detergent and protease inhibitors, and immediately subjected to electrophoresis (1). This suggests that the putative protease acts intracellularly (9). Furthermore, we have shown that the two receptor proteins are dissimilarly modified in their untransformed state. Since B is a doublet or triplet while A is a singlet in holoreceptors, one would have to postulate that if A is a proteolytic artifact, then the offending protease clips out a domain of B containing the site(s) responsible for this heterogeneity. However, such a protease cannot be invoked for the 30 min resident nuclear receptors, where protein B is a singlet while protein A is a doublet (5). Here different proteases would have to be involved that clip B at two sites 3000 daltons apart to generate the A doublet. Thus, we are left to conclude either that B is subject to degradation by a series of unusual intracellular proteases, or that A is a protein closely related to B that is formed intracellularly by other mechanisms. Since antigenic and hormone binding peptides below the size of the A-protein are similar for both A- and B-receptors, since B and A bind hormone (a site at the C-terminal end of the molecule) and DNA (in the center of the molecule), and since A/B-specific and B-specific antibodies exist, but no A-specific antibodies have been described, we postulate that B-receptors differ from A by having additional N-terminal sequences. Possible mechanisms for the synthesis of such partially homologous proteins include gene duplication, alternate transcription from a single gene, synthesis of multiple messages by alternate processing of a single precursor RNA, or use of alternate translation start sites from a single message. Two putative in-frame AUG codons, satisfying the Kozak rules (15) for translation initiation sites, are present 165 bases apart in the hPR message (16). These could theoretically code for two homologous proteins with the shorter protein truncated at the N-terminal end and ~18,000 daltons smaller. We have preliminary evidence that translation initiation from the downstream AUG leads to synthesis of A-receptors.

HUMAN PR PURIFICATION AND MONOCLONAL ANTIBODY PRODUCTION

In order to address the questions regarding the origins of the A- and B-proteins, we required antibodies specific to human PR. To this end, we purified B-receptors from T47D cells by immunoaffinity chromatography using an antibody designated PR-6 developed by D. Toft and colleagues (14) that binds the B-receptors of chick oviducts and cross-reacts with human B-proteins. Single step immunoaffinity chromatography resulted in enrichment of human B-receptors (identified by immunoblotting with PR-6 and by photoaffinity labeling with [^{3}H]R5020) from a specific activity of 0.71 to 1,915 pmol/mg protein (or 23% purity) with 27% yield (Table 1). Purity and yields as judged by gel electrophoresis and densitometric scanning of the silver-stained B-protein were approximately 1.7-fold higher due to partial loss of hormone binding activity at the elution step. A second purification step using DEAE chromatography gave further enrichment to 3,720 pmol/mg protein (or 44% purity) to yield only B-receptors plus one other component, a 72 kDa protein present in approximately equivalent amounts.

Based on physiochemical properties, single-step immunoaffinity purified B-receptors were in the native transformed state: isolated recep-

Table 1. Purification of human B receptors from T47D cells by single step immunoaffinity chromatography.

	Total Protein		B Receptors			
	(mg/ml)	(mg)	pmol[a]	yield (%)	sp. act. (pmol/mg)	purity[b] (%)
Cytosol	14.40	1,152.0	814	--	0.71	
pH eluate	0.021	0.132	221[c]	27.1	1,915.00	23

[a] B receptors in starting cytosol (estimated to be 50% of total receptors) were measured by steroid binding assay.
[b] Theoretical purity for B receptors based on MW of 120,000 = 8,352 pmol/mg protein.
[c] Receptor-hormone binding of the purified product was measured by hydroxylapatite assay with inclusion of 1% carrier albumin. Non-specific binding was determined with carrier albumin alone.
Values are average determinations from three separate purifications.

tors were maintained as undegraded 120 kDa doublets; they retained their hormone binding activity; and, they displayed the correct steroid specificity for PR. Isolated B-receptors also bound efficiently to DNA-cellulose requiring 0.25M salt for their release. They sedimented as 4S monomers on salt-containing sucrose gradients and as a 6S peak in the absence of salt. All these confirm their transformed state. In addition, under these conditions, purified B-receptors were free of the 90 kDa receptor-associated heat shock protein that is always observed to copurify with 8S untransformed receptors in other systems, and they were free also of the nonhormone binding 108 kDa antigen that copurifies with chick oviduct PR. However, in addition to the 120 kDa B-doublet, three silver stained bands are detected in the single-step purified preparations at 72, 62 and 58 kDa. These proteins are not reactive with PR-6 by immunoblotting, nor do they bind [^{3}H]R5020. Thus, they are not receptor fragments but unrelated proteins. The two smaller proteins are abundant cellular proteins that bind the immunomatrix nonspecifically, but the 72 kDa protein is receptor-associated since it cannot be purified from receptor-depleted cytosols. It may be similar to the GR-associated 72 kDa protein described by Gustafsson et al. (17) which is a heat shock protein (18).

The partially purified B-receptors from T47D cells were used to immunize mice, and three monoclonal antibodies (MAbs) against human PR were produced. They have been subcloned and are clonally stable. Their identifying codes and other properties are summarized in Table 2, and the monospecificity of the IgGs has been shown by immunoblotting. Although mice were injected only with B-receptors, the production of one antibody (AB-52) that cross-reacts with both A- and B-receptors again attests to the structural homology of these two proteins. The three IgGs are capable of shifting labeled PR on sucrose gradients and to demonstrate PR in cell and tumor samples by immunohistochemistry and flow cytometry. We have not yet determined whether B-30 and B-64 bind the same or different epitopes unique to B; clearly AB-52 binds a region common to both A- and B-proteins. The development of the monoclonals has been described in detail elsewhere (6).

IMMUNE ANALYSIS OF hPR STRUCTURE

Because it is B-specific and binds to native human PR, PR-6 was used to study the nature of the association between the A- and B-proteins in the untransformed 8S state, and in the transformed 4S state (7). This is of interest since there are conflicting models for the molecular interaction of the A- and B-proteins. One model holds that A and B dimerize and that they are subunits of a larger holoreceptor (19); the other model holds that A and B exist as separate 8S molecules (20,21).

Using PR-6 to immunoprecipitate B-receptors, we have been unable to co-precipitate A-receptors even in the presence of sodium molybdate. This should have been possible if A and B are tightly associated. We, therefore, tested the association of A and B more extensively using sucrose density gradient analysis and in situ photoaffinity labeling. We reasoned that if the dimeric subunit model is correct, addition of PR-6 to receptors stabilized in the 8S state would shift both A- and B-proteins to the bottom of sucrose density gradients, but that A would not be shifted if the two proteins form independent 8S holoreceptor complexes. A study was performed in which hPR, covalently labeled in situ with [^{3}H]R5020 by UV irradiation, were incubated with PR-6 or a control antibody and then sedimented on sucrose gradients in the continuous presence of molybdate and protease inhibitors to maintain intact and native PR conformation. Aliquots of every gradient fraction were counted to obtain the [^{3}H]R5020-binding profile and additional aliquots of the bottom fractions and peak

Table 2. Monoclonal antibodies to human PR.

MAb	Antibody Subtype	Reactivity* A	B
B-30	IgG_1	–	+
B-64	IgG_1	–	+
AB-52	IgG_1	+	+

*Reactivity with 94 kDa A- or 120 kDa B-receptor was determined by immunoblotting. See Estes et al., 1987, for details.

8S fractions were analyzed by gel electrophoresis and fluorography since they were photoaffinity labeled. The control antibody had no effect on 8S sedimentation of hPR, and electrophoretic analysis showed that 11 B- and A-receptors remained in the 8S peak. In contrast, after addition of PR-6, half of the 8S radioactivity was shifted to heavier sedimenting forms. Electrophoretic analysis showed only B present in the antibody-shifted fraction at the bottom of the gradient while A, separated from B, remained at 8S. We concluded that A and B do not dimerize but that each exists as a separate 8S multimeric receptor complex either because of selfassociation, or because of association with nonhormone binding proteins. Two such proteins of 90 and 72 kDa copurify with untransformed human B-receptors (6).

PR-6 can also separate B-receptors from A-receptors that have been transformed to the 4S species by treatment with salt. Approximately half of the radioactivity seen in the 4S peak in the presence of control antibody was shifted to heavier aggregates upon addition of PR-6 and a secondary antibody. The control 4S peak contained both A and B, but only A remained at 4S after PR-6 addition while the B-receptors were shifted to heavier sedimenting fractions. It appears, then, that antibody PR-6 cross-reacts both with the native 8S as well as the transformed 4S forms of B-receptors, and that like the case for 8S, there are two types of 4S species containing either A-protein or B-protein, but not both. The 72 kDa nonhormone binding protein copurifies with transformed 4S B-receptors (6).

Since A and B are not linked in transformed hPR, the two-stage nuclear binding model in which B is seen as a chromatin-specifying protein that guides A to appropriate DNA binding sites (19), is unlikely to be correct. The alternative model is that A- and B-proteins form independent receptor complexes, and that like other steroid receptors, each binds to DNA. While there appears to be consensus that A-receptors bind DNA, for B-receptors this point has been unsettled (11,19). We have tested the ability of immunopurified transformed human B-receptors to bind DNA-cellulose and find that they do so efficiently (6). In unpublished studies, we find that PR-negative cells transfected with a cDNA that encodes hPR_A synthesize only A-receptors and can respond to progestin treatment.

Our working model for the structure of native hPR is that there are two classes of untransformed 8S receptors, each associated with nonsteroid binding proteins of 72 kDa and 90 kDa. Transformation results from dissociation of the 90 kDa protein exposing DNA binding sites masked in the 8S receptor forms. Transformed 4S receptors which bind tightly to DNA may be heterodimers composed of one steroid binding protein and the 72 kDa protein. The A and B steroid binding proteins do not form A-B dimers but exist as separate 8S and 4S molecules (hPR_A and hPR_B) that are independent as DNA binding proteins and function independently to elicit a biological response.

ACKNOWLEDGMENTS

These studies were supported by grants from the National Institutes of Health, the National Science Foundation and the National Foundation for Cancer Research, and were performed in collaboration with D. P. Edwards, L. L. Wei and N. L. Krett. We are grateful to David Toft for his generous gift of PR-6.

REFERENCES

1. Horwitz KB, Wei LL, Sedlacek SM, d'Arville CN. Progestin action and progesterone receptor structure in human breast cancer: a review. Recent Prog Horm Res 1985; 41:249-316.
2. Herrmann W, Wyss R, Provider A, et al. The effects of an antiprogesterone steroid in women; interruption of the menstrual cycle and early pregnancy. CR Acad Sc Paris 1982; 294:933-8.
3. Horwitz KB, Mockus MB, Lessey BA. Variant T47D human breast cancer cells with high progesterone receptor levels despite estrogen and antiestrogen resistance. Cell 1982; 28:633-42.
4. Horwitz KB, Alexander PS. In situ photolinked nuclear progesterone receptors of human breast cancer cells; subunit molecular weights after transformation and translocation. Endocrinology 1983; 113: 2195-201.
5. Horwitz KB, Francis MD, Wei LL. Hormone-dependent covalent modification and processing of human progesterone receptors in the nucleus. DNA 1985; 4:451-60.
6. Estes PA, Suba EJ, Lawler-Heavner J, et al. Immunologic analysis of human breast cancer progesterone receptors. I. Immunoaffinity purification of transformed receptors and production of monoclonal antibodies. Biochemistry 1987 (in press).
7. Wei LL, Sheridan PL, Krett NL, et al. Immunologic analysis of human breast cancer progesterone receptors. II. Structure, phosphorylation and processing. Biochemistry 1987 (in press).
8. Loosfelt H, Logeat F, Hai MTV, Milgrom E. The rabbit progesterone receptor. Evidence for a single steroid-binding subunit and characterization of receptor mRNA. J Biol Chem 1984; 259:14196-202.
9. Birnbaumer M, Schrader WT, O'Malley BW. Assessment of structural similarities in chick oviduct progesterone receptor subunits by partial proteolysis of photoaffinity labeled proteins. J Biol Chem 1983; 255:1637-44.
10. Gronemeyer H, Harry P, Chambon P. Evidence for two structurally related progesterone receptors in chick oviduct cytosol. FEBS Lett 1983; 156:287-92.
11. Gronemeyer H, Govindan MV, Chambon P. Immunologic similarity between the chick oviduct forms A and B. J Biol Chem 1985; 260:6916-25.
12. Logeat F, Hai MTV, Fournier A, Legrain P, Buttin P, Milgrom E. Monoclonal antibodies to rabbit progesterone receptor: cross reaction with other mammalian progesterone receptors. Proc Natl Acad Sci USA 1983; 80:6456-9.
13. Logeat F, LeCunff M, Pamphile R, Milgrom E. The nuclear-bound form of the progesterone receptor is generated through a hormone-dependent phosphorylation. Biochem Biophys Res Comm 1985; 131:421-7.
14. Sullivan WP, Beito TJ, Proper J, Krco CJ, Toft DO. Preparation of

monoclonal antibodies to the avian progesterone receptor. Endocrinology 1986; 119:1549-57.

15. Kozak M. Bifunctional messenger RNAs in eukaryotes. Cell 1986;47: 481-3.

16. Misrahi M, Atger M, d'Auriol L, et al. Complete amino acid sequence of the human progesterone receptor deduced from cloned cDNA. Biochem Biophys Res Commun 1987; 143:740-8.

17. Gustafsson JA, Carlstedt-Duke J, Wrange O, Okret S, Wilkstrom AC. Functional analysis of the purified glucocorticoid receptor. J Steroid Biochem 1986; 24:63-8.

18. Welch WT, Feramisco JR. Rapid purification of mammalian 70,000-dalton stress proteins: affinity of proteins for nucleotides. Mol Cell Biol 1985; 5:1229-37.

19. Schrader WT, Birnbaumer ME, Hughes MR, Weigel NL, Grody WW, O'Malley BW. Studies on the structure and function of the chicken progesterone receptor. Recent Prog Horm Res 1981; 37:583-633.

20. Dougherty JJ, Toft DO. Characterization of two 8S forms of chick oviduct progesterone receptor. J Biol Chem 1982; 257:3113-9.

21. Renoir JM, Mester J. Chick oviduct progesterone receptor: structure, immunology, function. Mol Cell Endocrinol 1984; 37:1-13.

9

ANDROGEN REGULATION OF GENE EXPRESSION: STUDIES OF ORNITHINE DECARBOXYLASE IN MURINE KIDNEY

Olli A. Janne, Noreen J. Hickok, Mervi Julkunen,
Anne Crozat, Leonard Eisenberg, and Evie Melanitou

The Population Council and The Rockefeller University
1230 York Avenue, New York, New York 10021

INTRODUCTION

The action of androgenic steroids in their target tissues occurs in a receptor-mediated fashion similar to that of other steroid hormones. The details of steroid hormone action, as they are currently known, originate mainly from studies of glucocorticoids, estrogens, and progestins, despite the fact that the first and most convincing biological arguments for the importance of soluble receptors in the expression of steroid action are from studies of androgen resistance syndromes (1-3). There are several possible reasons that research on androgen action has lagged behind that of female sex steroids and glucocorticoids. These include problems in the measurement and purification of the androgen receptor; a relatively slow progress in isolation and characterization of androgen-responsive genes and their encoded products; and paucity of suitable experimental systems to study androgen action in cultured cells. Over the last several years, however, a number of gene products regulated by androgens have been characterized and their induction kinetics in vivo elucidated. The best defined of these genes/gene products fall, with regard to their tissues of expression, into three main categories: (i) α_{2u}-globulin and the major urinary protein (MUP) genes are regulated by androgens in rodent liver (4-11); (ii) prostatein and seminal vesicle basic protein genes are controlled by androgens in rat accessory sex organs (12-19), and (iii) ornithine decarboxylase (ODC), β-glucuronidase, RP2, and kidney androgen-regulated protein (KAP) genes exhibit androgen regulation in murine kidney (20-31).

There are some major differences in the expression of these genes, including the multi-hormonal control of rodent liver genes (7,9), the relatively high abundancy of the gene products in rat accessory sex organs (12,16), the genetically regulated androgen responsiveness of β-glucuronidase and ODC genes, and the induction kinetics of the genes (32). These different genes are, however, regulated by androgen in a similar manner in that increased accumulation of the respective mRNAs is always involved. Furthermore, at least in the case of murine renal genes, the induction is dependent on functional androgen receptors, as no change [except for some increase in KAP mRNA accumulation (31)] in their steady-state mRNA levels is elicited by androgens in testicular feminized (Tfm/Y) mice (20,32). An intriguing feature of androgen-regulated mRNA accumulation in murine kidney is the timing and sensitivity of the response; each gene exhibits a unique profile in terms of the lag for the initial increase to occur, the dose of androgen needed for the response, and the extent of the maximal response. We have recently reviewed these comparative aspects in the action of androgens on mouse renal cells (32). In this chapter, we concentrate mainly on the characteristics and regulation of ODC gene(s) in murine kidney.

ORNITHINE DECARBOXYLASE PROTEIN

ODC catalyzes conversion of L-ornithine to putrescine and is the first and one of the rate-controlling enzymes in polyamine biosynthesis. It is a constitutive enzyme probably present in all cells and tissues and requires pyridoxal 5'-phosphate for its catalytic activity (33). ODC activity appears to be indispensable for eukaryotic cells, as mutant cell lines devoid of the enzyme activity are polyamine auxotrophs (34,35). ODC concentration is very low in quiescent cells, but its activity is elevated manyfold within a few hours of exposure to a wide variety of trophic stimuli (33,36). Even after maximal stimulation, however, ODC forms a minute fraction of total cellular protein, ranging from 0.0001 to 0.04% of the soluble cytosol protein. For reasons not currently understood, the concentration of this enzyme in mouse kidney is relatively high under physiological conditions, and the renal tissue of androgen-treated mice appears to be one of the richest eukaryotic sources of ODC.

ODC protein has been purified to apparent homogeneity from a variety of tissues, including the murine kidney. The enzyme protein has a subunit molecular weight of approximately 50,000 under denaturing conditions, but appears to be a dimeric molecule in its active form (33,37,38). However, dimerization may not be required for catalytic activity, since the individual 50,000-dalton subunits bind covalently the active-site directed suicidal inhibitor, 2-difluoromethylornithine (38). On two-dimensional gel electrophoresis, the purified enzyme protein exhibits some charge heterogeneity (38), but the biochemical reason for this characteristic is currently not known.

In view of the crucial importance of ODC activity for the growth and survival of eukaryotic cells, it is not very surprising that the amino acid sequence of the enzyme is very well conserved among different species. Comparison of the amino acid sequences deduced from murine and human ODC cDNAs indicated that the enzymes of both species comprise 461 amino acids, with predicted molecular weights of 51,156 and 51,172 for the human and murine enzymes, respectively (39,40). The overall identity in the two amino acid sequences is about 90%, with 44 differences among their 461 residues. Of these changes in the sequences, 57% (25 of 44) are conservative. Interestingly, the distribution of amino acid differences between the two enzymes is uneven (Fig. 1) in that the amino-terminal and more hydrophobic half (residues 1-220) has only three nonconservative changes, and there are two stretches of 61 (residues 13-74) and 38 (residues 137-175) amino acids without any change. The most hydrophobic region in the two enzymes (residues 290-340) is flanked with identical sequences of 42 and 33 amino acids. On the basis of these similarities, it is tempting to speculate that the hydrophobic amino-terminal part and the hydrophilic region comprising residues 290-340 of the protein play an important role in the enzyme's catalytic function, such as binding of pyridoxal 5'-phosphate and L-ornithine. By contrast, the carboxy-terminal parts of the amino acid sequences are less well conserved and contain more than half of the nonconservative amino acid changes (Fig. 1). We and other investigators (41-43) have previously shown that cleavage of a 2,000- to 3,000-dalton peptide from the murine ODC does not abolish its catalytic activity. In view of the amino acid data, one can predict that this peptide is derived from the nonconserved region in the carboxyl terminus of the enzyme protein. This notion is supported by recent data from studies in which truncated murine ODC cDNA sequences were expressed in Escherichia coli; deletion of 38 carboxy-terminal amino acids from the enzyme protein changed its catalytic activity only very little (44).

A salient feature of ODC protein is its very fast turnover rate; the half-life of the enzyme is about 15 min in mouse kidney (38,45). Both the murine and human enzyme proteins contain two regions rich in proline, glutamic acid, serine, and threonine (so-called PEST sequences, Fig. 1), which seem to be typical of eukaryotic proteins exhibiting short half-lives (46). Interestingly, administration of testosterone at pharmacological doses for several days to mice altered the turnover rate of renal ODC by prolonging the half-life from 10-15 min to 100-150 min (38). The mechanisms responsible for this phenomenon remain to be elucidated. It may not have, however, any major physiological importance, since the half-life of the protein in intact male animals appears to be only 10-15 min (38).

A typical feature of ODC regulation by virtually all stimuli is the short-lived nature of the induction; the enzyme activity usually peaks within 4-8 h after the stimulus and subsides by 24 h after the inducer treatment (36,47). This phenomenon may occur due to a number of reasons, such as a short duration of action of the inducer itself, rapid turnover rate of ODC protein and/or ODC mRNA, and appearance of molecules that facilitate ODC inactivation after its maximal induction. In addition to these possibilities, recent studies in a number of laboratories have indicated that putrescine and other polyamines inhibit the translation of ODC mRNA, thereby controlling their own synthesis at this level (48,49). These latter findings also explain, at least in part, why androgen induction of ODC activity in murine renal cells is much longer-lived than in other tissues; in contrast to most other experimental systems, putrescine and other polyamines are excreted by the renal cells and do not accumulate in this tissue in concentrations commensurate with the extent of ODC activation (50). In keeping with this postulate, Sertich and Pegg (51) have recently shown that administration of exogenous putrescine to androgen-treated mice leads to an acute and dramatic reduction of renal ODC activity without affecting appreciably the ODC mRNA levels in the kidney.

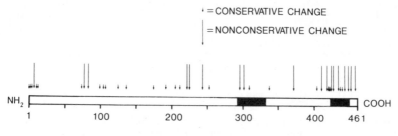

Fig. 1. Schematic comparison of human and murine ODC proteins sequences. The amino acid sequences used in the comparison are those deduced from the respective ODC cDNAs (39,40). Each enzyme has 461 residues in the primary amino acid sequence. The shaded areas depict regions that contain the so-called PEST sequences, the presence of which is possibly responsible for the enzyme's rapid turnover rate.

ODC mRNA SPECIES

Size Heterogeneity of ODC mRNAs

Mouse kidney contains at least two different ODC mRNA species of about 2.2 and 2.7 kb in size (20). The presence of two ODC mRNAs is not restricted to mouse kidney, but multiple mRNAs are also expressed in several other murine, rat and hamster tissues. By contrast, human tissues and cell lines appear to express only one ODC mRNA species of 2.3 kb in length (39). DNA sequencing of ODC cDNA clones has indicated that the size difference of these two mRNA species is due to a longer 3'-non-translated region in the 2.7-kb ODC mRNA (23,40,52). The longer mRNA contains two polyadenylylation signals (AAUAAA); the second one is 422 nucleotides downstream from the first one, resulting in a 3'-noncoding region of 748 nucleotides in this mRNA as opposed to a 329-nucleotide long 3'-noncoding sequence in the 2.2-kb ODC mRNA (23). In view of these data, it is obvious that the main size heterogeneity of ODC mRNAs is due to their dissimilar 3'-ends. It also appears that no appreciable heterogeneity exists at the 5'-end of the messages, as judged by primer extension experiments (40, and our unpublished observations). However, additional mRNA species may be present in murine tissues. For example, we have identified and partially sequenced one ODC cDNA clone from a mouse kidney cDNA library, which has the poly(A)-tail added 5 nucleotides downstream from that in the 2.2-kb mRNA. That this cDNA represents an authentic mRNA sequence is supported by the presence of a corresponding ODC pseudogene in the mouse genome.

There are multiple ODC gene sequences in the murine genome (21,22, 52), but whether or not more than one of these is expressed has not so far been proven. Comparison of the partial nucleotide sequences of the two cDNAs corresponding to the 2.2- and 2.7-kb ODC mRNAs revealed some mis-matches, suggesting that they may originate from two very similar, yet different ODC genes. Alternatively, these minor sequence mismatches may represent allelic variations in a single expressed gene, in particular since the initial cloning of the cDNAs was performed using ODC mRNA purified from kidneys of randomly-bred mice (20). It remains to be elucidated whether the presence of multiple ODC mRNAs in murine kidney has any bearing on the charge heterogeneity of the enzyme protein present in the same tissue (38).

As mentioned above, human tissues express only one ODC mRNA species that is slightly longer than the 2.2-kb mRNA in murine cells. The human genome contains at least two ODC gene loci (39,53) that were mapped to chromosomes 2 and 7. In keeping with the presence of a single mRNA species, our recent isolation and sequencing of the expressed human chromosomal ODC gene has indicated that its 3'-end contains only one polyadenylylation/termination signal.

Androgen Regulation of ODC mRNA Accumulation

There is a clear sexual dimorphism in ODC activity, immunoreactive enzyme protein concentration, and ODC mRNA content in renal tissue of most mouse strains so far studied, indicating that physiological androgen concentrations regulate the expression of the ODC gene(s) in the kidney (20,38,50,54). The physiological significance of this phenomenon is unclear at present. It is of interest to note, however, that the ODC gene has maintained its androgen regulation in the kidney throughout the evolution of the Mus species as opposed to most other androgen-induced renal gene products (F. G. Berger, personal communication). In contrast to the wild-type animals, androgen-insensitive (Tfm/Y) mice show no change in ODC gene expression during prolonged testosterone administration,

indicating that androgen receptors are required for this regulation
(20,54). ODC activities, immunoreactive enzyme protein concentrations,
and ODC mRNA levels are all very similar in kidneys of Tfm/Y animals,
intact females, and castrated males. These values thus appear to result
from a constitutive expression of the ODC gene, which is needed for the
basal functions of the renal cells.

Administration of testosterone at pharmacological doses increases the
accumulation of the two ODC mRNA species in a coordinate fashion with
relatively rapid kinetics. After a single dose of androgen, the induction
of ODC mRNA parallels very closely to that of the immunoreactive enzyme
protein, with the initial increase in the mRNA content being detected
between 2 and 6 h after steroid administration (20,38). When cycloheximide, a protein synthesis inhibitor, is administered with testosterone,
no induction of the enzyme protein occurs. These data thus indicate that
the androgenic induction of ODC activity takes place through de novo
synthesis of the enzyme protein, rather than via activation of existing
inactive forms of the enzyme (54). In addition, the increase in ODC
synthesis appears to be the result of enhanced ODC mRNA accumulation after
a single dose of testosterone.

Long-term administration of androgen using steroid-releasing implants
elicits changes in ODC activity, immunoreactive protein concentration, and
ODC mRNA accumulation in a fashion similar to that in acute single-dose
studies. In all these investigations, the changes in ODC activity and
enzyme protein concentration have always been identical, indicating that
posttranslational modifications of the protein play a minor, if any, role
in the androgen regulation of ODC activity in murine kidney (38). Implantation of female mice for 7 days with Silastic rods releasing 10, 20, 40,
80, and 200 µg testosterone per day resulted in a dose-dependent increase
in renal ODC activity, with the maximal enzyme protein concentration being
200- to 500-fold higher than that in intact female animals. Under these
conditions, the extent of induction of ODC activity was directly proportional to the nuclear androgen receptor concentration (J. Bertolini, C. W.
Bardin and O. A. Janne, unpublished observations). These data again
emphasize the importance of androgen receptors in the mechanisms regulating ODC gene expression.

Administration of androgens at pharmacological doses for several days
increases ODC mRNA accumulation 10- to 50-fold over the values in intact
females or castrated males (20,23). The relative induction is, however,
dependent on the mouse strain used (see below). Although ODC mRNA
measurements have been only semiquantitative, it appears that the
increases in the enzyme activity and the immunoreactive ODC concentration
(200- to 500-fold) are relatively greater than those in the mRNA accumulation. This notion is in agreement with the findings that prolonged
androgen treatment decreases the rate of ODC turnover (38,45) and that the
rate of enzyme protein synthesis is increased about 25-fold by androgen
administration in murine kidney (42). Despite the dual mechanism leading
to increased ODC protein content (increased synthesis and decreased
degradation), the enzyme activation after androgen administration is
always accompanied by enhanced mRNA accumulation. These results along
with those on nuclear androgen receptors do not, however, prove that
androgens stimulate directly the rate of transcription of the renal ODC
gene(s). The possibility that accumulation of ODC mRNAs would occur
mainly through mechanisms not requiring an increased rate of ODC gene
transcription has been inferred from some recent studies in our and other
laboratories.

As illustrated in Figure 2, administration of testosterone to female
mice fails to elicit a significant increase in the rate of transcription

of the ODC gene, as measured by nuclear run-on assays. In this study, single-stranded RNA sequences covering the entire protein coding sequence and most of the the the 5'- and 3'-nontranslated regions of the ODC mRNA were immobilized to nitrocellulose and used to hybridize with [^{32}P]UTP-labeled nuclear RNA. Antisense and sense RNA sequences were immobilized separately to assure the specificity of the RNA-RNA hybridization. The data in Fig. 2 indicate that both strands of the ODC gene are actively transcribed in renal cell nuclei, the transcription of the opposite strand being somewhat less active than that coding for ODC mRNA (+, mRNA strand synthesis; -, opposite strand synthesis in Fig. 2). However, in view of the presence of multiple ODC gene sequences in the mouse genome, it is possible that the two hybridizable RNAs do not originate from the same transcription unit. In a similar study using double-stranded DNA sequences as hybridization probes for three different renal gene products (ODC, KAP, and RP2 mRNAs), Berger et al. (55) showed that androgens had little or no effect on the synthesis of these mRNAs, despite their 10- to 20-fold increased steady-state levels. Taken together, these data suggest that induction of ODC mRNA (and some other renal mRNAs) by androgens is not fully accounted for by stimulation of gene transcription but must be generated predominantly at the level of mRNA processing and/or turnover. This notion seems to apply also to other androgen-regulated mRNAs, such as those encoded in rat prostate by prostatein genes (13).

Androgen-induced accumulation of ODC mRNA species can be seen not only in cytoplasmic but also in nuclear RNA (Fig. 3). No preferential accumulation of ODC mRNA precursors takes place in nuclei of intact or androgen-treated female animals, suggesting that processing of the primary transcripts of the ODC gene is neither a rate-limiting nor an androgen-regulated event. The RNA samples shown in Figure 3 are those enriched by oligo(dT)-cellulose column chromatography (i.e., polyadenylylated RNAs); however, simultaneous Northern blotting of nuclear and cytoplasmic RNAs that failed to bind to oligo(dT)-cellulose column did not reveal marked changes in any specifically hybridizable RNA species. Comparison of the relative quantities of nuclear and cytoplasmic ODC mRNA species indicated that there are about 50 times more ODC mRNA sequences in the cytoplasmic

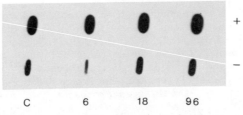

Fig. 2. Effect of androgen administration on the rate of transcription of the renal ODC gene(s). Nuclei were isolated from kidneys of intact female mice (C), female mice treated with single 5-mg doses of testosterone for 6 or 18 hours, and females implanted with testosterone-releasing rods (200 μg steroid/day) for 96 hours. Nuclear RNA synthesis in the presence of [^{32}P]UTP was carried out at 25°C for 20 min, nuclear RNA isolated and hybridized to nitrocellulose filter-bound antisense (+) and sense (-) ODC RNAs. After treatment with single-strand specific RNase, the filter was exposed to Kodak XAR film. Hybridization of labeled ODC mRNA sequences is detected in the (+) lane, whereas transcripts originating from the opposite strand hybridize to the (-) lane.

than nuclear compartment; this ratio is not significantly different between the intact and androgen-treated female animals.

If the major regulatory site of androgen action is at the posttranscriptional level, as illustrated by studies cited above, it suggests that the principal function of the androgen receptor may be different from that of other steroid receptors. This type of steroid hormone action is not, however, totally unknown, since both transcriptional and posttranscriptional regulation has been reported for other experimental systems (56-59). A corollary to the above notion is that gene-specific responses in mouse kidney may reflect a direct interaction of the androgen receptor with induced mRNAs or processes responsible for their degradation/stabilization. Alternatively, androgen action may involve a receptor-mediated production of a <u>trans</u>-acting factor in renal cells during the hormone response, which, in turn, brings about its action via posttranscriptional mechanisms. It should be kept in mind, however, that most of the current data originate from investigations in vivo and that no direct studies of the regulatory regions in the renal androgen-responsive genes have been performed. In the case of the ODC gene(s), these kinds of studies seem to be possible in the near future, since several laboratories including ours have recently isolated an authentic ODC gene, and elucidation of its regulatory regions is in progress.

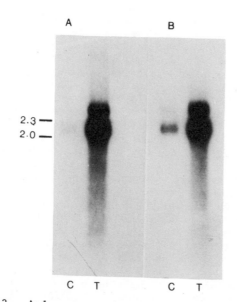

Fig. 3. Androgen regulation of nuclear (A) and cytoplasmic (B) ODC mRNA species. Nuclear and cytoplasmic RNAs were isolated from kidneys of intact female mice (C) and females treated with testosterone-releasing implants (200 μg steroid/day) for 96 hours (T), enriched for poly(A)-containing RNA by oligo(dT)-cellulose chromatography, separated by electrophoresis on 1% agarose gel containing 2.2 M formaldehyde, and transferred to nitrocellulose. Hybridization was performed using a 1.7-kb long ^{32}P-labeled ODC cRNA. After treatment with RNase, the filters were exposed to Kodak XAR film for 24 h (A) or 3 h (B).

A number of tissue functions and/or specific gene products are expressed in a genetically-regulated manner in inbred strains of mice. Among the specific, hormone-regulated genes are those coding for renal β-glucuronidase (25,27,32) and RP2 mRNAs (29,30), submaxillary gland renin mRNAs (60), and hepatic MUP mRNAs (9,10,61). These examples have revealed that several mechanisms may account for the genetic differences, such as polymorphism in the structural gene, differential expression of two non-allelic structural genes, and presence of a cis-acting regulatory locus in close proximity to the structural gene. Our recent studies have demonstrated that the renal ODC gene(s) can be included in the list of these genes, the control of which is regulated by the genetic background of the animals.

Renal ODC activity and ODC mRNA concentration among eight inbred strains of mice (A/J, C57BR/cdJ, 129/J, C57L/J, BALB/cJ, SM/J, RF/J, and C57BL/6J) do not exhibit significant differences in intact females; however, there is a marked strain-dependent variation in intact males (62). Male animals of three strains (RF/J, SM/J, and C57BR/cdJ) have 5- to 20-fold higher enzyme activities than other strains, and similar differences are present in the renal ODC mRNA concentrations (Table 1). As mentioned previously, two ODC mRNA species (2.2 and 2.7 kb in size) are constitutively expressed and androgen-regulated in murine kidney. The relative amounts of these mRNAs varied among the eight strains studied, with the 2.7-kb mRNA representing 3.3%-19.2% and 2.9%-23.9% of total ODC mRNA content in kidneys of females and males, respectively. This variation appears to be, however, unrelated to the genetic regulation that governs the extent of androgen responsiveness of the ODC gene(s). In addition to the three high-responsive strains, there are two strains of mice (A/J and C57BL/6J) with a low male-to-female ratio in the basal ODC activity and a blunted increase in the enzyme activity after administration of superphysiological doses of testosterone (40 μg/day for 7 days). As illustrated in Table 1, a similar diminished induction is seen in the accumulation of ODC mRNA in these two strains of mice. In contrast to their high enzyme activity and ODC mRNA content in the males, C57BR/cdJ, SM/J and RF/J strains did not exhibit a greater response to exogenous testosterone administration than other strains except A/J and C57BL/6J (Table 1). These data are interpreted to indicate that the major genetic regulation of ODC gene expression is at the level of androgen sensitivity, as illustrated by the strain-dependent variation in the response to endogenous androgens in intact males. By contrast, six out of eight strains had a very similar maximal response, which may not be controlled by the same mechanism as the androgen sensitivity.

Studies of reciprocal F_1 hybrids of mice which exhibited a sex difference in the ODC mRNA concentration (C57BR/cdJ) and of those which did not (C57BL/6J) showed that the androgen sensitivity in these crosses is inherited in an autosomal dominant manner (62). In agreement with other studies using superphysiological doses of exogenous testosterone, the F_1 progeny of both hybrid strains had similar maximal responses in the accumulation of ODC mRNA species.

The factors responsible for the genetic control of the ODC gene(s) in murine kidney are not known at present. The strain-dependent variation in the males cannot be explained by differences in serum testosterone concentrations, since no systematic correlation between renal ODC activity and serum testosterone level is found in individual male mice (62). Similarly, differences in nuclear androgen receptors among the strains do not relate to the renal ODC concentration or ODC mRNA content (Table 1). We infer from these data that it is the renal ODC gene, or its regulator,

Table 1. Relative ODC mRNA and nuclear androgen receptor (AR) concentrations in kidneys of different inbred mouse strains.*

Mouse strain	Males	Testosterone treatment	Nuclear AR
A/J	1.1	4.4	246 ± 62
C57BR/cdJ	5.1	14.7	412 ± 71
129/J	3.2	11.2	463 ± 92
C57L/J	1.4	14.0	532 ± 182
BALB/cJ	1.8	20.2	132 ± 43
SM/J	2.9	24.6	396 ± 120
RF/J	14.2	22.6	246 ± 32
C57BL/6J	0.8	8.1	299 ± 198

The ODC mRNA concentrations are expressed relative to untreated females whose values are not significantly different between the strains. Testosterone treatment of female mice lasted for 7 days with implants releasing 40 μg steroid/day. Nuclear androgen receptor concentrations in intact males are expressed as receptors/cell. Data adapted from Melanitou et al. (62).

whose androgen responsiveness is controlled by the genetic background of the mice, rather than genetic regulation of testicular androgen production or nuclear androgen receptor occupancy. The genetic control of ODC gene expression appears to be distinctly different from that of β-glucuronidase, but somewhat similar to that seen in the control of KAP mRNA accumulation (32).

CONCLUDING REMARKS

Androgenic regulation of ODC in murine kidney has a number of characteristics that render this system an attractive model to study steroid hormone action. First, there are several levels of regulation of ODC activity by androgens, including increased mRNA accumulation, enhanced rate of enzyme protein synthesis, and decreased rate of degradation of the protein. An additional control seems to be exerted by polyamines themselves at the level of ODC mRNA translation. Second, at least two ODC mRNA species are expressed and androgen-regulated in the murine kidney. These two mRNAs differ in the length of their 3'-noncoding regions and possess some additional sequence differences, which may indicate that they are encoded by two different ODC genes. Third, there are multiple copies of the ODC gene in the murine genome. Although we have tacitly assumed that androgen regulation does not involve activation of previously silent genes, this question has not been answered by direct experiments. Fourth, androgen induction of ODC mRNA accumulation seems to involve mainly stabilization of the mRNA as opposed to enhancement of the rate of ODC gene transcription. Whatever is the mechanism, it is androgen receptor-dependent, as it does not occur in receptor deficient Tfm/Y animals and can be abolished by a concomitant antiandrogen treatment. Fifth, androgen sensitivity of ODC induction is dependent on the genetic background of the animals, as is the relative abundance of the 2.2- and 2.7-kb ODC mRNA species. Finally, ODC gene sequences are easily amplified in cultured cells under a selective metabolic pressure. The significance of this feature is currently unknown, but it may be a useful property to be exploited in evaluating the importance of polyamines for the expression of other androgen-regulated genes.

ACKNOWLEDGMENT

This work was supported by the National Institutes of Health (Grant No. HD-13541).

REFERENCES

1. Bardin CW, Catterall JF. Testosterone, a major determinant of extra-genital sexual dimorphism. Science 1981; 211:1285-94.
2. Griffin JE, Leshin M, Wilson JD. Androgen resistance syndromes. Am J Physiol 1982; 243:E81-7.
3. Kontula KK, Janne OA, Bardin CW. Intracellular hormone receptor defects and disease. In: Conn PM, ed. Receptors IV. Orlando: Academic Press, 1986:37-74.
4. Roy AK, Chatterjee B, Prasad MSK, Unakar NJ. Role of insulin in the regulation of the hepatic messenger RNA for α_{2u}-globulin in diabetic rats. J Biol Chem 1980; 255:11614-8.
5. Nakhasi HL, Lynch KR, Dolan KP, Unterman R, Antakly T, Feigelson P. Modification in α_{2u}-globulin gene structure, transcription, and mRNA translation in hepatomas. J Biol Chem 1982; 257:2726-9.
6. Roy AK, Nath TS, Matwani NM, Chatterjee B. Age-dependent regulation of the polymorphic forms of α_{2u}-globulin. J Biol Chem 1983; 258: 10123-7.
7. Kulkarni AB, Gubito RM, Feigelson P. Developmental and hormonal regulation of α_{2u}-globulin gene transcription. Proc Natl Acad Sci USA 1985; 82:2579-82.
8. Derman E. Isolation of a cDNA clone for mouse urinary proteins: age- and sex-related expression of mouse urinary protein genes is transcriptionally controlled. Proc Natl Acad Sci USA 1981; 78: 5425-9.
9. Kuhn NJ, Woodworth-Gutai M, Gross KW, Held WA. Subfamilies of the major mouse urinary protein (MUP) multi-gene family: sequence analysis of cDNA clones and differential regulation in the liver. Nucleic Acids Res 1984; 12:6073-90.
10. Clark AJ, Hickman J, Bishop J. A 45-kb DNA domain with two diver-gently orientated genes is the unit of organisation of the murine major urinary protein genes. EMBO J 1984; 3:2055-64.
11. Hastie ND, Held WA, Toole JJ. Multiple genes coding for the an-drogen-regulated major urinary proteins of the mouse. Cell 1979; 17:749-57.
12. Parker MG, White R, Williams JG. Cloning and characterization of androgen-dependent mRNA from rat ventral prostate. J Biol Chem 1980; 255:6996-7001.
13. Page MJ, Parker MG. Effect of androgen on the transcription of rat prostatic binding protein genes. Mol Cell Endocrinol 1982; 27:343-55.
14. Viskochil DH, Perry ST, Lea OA, Stafford DW, Wilson EM, French FS. Isolation of two genomic sequences encoding the Mr=14,000 subunit of rat prostatein. J Biol Chem 1983; 258:8861-6.
15. Parker M, Hurst H, Page M. Organization and expression of prostatic steroid binding protein genes. J Steroid Biochem 1984; 20:67-71.
16. Kistler MK, Taylor RE Jr, Kandala JC, Kistler WS. Isolation of recombinant plasmids containing structural gene sequences for rat seminal vesicle secretory proteins IV and V. Biochem Biophys Res Commun 1981; 99:1161-6.
17. Kandala JC, Kistler WS, Kistler MK. Methylation of the rat seminal

vesicle secretory protein IV gene. Extensive demethylation occurs in several male sex accessory glands. J Biol Chem 1985; 260:15959–64.

18. Harris SE, Mansson P-E, Tully DB, Burkhart B. Seminal vesicle secretion IV gene: allelic differences due to a series of 20-base-pair direct tandem repeats within an intron. Proc Natl Acad Sci USA 1983; 80:6460–4.

19. Fawell SE, McDonald CJ, Higgins SJ. Comparison of seminal vesicle secretory proteins of rodents using antibody and nucleotide probes. Mol Cell Endocrinol 1987; 50:107–14.

20. Kontula KK, Torkkeli TK, Bardin CW, Janne OA. Androgen induction of ornithine decarboxylase mRNA in mouse kidney as studied by complementary DNA. Proc Natl Acad Sci USA 1984; 81:731–5.

21. McConlogue L, Gupta M, Wu L, Coffino P. Molecular cloning and expression of the mouse ornithine decarboxylase gene. Proc Natl Acad Sci USA 1984; 81:540–4.

22. Berger FG, Szymanski P, Read E, Watson G. Androgen regulated ornithine decarboxylase mRNAs of mouse kidney. J Biol Chem 1984; 259:7941–6.

23. Hickok NJ, Seppanen PJ, Kontula KK, Janne PA, Bardin CW, Janne OA. Two ornithine decarboxylase mRNA species in mouse kidney arise from size heterogeneity at their 3' termini. Proc Natl Acad Sci USA 1986; 83:594–8.

24. Swank RT, Paigan K, Davey R, Chapman V, Labarca C, Watson G, Ganschow R, Brandt EJ, Novak E. Genetic regulation of mammalian glucuronidase. Recent Prog Horm Res 1978; 34:401–36.

25. Palmer R, Gallagher PM, Boyko WL, Ganschow RE. Genetic control of levels of murine kidney glucuronidase mRNA in response to androgen. Proc Natl Acad Sci USA 1983; 80:7596–600.

26. Catterall JF, Leary SL. Detection of early changes in androgen-induced mouse renal β-glucuronidase mRNA using cloned cDNA. Biochemistry 1983; 22:6049–53.

27. Watson CS, Catterall JF. Genetic regulation of androgen-induced accumulation of mouse renal β-glucuronidase mRNA. Endocrinology 1986; 118:1081–6.

28. Berger FG, Gross KW, Watson G. Isolation and characterization of a DNA sequence complementary to an androgen-inducible messenger RNA from mouse kidney. J Biol Chem 1981; 256:7006–13.

29. Elliott RW, Berger FG. DNA sequence polymorphism in an androgen-regulated gene is associated with alteration in the encoded RNAs. Proc Natl Acad Sci USA 1983; 80:501–4.

30. King D, Snider LD, Lingrel JB. Polymorphism in an androgen-regulated mouse gene is the result of the insertion of B1 repetitive element into the transcription unit. Mol Cell Biol 1986; 6:209–17.

31. Watson CS, Salomon D, Catterall JF. Structure and expression of androgen-regulated genes in mouse kidney. Ann NY Acad Sci 1984; 438:101–14.

32. Catterall JF, Kontula KK, Watson CS, Seppanen PJ, Funkenstein B, Melanitou E, Hickok NJ, Bardin CW, Janne OA. Regulation of gene expression by androgens in murine kidney. Recent Prog Horm Res 1986; 42:71–109.

33. Pegg AE, McCann PP. Polyamine metabolism and function. Am J Physiol 1982; 243:C212–21.

34. Steglich C, Scheffler IE. An ornithine decarboxylase-deficient mutant of Chinese hamster ovary cells. J Biol Chem 1982; 257:4603–9.

35. Pohjanpelto P, Holtta E, Janne OA. Mutant strain of Chinese hamster ovary cells with no detectable ornithine decarboxylase activity. Mol Cell Biol 1985; 5:1385–90.

36. Janne J, Poso H, Raina A. Polyamines in rapid growth and cancer. Biochim Biophys Acta 1978; 473:241–93.

37. Seely JE, Poso H, Pegg AE. Purification of ornithine decarboxylase from kidneys of androgen treated mice. Biochemistry 1982; 21:3394–9.

38. Isomaa VV, Pajunen AEI, Bardin CW, Janne OA. Ornithine decarboxylase in mouse kidney. Purification, characterization and radioimmunological determination of the enzyme protein. J Biol Chem 1983; 258: 6735-40.

39. Hickok NJ, Seppanen PJ, Gunsalus GL, Janne OA. Complete amino acid sequence of human ornithine decarboxylase deduced from complementary DNA. DNA 1987; 6:179-87.

40. Gupta M, Coffino P. Mouse ornithine decarboxylase. Complete amino acid sequence deduced from cDNA. J Biol Chem 1985; 260:2941-4.

41. Janne OA, Kontula KK, Isomaa VV, Torkkeli TK, Bardin CW. Androgen receptor-dependent regulation of ornithine decarboxylase gene expression in mouse kidney. In: Eriksson H, Gustafsson J-A, eds. Steroid hormone receptors: structure and function. Amsterdam: Elsevier Science Publishers BV, 1983:461-76.

42. Persson L, Seely JE, Pegg AE. Investigation of structure and rate of synthesis of ornithine decarboxylase protein in mouse kidney. Biochemistry 1984; 23:3777-83.

43. Pulkka A, Taskinen T, Aaltonen H, Ramberg J, Pajunen AEI. Studies on the degradation of ornithine decarboxylase by the immunoblotting technique. Biochem Int 1985; 11:845-51.

44. Macrae M, Coffino P. Complementation of a polyamine-deficient Escherichia coli mutant by expression of mouse ornithine decarboxylase. Mol Cell Biol 1987; 7:564-7.

45. Seely JE, Pegg AE. Changes in mouse kidney ornithine decarboxylase activity are brought about by changes in the amount of enzyme protein as measured by radioimmunoassay. J Biol Chem 1983; 258:2496-500.

46. Rogers S, Wells R, Rechsteiner M. Amino acid sequences common to rapidly degraded proteins: the PEST hypothesis. Science 1986; 234:364-8.

47. Tabor CW, Tabor H. Polyamines. Annu Rev Biochem 1984; 53:749-90.

48. Kahana C, Nathans D. Translational regulation of mammalian ornithine decarboxylase by polyamines. J Biol Chem 1985; 260:15390-3.

49. Holtta E, Pohjanpelto P. Control of ornithine decarboxylase in Chinese hamster ovary cells by polyamines. Translational inhibition of synthesis and acceleration of degradation of the enzyme by putrescine, spermidine, and spermine. J Biol Chem 1986; 261:9502-8.

50. Pajunen AEI, Isomaa VV, Janne OA, Bardin CW. Androgenic regulation of ornithine decarboxylase activity and its relationship to changes in cytosol and nuclear androgen receptor concentrations. J Biol Chem 1982; 257:8190-8.

51. Sertich GJ, Pegg AE. Polyamine administration reduces ornithine decarboxylase activity without affecting the mRNA content. Biochem Biophys Res Commun 1987; 143:424-30.

52. Kahana C, Nathans D. Nucleotide sequence of murine ornithine decarboxylase mRNA. Proc Natl Acad Sci USA 1985; 82:1673-7.

53. Winqvist R, Makela TP, Seppanen P, Janne OA, Alhonen-Hongisto L, Janne J, Grzeschik K-H, Alitalo K. Human ornithine decarboxylase sequences map to chromosome regions 2pter-->p23 and 7cen-->qter but are not co-amplified with the NMYC oncogene. Cytogenet Cell Genet 1986; 42:133-40.

54. Janne OA, Kontula KK, Isomaa VV, Bardin CW. Ornithine decarboxylase mRNA in mouse kidney: a low abundancy gene product regulated by androgens with rapid kinetics. Ann NY Acad Sci 1984; 438:72-84.

55. Berger FG, Loose D, Meisner H, Watson G. Androgen induction of messenger RNA concentrations in mouse kidney is posttranscriptional. Biochemistry 1986; 25:1170-5.

56. Brock ML, Shapiro DJ. Estrogen stabilizes vitellogenin mRNA against cytoplasmic degradation. Cell 1983; 34:207-14.

57. Brock ML, Shapiro DJ. Estrogen regulates the absolute rate of transcription of the Xenopus levis vitellogenin genes. J Biol Chem 1983; 258:5449-55.

58. Vannice JL, Taylor JM, Ringold GM. Glucocorticoid-mediated induction of α_1-acid glycoprotein: evidence for hormone-regulated RNA processing. Proc Natl Acad Sci USA 1984; 81:4241-5.

59. Paek I, Axel R. Glucocorticoids enhance stability of human growth hormone mRNA. Mol Cell Biol 1987; 7:1496-1507.

60. Field LJ, Gross KW. Ren-1 and Ren-2 loci are expressed in mouse kidney. Proc Natl Acad Sci USA 1985; 82:6196-200.

61. Bishop JO, Clark AJ, Clissold PM, Hainy S, Franke V. Two main groups of mouse major urinary protein genes, both largely located on chromosome 4. EMBO J 1982; 1:615-20.

62. Melanitou E, Cohn DA, Bardin CW, Janne OA. Genetic variation in androgen regulation of ornithine decarboxylase gene expression in inbred strains of mice. Mol Endocrinol 1987; 1:266-73.

10

ADVANCES IN UTERUS ESTRADIOL RECEPTOR PHOSPHORYLATION ON TYROSINE AND PRELIMINARY EVIDENCES THAT LIVER GLUCOCORTICOID RECEPTOR MIGHT BE PHOSPHORYLATED ON TYROSINE

G. Castoria, A. Migliaccio, M. Di Domenico, M. Pagano,
A. Rotondi, E. Nola,* and F. Auricchio

II Cattedra di Patologia Generale
*I Cattedra di Istituzioni di Patologia Generale
Istituto di Patologia Generale, I Facolta di Medicina
e Chir, Universita di Napoli, Italy

Our group has been working since 1979 on the process which reversibly regulates hormone binding of the uterus estradiol receptor. The possibility that phosphorylation of proteins is responsible for the hormone binding to steroid receptors was proposed for the first time for the glucocorticoid receptor when it was observed that ATP shortage of thymocytes decreases their ability to bind hormone whereas ATP recovery parallels recovery of this binding (1). Subsequently, it was observed that hormone binding to different steroid receptors is inactivated by exogenous phosphatases and reactivated by processes requiring ATP (2-4). Unfortunately, neither in the case of glucocorticoid receptor nor in the case of other steroid receptors was it proved that the observed fluctuations of hormone binding were due to phosphorylation-dephosphorylation of either receptors or receptor-related proteins.

In 1981 we succeeded in identifying and partially purifying two uterus enzymes that subsequently were identified as a phosphatase and a kinase (5-7). The phosphatase inactivates the hormone binding of the uterus estradiol receptor (5,6), the kinase reactivates the phosphatase-inactivated binding (7). After using these enzymes in sequence on the purified receptor, it has been demonstrated that estradiol receptor binding in the cell-free system requires phosphorylation on tyrosine of the receptor (8,9). Phosphorylation of proteins on tyrosine is about a thousandfold less frequent than phosphorylation on serine and threonine (10) and seems to be involved in important processes like growth factor induced cell multiplication, cell transformation and cell differentiation (11-13). Phosphorylation on tyrosine of a steroid receptor and its involvement in hormone binding is a new finding. We will review in this chapter recently observed properties of the two enzymes regulating the hormone binding of the estradiol receptor, the effect of antiestrogens on these enzymes and the evidence that estradiol receptor is phosphorylated on tyrosine in whole uterus (14). We will also report that the rat liver glucocorticoid receptor interacts with high affinity and specificity with antiphosphotyrosine antibodies. This finding also suggests that this receptor is phosphorylated on tyrosine (15).

REGULATION OF ESTRADIOL RECEPTOR-TYROSINE KINASE BY
Ca^{2+}-CALMODULIN AND ESTRADIOL

This enzyme converts the nonhormone binding into hormone binding receptor through phosphorylation of the receptor on tyrosine (9). It is routinely purified from calf uterus cytosol and assayed from its ability to reactivate the binding or to rephosphorylate the calf uterus estradiol receptor inactivated and dephosphorylated by the calf uterus nuclear phosphatase (16). It is unstable during and after purification (16). The Michaelis constant for the dephosphorylated receptor in optimal conditions is 0.3 nM (7). This extraordinary affinity is strong evidence that nonphosphorylated, nonhormone binding receptor is the natural substrate of this kinase.

Regulation of the activity of this enzyme is rather complex. In fact, the kinase is stimulated by Ca^{2+}-calmodulin (9) as well as by estradiol-receptor complex (17). It was initially observed that Ca^{2+} stimulates the kinase activity which was followed by the hormone-binding activation assay performed with crude substrate (7). To assess whether Ca^{2+} stimulation is mediated by calmodulin, homogeneous, calmodulin-free, and partially inactivated by the purified nuclear receptor-phosphatase receptor was used as substrate in the hormone-binding activation assay (9). It was found that combined Ca^{2+} and calmodulin is required for kinase stimulation by Ca^{2+} (9). Alone, neither substance produces a stimulatory effect. Dose-response curves for calmodulin and for Ca^{2+} stimulation of hormone-binding activation by the kinase have been calculated. The half-maximal and maximal rates of activation are reached at approximately 60 and 600 nM calmodulin and 0.8 and 1 µM Ca^{2+}, respectively (9). The high affinity of the kinase for calmodulin prompted us to use calmodulin-Sepharose to purify the kinase further (16). Ca^{2+}-calmodulin stimulates binding activation as well as phosphorylation on tyrosine of the estradiol receptor in parallel fashion (9), confirming that receptor phosphorylation is required for hormone binding.

As regard to stimulation of the kinase by estradiol in a preliminary experiment using a crude system, it was observed that the ability of the kinase to activate estradiol specific binding sites of phosphatase inactivated receptor, barely detectable in the absence of exogenous estradiol, is drastically stimulated by receptor preincubated with exogenous hormone (18). Since activation of binding sites is linked with receptor phosphorylation, it was expected that estradiol also stimulates phosphorylation of its own receptor. Our recent experiments reported in the following paragraph prove this point.

The receptor purified from calf uterus by ammonium sulphate precipitation and heparin-Sepharose chromatography was partially inactivated by the phosphatase and preincubated in the absence or in presence of 4 nM ^3H estradiol, then incubated with partially purified kinase and γ-^{32}P ATP. Control receptor-less or kinase-less samples preincubated with hormone were also run. After incubation with monoclonal antibody against estradiol receptor (19), all the samples were treated with protein A-Sepharose (Pansorbin) to precipitate the antibodies and proteins associated with antibodies. The proteins eluted from the pellets were submitted to SDS-PAGE followed by autoradiography (Fig. 1), and in a different experiment, to phosphoaminoacid analysis (panel A of Fig. 2). In the incubation mixture containing estradiol receptor incubated with hormone and kinase (lane 4 of Fig. 1), the receptor has clearly been phosphorylated. In fact, autoradiography of this lane shows a more phosphorylated band migrating as a 68 Kd protein and lighter and less phosphorylated proteins, probably proteolytic products of the 68 Kd receptor (14,20-22). In contrast, when the same incubation was performed with receptor preincubated without estradiol, very faint phosphorylation of the receptor is detectable (lane 3 of Fig. 1). Comparison of lane 3 with lane 4 and activation of binding sites by the kinase with and without hormone assayed in parallel samples (0.011 and 0.107 pmol, respectively) shows that estradiol strongly stimulates phosphorylation of receptor as well as activation of hormone binding. No phosphorylation is detected by pre-incubation of the receptor with hormone followed by incubation in the absence of kinase (lane 2). This shows that the kinase is required for the phosphorylation of the phosphatase-inactivated receptor observed in lane 4. Almost undetectable phosphorylation of the 68 Kd band of the receptor is present in the sample containing kinase preincubated with hormone and incubated in the absence of receptor (lane 1). This phosphorylation was not observed with every kinase preparation and is due to the copurification with the partially purified kinase of small amounts of dephosphorylated as well as hormone binding receptor from calf uterus cytosol (17). Lane 5 shows a sample identical to that shown by lane 4 except for incubation with N6 control antibody. No ^{32}P phosphorylated protein is immunoprecipitated in this sample, confirming the specificity of the receptor immunoprecipitation by JS 34/32 antibody. In conclusion, the experiment in Figure 1 shows that estradiol strongly stimulates phosphorylation of the phosphatase-inactivated receptor by the kinase. Similar experiments using sucrose gradient centrifugation to detect interaction between ^{32}P phosphorylated receptor and the monoclonal antibody against the receptor confirmed that the hormone stimulates receptor phosphorylation as well as hormone binding activation by the kinase (17).

Several findings prove that estradiol stimulation of the kinase on the phosphatase-inactivated receptor is mediated by the phosphorylated, hormone binding receptor: tamoxifen inhibits at a similar extent hormone binding to the receptor and stimulatory effect of estradiol on the kinase; other steroid hormones do not stimulate the kinase; estradiol stimulates the kinase at physiological concentrations (17). In addition, the possibility that estradiol directly stimulates the kinase is excluded by the lack of estradiol binding to the purified kinase at physiological concentrations (17).

Phosphoaminoacid analysis of the receptor reactivated and ^{32}P phosphorylated by the kinase in the absence and in the presence of estradiol has been performed either on the receptor immunoprecipitated (panel A of Fig. 2), or on the 68 Kd protein band eluted from the SDS-PAGE of the immunoprecipitated receptor (panel B of Fig. 2). In the first case (panel A), the phosphoaminoacid electrophoresis was run at pH 3.5 in one direction; in the second case (panel B), it was run at pH 1.9 in the first direction, and at pH 3.5 in the second direction. In both cases, phosphoaminoacid analysis shows that the receptor has been phosphorylated exclusively on tyrosine, confirming previous reports on estradiol receptor phosphorylation in cell-free system (9) as well as in whole uterus (14).

Figure 2 also shows that estradiol stimulates phosphorylation on tyrosine of the receptor. In the experiment of panel A, phosphorylation is observed also in the absence of exogenous hormone. Conversely, in the panel B experiment, in the absence of estradiol, no phosphorylation of the immunoprecipitated receptor submitted to SDS-PAGE (as well as no significant reactivation of binding) was detectable. Actually, the extent of stimulation of the kinase by estradiol is different in the different experiments, and this might be due to different amounts of endogenous estradiol complexed with the purified receptor preparations.

About the relationship between stimulation of the kinase by Ca^{2+}-calmodulin and that by estradiol-receptor complex, it should be stressed that we have measured stimulation by Ca^{2+}-calmodulin in the presence of

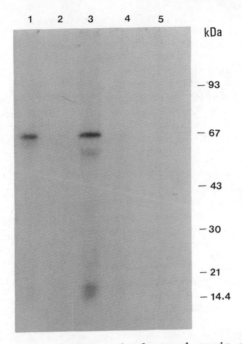

Fig. 1. SDS-polyacrylamide gel electrophoresis of the immuno-precipitated estradiol receptor phosphorylated in absence and in presence of hormone. 300 μl samples containing receptor par-tially inactivated by the phosphatase (0.4 pmol of hormone bind-ing sites) were preincubated at $0°C$ for 3 h in the absence (lane 3) and in the presence of 4 nM ^3H estradiol (lanes 4 and 5). Samples were then incubated with the kinase at 15°C in TGD-buffer (50 mM Tris-HCl, 0.2 mM EGTA, 1 mM DTT; pH 7.4) contain-ing 5 mM $MgCl_2$, 10 mM Na_2MoO_4, 0.8 mM $CaCl_2$, 10 μg/ml calmodulin and 0.15 mM $\gamma-^{32}P$ ATP (10 Ci/mmol). Receptor-less and kinase-less controls were run in parallel after preincubation at 0°C for 3 h in the presence of 4 nM ^3H estradiol (lane 1 and lane 2, respectively). At the end of incubation, each sample was added with 20 μl rat ascites containing either JS 34/32 antireceptor (lanes 1-4) or control antibodies (lane 5) and 15 μl of 1% pansorbin suspension (Calbiochem) and incubated overnight at 4°C under gentle shaking. Samples were centrifuged and their pellets were washed twice with ice-cold PBS buffer (1 ml) and proteins eluted by boiling the pellets in 50 μl of 0.2% SDS-PAGE sample buffer for 5 min. Thirty μl sample aliquots were submit-ted to SDS-PAGE and the gel dried and autoradiographed. Activa-tion of estradiol specific binding sites by the kinase in the absence and presence of hormone was measured in parallel samples (0.011 pmoles and 0.107 pmol, respectively, the latter value corresponding to a complete reactivation of the phosphatase-inactivated binding sites) (17).

hormone-receptor complex because in the absence of hormone the kinase activity frequently is very low (17,18). Therefore, we do not know yet whether in the absence of estradiol, Ca^{2+}-calmodulin still stimulates the kinase.

Regulation of the estradiol receptor tyrosine kinase is similar to that of the insulin receptor-associated tyrosine kinase since both tyrosine kinases are stimulated by Ca^{2+}-calmodulin (23,24) as well as by

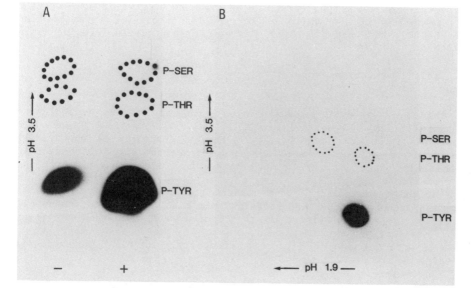

Fig. 2. Phosphoaminoacid analysis of the estradiol receptor phosphorylated by the kinase in the absence and in the presence of hormone. <u>Panel A</u>: 200 µl samples containing partially purified receptor partially inactivated by the phosphatase (0.35 pmoles of hormone binding receptor and 0.15 pmoles of phosphatase inactivated receptor) were preincubated at 0°C for 3 h in the absence and presence of 4 nM ^{3}H estradiol and incubated at 15°C with partially purified kinase and $\gamma-^{32}$P ATP, as described in the legend to Figure 1. Parallel samples were incubated in the same conditions in the absence and presence of radioinert ATP to measure the activation of estrogen binding sites by the kinase. Aliquots containing 0.039 pmoles of binding sites were activated in the absence of hormone and 0.145 pmoles, corresponding to 97% of the phosphatase-inactivated binding sites, in presence of hormone. Samples incubated with $\gamma-^{32}$P ATP were mixed with 15 µl rat ascites containing JS 34/32 anti-receptor antibody and 10 µl 1% Pansorbin. The suspensions were incubated at 4°C, then centrifuged and pellets eluted by 30 µl of 0.2% SDS-PAGE sample buffer after washing as described in the previous figure. Samples were centrifuged again and 25 µl supernatant diluted to 250 µl with water and added with 5 vol of cold acetone (-20°C) after addition of bovine serum albumin as a carrier. Samples were centrifuged and pellets washed twice with acetone, dried and submitted to phosphoaminoacid analysis. Sample phosphorylated without hormone: lane -; sample phosphorylated with hormone: lane +. <u>Panel B</u>: 300 µl sample containing receptor partially inactivated by the phosphatase (0.55 pmoles of active, hormone binding receptor and 0.31 pmoles of inactivated receptor) were preincubated at 0°C for 3 h with and without hormone and then incubated at 15°C with partially purified kinase in the presence of $\gamma-^{32}$P ATP as in the experiment of panel A. Parallel samples were incubated with radioinert ATP to measure the activation of estrogen binding sites. 0.01 pmoles were reactivated by the kinase in absence of hormone and 0.30 pmoles (corresponding to 97% of the phosphatase-inactivated binding sites) reactivated in presence of hormone. Samples incubated with $\gamma-^{32}$P ATP were incubated with antireceptor antibody and Pansorbin as reported in legend to panel A, pellets were eluted by 75 µl of SDS-PAGE sample buffer, and each sample was divided in two aliquots of (continued on next page)

hormone occupancy of the corresponding receptor (25). Hormone occupancy of receptors also stimulates other receptor-associated tyrosine kinase like the EGF, PDGF and somatomedin C receptor-associated tyrosine kinases (26-28).

Table 1 summarizes some of the properties of the estradiol receptor kinase.

There are several reports suggesting that steroid receptors are kinases (29a,29b). Nevertheless, it is unlikely that the receptor is a kinase since it does not bind ATP analog (unpublished observation). Finally, we cannot exclude that the receptor and the kinase are associated in the cell. In fact, the tissue homogenization and ammonium sulphate fractionation used to partially separate the receptor from the kinase, and the chaotropic salts and heparin utilized to purify the receptor, dissociate the receptor from other proteins. It might be that in intact cells estradiol receptor and kinase are associated, and that this association favors stimulation of the kinase activity by hormone occupancy of the receptor with consequent increased phosphorylation of endogenous substrate(s) on tyrosine.

THE PHOSPHATASE INACTIVATING THE HORMONE BINDING OF THE RECEPTOR IS AN ESTRADIOL RECEPTOR-PHOSPHOTYROSINE PHOSPHATASE

The phosphatase assayed as estradiol receptor hormone binding inactivating activity has been found in the nuclei of mouse mammary gland and calf, rat and mouse uterus (5). It is not present in mouse quadriceps muscle nuclei (5). It is completely inhibited by several phosphatase inhibitors including protein-phosphotyrosine phosphatase-like zinc and orthovanadate (5,14). In vitro, the enzyme inactivates the hormone binding of crude and pure cytosol receptor (6). In vivo, inactivation and dephosphorylation of estradiol receptor has been observed as a consequence of receptor "translocation" into nuclei of mouse uterus injected with estradiol and attributed to this phosphatase (30). This enzyme inactivates hormone-free as well as hormone-bound receptor (6).

The extraordinary affinity of the hormone binding inactivating activity of the phosphatase for the receptor (~1 nM) (6) lends weight to our hypothesis that the receptor is a physiological substrate of this enzyme.

That the phosphatase inactivating the hormone binding of the estradiol receptor dephosphorylates phosphotyrosyl residue(s) of the receptor is proved by the following two findings.

Phosphorylation by the kinase of phosphatase-inactivated receptor using γ-^{32}P ATP produces reactivated receptor which is ^{32}P-phosphorylated exclusively on tyrosine (9). Incubation of the ^{32}P-receptor in the

---

(Fig. 2 continued) 15 and 55 µl, respectively. The aliquots were separately submitted to SDS-PAGE. The lanes loaded with 15 µl aliquots were dried and submitted to autoradiography. No phosphorylated receptor was detected in the sample incubated in absence of hormone and therefore no phosphoaminoacid analysis was performed on this sample. The 68 Kd phosphorylated protein was extracted from the SDS-PAGE loaded with the 55 µl aliquot of the sample incubated in the presence of hormone, hydrolyzed, lyophilized and submitted to phosphoaminoacid analysis (17).

Table 1. Properties of the estradiol receptor-kinase.

It is purified from calf uterus cytosol.

It phosphorylates the receptor exclusively on tyrosine converting the nonhormone-binding into hormone-binding receptor.

It interacts with calmodulin-Sepharose and is stimulated by Ca^{2+}-calmodulin.

It is stimulated by estradiol-receptor complex.

K_m for the nonphosphorylated receptor: 0.3 nM.

presence of the phosphatase removes significant amount of ^{32}P incorporated into the receptor as shown by SDS-PAGE in Figure 3 (31).

Calf uterus estradiol receptor interacts with high affinity with 2G8 and 1G2 antiphosphotyrosine antibodies coupled to Sepharose beads (Kd 0.28 and 1.11 nM respectively), whereas it does not interact with bovine serum albumin- or bovine immunoglobulin-Sepharose (14,15). Incubation of calf uterus cytosol receptor with homologous nuclei containing the receptor-phosphatase inactivates a portion of the receptor. Table 3 shows that this portion does not bind to antiphosphotyrosine and can be reactivated by phosphorylation (14). This observation confirms with a different approach that phosphatase hydrolyses receptor phosphotyrosine since it abolishes interaction of the receptor with antiphosphotyrosine antibody (14). In addition, it is clear that phosphorylation on tyrosine of the calf uterus receptor is required for hormone binding since loss of interaction with antiphosphotyrosine antibody parallels loss of hormone binding.

Table 2. Properties of the estradiol receptor-phosphotyrosine phosphatase.

Localized in nuclei of estrogen target tissues.

Purified from calf uterus.

Stimulated by dithiothreitol.

Inhibited by zinc, molybdate, fluoride, phosphate, pyrophosphate, p-nitrophenyl phosphate and orthovanadate.

It inactivates in vitro the hormone binding of crude and pure cytosol and nuclear receptor.

K_m for estrogen-free receptor: 1.5 nM.

K_m for estrogen-bound receptor: 0.8 nM.

It apparently inactivates in vivo the hormone binding of the nuclear estradiol-receptor complex.

It does not inactivate in vitro the hormone binding of the receptor complexed with antiestrogens like tamoxifen and nafoxidine.

It dephosphorylates the estradiol receptor phosphorylated exclusively on tyrosine by the receptor tyrosine-kinase.

It abolishes the interaction of estradiol receptor with antiphospho-tyrosine antibody.

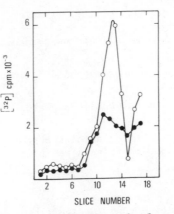

Fig. 3. SDS-polyacrylamide gel electrophoresis of the phosphorylated receptor before and after incubation with the phosphatase. Pure estradiol-17β receptor binding 8.71 pmol of hormone was partially inactivated by incubation with the nuclear phosphatase and used as substrate of the kinase. The binding of the receptor was activated in TGD-buffer under the following conditions: the temperature was 15°C; 5 mM $MgCl_2$, 10 mM Na_2MoO_4, 0.15 mM γ-^{32}P ATP (6 Ci/mmol), 27 arbitrary units of purified kinase were added together with 1 μM Ca^{2+} and 0.6 μM calmodulin in a final volume of 1.5 ml. Two aliquots of 100 μl were incubated in the absence and presence of purified phosphatase, respectively, for 20 min at 25°C (final volume 150 μl). The samples were extensively dialyzed against TGD-buffer. One hundred μl aliquots of the samples were submitted to SDS-gel electrophoresis. Then the gel lanes were sliced and counted for ^{32}P radioactivity. Open symbols: receptor incubated in absence of phosphatase. Closed symbols: receptor incubated in presence of phosphatase (31).

NONSTEROIDAL ANTIESTROGENS: INHIBITION OF IN VITRO INACTIVATION—REACTIVATION OF ESTRADIOL RECEPTOR

In a previous report we observed that nonsteroidal antiestrogens like tamoxifen and nafoxidine once complexed either in vitro or in vivo with uterus estradiol receptor protect the hormone binding of the receptor from the in vitro inactivation by the nuclear phosphatase (32). To complex antihormone with the receptor in vitro calf uterus cytosol receptor was incubated with the antihormones and subsequently incubated with the phosphatase. To complex antihormones with receptor in vivo mice were injected with antihormones and nuclei containing antihormone-receptor complexes were isolated from uterus and incubated in conditions in which the nuclear phosphatase inactivates the hormone-receptor complex (32). In both cases the antiestrogen receptor complex, unlike the hormone-receptor complex, is refractory to the phosphatase activity. These findings, when related to the observation that nonsteroidal antiestrogen-receptor complexes, in contrast with estrogen receptor complex, are slowly lost in nuclei of intact cells (33), support the possibility that the nuclear phosphatase is responsible for the loss of receptor "translocated" into nuclei by the hormone in vivo.

Table 3. Lack of interaction of nonhormone binding estradiol receptor with 2G8 anti-P-tyrosine antibody coupled to Sepharose.

	Hormone binding receptor		Nonhormone binding receptor	
	fmol	%	fmol	%
Cytosol after incubation with nuclei	2794	100	1164	100
Anti-P-tyr-Sepharose supernatant	147	5	1081	93

Calf uterus cytosol (2 ml) ^{3}H estradiol-receptor complex preparation containing 3958 fmol of the complex were incubated at 25°C for 20 min with homologous nuclei in TGD buffer. During the incubation, nuclear receptor phosphatase inactivated 1164 fmol of the ^{3}H estradiol specific binding sites of the receptor. This cytosol, containing hormone binding receptor (2794 fmol) and nonhormone binding receptor was incubated overnight at 0°C with 0.2 ml of 2G8 anti-P-tyr-Sepharose under gentle shaking. The suspensions were centrifuged and supernatant assayed for estradiol-specific binding sites under standard conditions (hormone binding, phosphorylated receptor) and after incubation at 15°C in the absence and presence of ATP (to assay the nonhormone binding, dephosphorylated receptor).

As previously reported in this chapter, estradiol in complex with its hormone binding receptor stimulates the receptor-tyrosine kinase which activates the hormone binding of the dephosphorylated, nonhormone binding receptor. Tamoxifen at a concentration which reduces the occupancy of the receptor by estradiol by 50% also reduces the stimulatory effect of the hormone on the kinase, assayed by receptor hormone binding activation, by 45% (17). This experiment shows that tamoxifen by its interaction with the receptor prevents the stimulation of the kinase by estradiol.

In synthesis in cell-free systems antiestrogens inhibit inactivation as well as activation of hormone binding of the receptor. Both effects are reached through the formation of the receptor-antihormone complex since this complex, unlike the receptor-hormone complex, is recognized neither as a substrate by the phosphatase nor as an activator by the kinase.

PHOSPHORYLATION OF ESTRADIOL RECEPTOR IN WHOLE UTERUS

To prove that estradiol receptor is phosphorylated on tyrosine not only in cell-free systems but also in whole tissues, uteri from intact adult rats were incubated with ^{32}P-orthophosphate at 39°C for 1 h. 80 μM Na$_3$VO$_4$ was added to the incubation buffer. The uteri were mixed with carrier uteri and homogenized (14) to prepare high speed supernatant. This supernatant was used to purify estradiol receptor by cycling it through diethylstilbestrol (DES) Sepharose column (20). The receptor was eluted from the affinity resin with ^{3}H estradiol, cycled through heparin-Sepharose column and finally eluted from this resin by a buffer containing heparin (20).

Two samples of the estradiol receptor eluted from heparin-Sepharose were equilibrated with 12 nM ^{3}H estradiol and incubated with an excess of immunoglobulins. These immunoglobulins were purified either from a control hybridoma derived from the fusion of myeloma cells with spleen cells from nonimmunized mice or from the JS 34/32 clone produced by fusion

141

of myeloma cells with spleen cells from mice immunized with purified estradiol receptor (19). The two samples were analyzed by centrifugation through high salt sucrose gradients. The ^{3}H estradiol peak bound to the receptor incubated with control immunoglobulins co-sediments at 4.5 S with a peak of [32]P. Preincubation of the receptor preparation with JS 34/32 antibodies against purified receptor causes both peaks to shift to 7.5 S. Since this shift is due to the formation of an antibody-receptor complex in a 1:1 molar ratio (19), it is clear that the ^{32}P peak shifted to 7.5 S by the antibodies belongs to the receptor (14).

The receptor eluted from heparin-Sepharose was further purified by chromatography through a column of Sepharose to which JS 34/32 monoclonal antibodies against the receptor have been linked (34). The receptor sample eluted from the antibody-Sepharose column at alkaline pH and neutralized immediately after the elution was concentrated by acid precipitation using myoglobin as a carrier. The pellet was dissolved and submitted to SDS-polyacrylamide gel electrophoresis (Fig. 4). Silver nitrate stained several protein bands; only two of them (those indicated by arrows in Fig. 4) belong to the receptor preparation since they were not detectable in the control sample of myoglobin. The molecular weights of these two proteins were 68 and 48 Kd, respectively. Autoradiography showed a heavily phosphorylated band coincident with the 68 Kd protein and a barely phosphorylated band coincident with the lighter protein that is probably a proteolytic product of the 68 Kd receptor (14,20-22).

A sample of the immunopurified receptor was subjected to acid hydrolysis, concentrated by lyophilization, dissolved in a small volume of water, and analyzed by one-dimensional electrophoresis at pH 3.5. The electrophoresis plate was exposed for autoradiography. The only phosphorylated aminoacid detectable was phosphotyrosine (Fig. 5). This is the first demonstration of a steroid receptor phosphorylation on tyrosine in whole tissues.

INTERACTION OF RAT LIVER GLUCOCORTICOID RECEPTOR WITH ANTIPHOSPHOTYROSINE ANTIBODY

2G8 monoclonal antibodies have been raised against the hapten azobenzylphosphonate, a close phosphotyrosine analog (35). These antibodies have been covalently coupled to Sepharose beads and previously used to purify proteins phosphorylated on tyrosine, e.g., the phosphotyrosyl proteins from cells transformed by Abelson murine leukemia virus (36) and the platelet-derived growth factor receptor (37). These antibodies react with high affinity and specificity with the phosphorylated form of the calf uterus estradiol receptor and have been used to purify this receptor (14,15).

We observed that the rat liver glucocorticoid receptor interacts with a high affinity and specificity with 2G8 antiphosphotyrosine antibodies. This fact suggests that glucocorticoid receptor from rat liver is phosphorylated on tyrosine. This possibility is supported by the recent evidence that glucocorticoid receptor in human breast epithelial cells is also phosphorylated on tyrosine (38).

Rat liver cytosol was obtained from adrenalectomized male adult (15) and the ^{3}H triamcinolone-receptor complex was purified from the cytosol by heparin-Sepharose chromatography (39). Three 0.3 ml samples of ^{3}H triamcinolone-receptor complex were separately incubated with either BSA-Sepharose, or IgG-Sepharose or 2G8 anti-P-tyr-Sepharose at 0°C for 2 h. Suspensions were centrifuged and supernatants assayed for specific hormone binding sites. Receptor bound to Sepharose was calculated from the

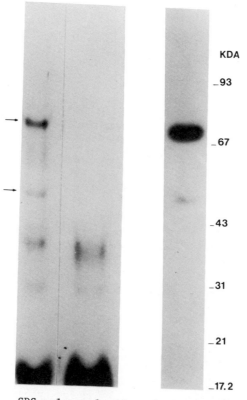

Fig. 4. SDS-polyacrylamide gel electrophoresis of the estradiol receptor purified from rat uteri incubated with ^{32}P-orthophosphate. Receptor was purified by DES-Sepharose, heparin-Sepharose and antireceptor antibody-Sepharose chromatography. Receptor preparation (0.6 ml) was added with 10% TCA using myoglobin as a carrier. The pellet was washed twice with ether:ethanol (1:1) and dissolved with 60 μl of SDS-PAGE sample buffer, then heated at 100°C for 3 min. A 50 μl aliquot was submitted to SDS-PAGE. After the run, the gel was stained with silver stain (Bio-Rad), dried and exposed to autoradiography. Lane A: silver staining of the receptor sample added with myoglobin. Lane B: silver staining of myoglobin control sample. Lane C: autoradiography of lane A. The arrows show the two protein bands present only in the receptors sample (14).

difference between specific binding sites present in the samples before and after incubation with Sepharose. Only 10% of the glucocorticoid receptor bound to BSA- or IgG-Sepharose, whereas all the receptor bound to anti-P-tyr-Sepharose (15). This experiment shows that glucocorticoid receptor interacts with antiphosphotyrosine antibody and this interaction is specific.

In another experiment, the receptor bound to anti-P-tyr-Sepharose was eluted with buffer containing different compounds. The results are reported in Table 4. Buffer containing NaSCN (control) eluted 3% of the receptor bound to Sepharose. Addition of P-serine, P-threonine and

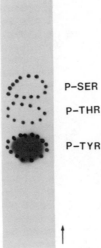

P-SER

P-THR

P-TYR

Fig. 5. Phosphoaminoacid analysis of the estradiol receptor purified from rat uteri incubated
with ^{32}P-orthophosphate. Receptor was purified by
DES-Sepharose, heparin-Sepharose and antireceptor
antibody-Sepharose chromatography. Receptor
preparation (0.3 ml) was subjected to acid hydrolysis by incubation under vacuum of 6 N HCl at
110°C for 3 h. The sample was diluted with water
to 4 ml, then lyophilized and solubilized with 30
μl of water containing 30 μg of phosphoserine
(P-ser), phosphothreonine (P-thr) and phosphotyrosine (P-tyr). 20 μl of this sample were subjected
to electrophoresis at pH 3.5. The plate was
stained with ninhydrin and then exposed to autoradiography. The dotted lines represent the
standard superimposed on autoradiography (14).

tyrosine to the buffer containing NaSCN does not increase the amount of
eluted receptor. P-tyrosine, and to a greater extent phenyl phosphate, a
very close analog of hapten azobenzylphosphonate, eluted significant
amount of specific binding sites in the presence of NaSCN: 18 and 48%,
respectively (15). This fact shows that the antiphosphotyrosine antibody
recognizes phosphotyrosine whereas it does not recognize other phospho-
aminoacids and nonphosphorylated tyrosine.

To measure the affinity of the glucocorticoid receptor for the 2G8
antibody, ^{3}H triamcinolone-receptor complex was incubated with BSA-
Sepharose for 2 h at 0°C to remove nonspecific binding, then centrifuged.
The supernatant was divided into fractions containing from 39 to 400 fmol
of ^{3}H triamcinolone specific binding sites. Each fraction was diluted to
0.5 ml with TGD glycerol buffer (50 mM Tris-HCl, 0.2 mM EGTA, 1 mM DTT,
10% glycerol; pH 7.4), incubated for 12 h at 0°C with 30 μl of 2G8 anti-
P-tyr-Sepharose, and then centrifuged. The supernatants were assayed for
specific binding sites and these served as a measure of free ^{3}H triamcinolone-receptor complex. The bound ^{3}H triamcinolone-receptor complex
was calculated from the difference between specific binding sites present
in samples before and after incubation with anti-P-tyr-Sepharose. Data
are plotted in Figure 6. The Kd value, 0.21 nM, shows that glucocorticoid
receptor, like estradiol receptor, interacts with a very high affinity
with the monoclonal antibody.

Table 4. Effect of different compounds on the elution of rat liver glucocorticoid receptor bound to antiphosphotyrosine antibody coupled to Sepharose (15).

	Specific ^{3}H triamcinolone binding sites eluted from anti-P-tyr-Sepharose	
	fmol	% sites bound to anti-P-tyr-Sepharose
Control	2.9	2.7
+ P-serine	2.6	2.4
+ P-threonine	2.6	2.4
+ tyrosine	2.5	2.3
+ P-tyrosine	20.0	18.3
+ phenyl phosphate (hapten buffer)	52.0	48.0

Specificity of interaction and elution from antiphosphotyrosine antibody together with the high affinity interaction of the glucocorticoid receptor with the 2G8 antibody suggest that this receptor is phosphorylated on tyrosine. Interaction of glucocorticoid and estradiol receptors with antiphosphotyrosine antibody coupled to Sepharose has been utilized to efficiently purify these receptors (15).

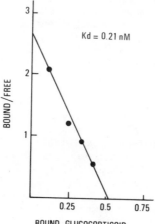

Fig. 6. Measurement of the affinity of ^{3}H triamcinolone receptor complex for antiphosphotyrosine antibodies coupled to Sepharose. Rat liver ^{3}H triamcinolone-receptor complex purified by heparin-Sepharose was employed. Increasing amounts of the hormone-receptor complex were added to a fixed amount of 2G8 anti-P-tyr-Sepharose and gently shaken at 0°C overnight. Suspensions were centrifuged and the hormone-receptor complex remaining in the supernatants assayed. B/F, bound/free hormone-receptor complex (15).

ACKNOWLEDGMENTS

The authors gratefully acknowledge Mr. Gian Michele La Placa for editorial work. This research was supported by grants from Associazione Italiana per la Ricerca sul Cancro, from Italian National Research Council, Special Project Oncology, contract No. 86.00295.44 and from Ministero Pubblica Istruzione, Italy.

REFERENCES

1. Munck A, Brinck-Johnsen T. Specific and non-specific physiological interaction of glucocorticoids and related steroids with rat thymus cells in vitro. J Biol Chem 1968; 243:5556-65.
2. Sando JJ, Hammond ND, Stratford CA, Pratt WB. Activation of thymocyte glucocorticoid receptors to the steroid binding form. J Biol Chem 1979a; 254:4779-89.
3. Sando JJ, La Forest AC, Pratt WB. ATP-dependent activation of cell glucocorticoid receptors to the steroid binding form. J Biol Chem 1979b; 254:4772-8.
4. Liao S, Rossini GP, Hiipakka RA, Chen C. Factors that can control the interaction of the androgen-receptor complex with the genomic structure in the rat prostate. In: Bresciani F, ed. Perspectives in steroid receptor research. 1980;99-112.
5. Auricchio F, Migliaccio A. Inactivation of estradiol receptor by nuclei: prevention by phosphatase inhibitors. FEBS Lett 1980; 117:224-6.
6. Auricchio F, Migliaccio A, Rotondi A. Inactivation of oestrogen receptor "in vitro" by nuclear dephosphorylation. Biochem J 1981; 194:569-74.
7. Auricchio F, Migliaccio A, Castoria G, Lastoria S, Schiavone E. ATP dependent enzyme activating hormone binding of estradiol receptor. Biochem Biophys Res Commun 1981; 101:1171-8.
8. Migliaccio A, Lastoria S, Moncharmont B, Rotondi A, Auricchio F. Phosphorylation of calf uterus 17β-estradiol receptor by endogenous Ca^{2+}-stimulated kinase activating the hormone binding of the receptor. Biochem Biophys Res Commun 1982; 109:1002-10.
9. Migliaccio A, Rotondi A, Auricchio F. Calmodulin stimulated phosphorylation of 17β-estradiol receptor on tyrosine. Proc Natl Acad Sci USA 1984; 81:5921-5.
10. Hunter T, Cooper JA. Protein tyrosine kinase. Annu Rev Biochem 1985; 54:897-930.
11. Bishop M. Viral oncogenes. Cell 1985; 42:23-38.
12. Hunter T, Sefton B. Transforming gene product of Rous sarcoma virus phosphorylates tyrosine. Proc Natl Acad Sci USA 1980; 77:1311-5.
13. Hafen E, Basler K, Edstrom JE, Rubin GM. Sevenless, a cell-specific homeotic gene of Drosophila, encodes a putative transmembrane receptor with a tyrosine kinase domain. Science 1987; 236:55-63.
14. Migliaccio A, Rotondi A, Auricchio F. Estradiol receptor: phosphorylation on tyrosine in uterus and interaction with antiphosphotyrosine antibody. EMBO J 1986; 5:2867-72.
15. Auricchio F, Migliaccio A, Castoria G, et al. Phosphorylation on tyrosine of oestradiol-17β receptor in uterus and interaction of oestradiol-17β and glucocorticoid receptors with antiphosphotyrosine antibodies. J Steroid Biochem 1987 (in press).
16. Auricchio F, Migliaccio A, Castoria G, Rotondi A, Di Domenico M. Calmodulin-stimulated estradiol receptor-tyrosine kinase. Methods Enzymol 1987; 139:731-44.
17. Auricchio F, Migliaccio A, Di Domenico M, Nola E. Oestradiol stimulates phosphorylation of its own receptor in a cell-free system. EMBO J 1987 (in press).

18. Auricchio F, Migliaccio A, Castoria G, Rotondi A, Di Domenico M, Pagano M. Activation-inactivation of hormone binding sites of the oestradiol 17β-receptor is a multiregulated process. J Steroid Biochem 1986; 24:39-43.

19. Moncharmont B, Su JL, Parik I. Monoclonal antibodies against estrogen receptor: interaction with different molecular forms and functions of the receptor. Biochemistry 1982; 21:6916-21.

20. Van Osbree TR, Kim UH, Mueller GC. Affinity chromatography of estrogen receptors on diethylstilbestrol-agarose. Anal Biochem 1984; 136:321-7.

21. Katzenellenbogen JA, Carlson KE, Heiman DF, Robertson DW, Wei LL, Katzenellenbogen BS. Efficient and highly selective covalent binding labeling of the estrogen receptor with ^{3}H-tamoxifen aziridine. J Biol Chem 1983; 258:3487-59.

22. Walter P, Green S, Greene G, et al. Cloning of the human estrogen receptor cDNA. Proc Natl Acad Sci USA 1985; 82:7889-93.

23. Graves CB, Gale RD, Laurino JP, McDonald JM. The insulin receptor and calmodulin. Calmodulin enhance insulin-mediated receptor kinase activity and insulin stimulates phosphorylation of calmodulin. J Biol Chem 1986; 261:10429.

24. Graves CB, Goewert RR, McDonald JM. The insulin receptor contains a calmodulin-binding domain. Science 1985; 230:827-9.

25. Kasuga M, Karlsson FA, Kahn CR. Insulin stimulates the phosphorylation of the 95,000 dalton subunit of its own receptor. Science 1982; 215:185-7.

26. Cohen S, Carpenter G, King L. Epidermal growth-factor receptor protein kinase interactions: co-purification of receptor and epidermal growth factor enhanced phosphorylation. J Biol Chem 1980; 255:4834.

27. Ek B, Heldin CH. Characterization of a tyrosine specific kinase activity in human fibroblast membranes stimulated by platelet derived growth factor. J Biol Chem 1982; 257:10486.

28. Jacobs S, Kull FC, Earp HS, Svoboda ME, Van Wyk JJ, Cuatrecasas P. Somatomedin-C stimulates the phosphorylation of the B subunit of its own receptor. J Biol Chem 1983; 258:9581-4.

29a. Singh VB, Moudgil VK. Protein kinase activity of purified rat liver glucocorticoid receptor. Biochem Biophys Res Commun 1984; 1067-73.

29b. Miller-Diener A, Schmidt TJ, Litwack G. Protein kinase activity associated with the purified rat hepatic glucocorticoid receptor. Proc Natl Acad Sci USA 1985; 82:4003-7.

30. Auricchio F, Migliaccio A, Castoria G, Lastoria S, Rotondi A. Evidence that "in vivo" estradiol receptor translocated into nuclei is dephosphorylated and released into cytoplasm. Biochem Biophys Res Commun 1982; 106:149-57.

31. Auricchio F, Migliaccio A, Castoria G, Rotondi A, Lastoria S. Direct evidence of "in vitro" phosphorylation-dephosphorylation of the estradiol-17β receptor. Role of Ca^{2+}-calmodulin in the activation of hormone binding sites. J Steroid Biochem 1984; 20:31-5.

32. Auricchio F, Migliaccio A, Castoria G. Dephosphorylation of oestradiol nuclear receptor in vitro. A hypothesis on the mechanism of action of non-steroidal anti-oestrogens. Biochem J 1981; 198:699-702.

33. Horwitz KB, McGuire WL. Nuclear mechanism of estrogen action: effect of estradiol and anti-estrogens on estrogen receptors and nuclear receptor processing. J Biol Chem 1978; 23:8185-91.

34. Cuatrecasas P. Protein purification by affinity chromatography. Derivatization of agarose and polyacrylamide beads. J Biol Chem 1970; 245:3059-65.

35. Ross AH, Baltimore D, Eisen HH. Phosphotyrosine containing proteins isolated by affinity chromatography with antibodies to a synthetic hapten. Nature 1981; 294:654-6.

36. Foulkes JG, Chow M, Gorka C, Frackelton AR, Baltimore D. Purification and characterization of a protein-tyrosine kinase encoded by the Abelson murine leukemia virus. J Biol Chem 1985; 260:8070-7.

37. Daniel TD, Tremble AR, Frackelton AR, Williams LT. Purification of the platelet-derived growth factor receptor by using an anti phosphotyrosine antibody. Proc Natl Acad Sci USA 1985; 82:2684-7.

38. Rao KVS, Fox F. Epidermal growth factor stimulates tyrosine phosphorylation of human glucocorticoid receptor in cultured cells. Biochem Biophys Res Commun 1987; 144:512-9.

39. Weisz A, Puca GA, Masucci MT, et al. Interaction of rat liver glucocorticoid receptor with heparin. Biochemistry 1984; 23:5393-7.

IV. RECEPTOR GENE STRUCTURE AND FUNCTION

11

FUNCTIONAL ANALYSIS OF THE ESTROGEN AND PROGESTERONE RECEPTORS

H. Gronemeyer, M. Berry, M. T. Bocquel, J. Eul, S. Green,
J. M. Jeltsch, A. Krust, V. Kumar, M. E. Meyer, G. Stack,
C. Stricker, B. Turcotte, and P. Chambon

Laboratoire de Genetique Moleculaire des Eucaryotes du
C.N.R.S.. Unite 184 de Biologie Moleculaire et de Genie
Genetique de l'INSERM, Institut de Chimie Biologique,
Faculte de Medecine 11, rue Humann,
67085 Strasbourg Cedex, France

INTRODUCTION

The molecular basis for the regulation of patterns of gene expression, both during the development of eukaryotic organisms and in terminally differentiated cells, is one of the major subjects of molecular biology. At the level of transcription, this regulation appears to be achieved through positive and negative effects mediated by trans-acting proteins interacting with cis-acting DNA promoter elements. Steroid hormones trigger complex developmental and physiological processes. The structural information provided by a given steroid hormone is converted into a regulatory signal by its interaction with specific receptor proteins. Upon binding of the hormone, the receptor gains the ability to specifically alter gene transcription; a process which appears to result from the binding of the hormone-receptor complex to "enhancer" elements of target gene promoters. Thus, understanding (i) how the receptor protein is able to specifically recognize its cognate hormone; (ii) how this binding results in the interaction of the receptor with target gene promoter elements; (iii) how this interaction leads to initiation of specific gene transcription; and, (iv) what the role of the hormone is in these processes, is essential in order to understand the molecular mechanism of steroid hormone-controlled gene activity. Such an analysis has now become possible following the recent cloning of several members of the steroid/thyroid hormone superfamily of nuclear receptor genes (for reviews and references, see reference 1).

STRUCTURE

Amino Acid Sequence Comparison Between Estrogen and Progesterone Receptors of Different Species Reveals a Segmented Structure

An alignment of the primary amino acid sequences of the human (2), chicken (3), rat (4) and Xenopus (5) estrogen receptor (ER) is shown in Figure 1. There are apparently two regions, C and D, which exhibit a high degree of conservation flanked by regions B, D and F of low homology. The

N-terminal region A of the mammalian ERs also shows an increased homology, but this segment is not conserved in the frog receptor. It is striking that region C is 100% conserved for the mammalian ERs and that there is only one amino acid difference in the Xenopus ER region C. Apparently, during evolution, a selective pressure has conserved this domain during the last 350 million years since the ancestors of frogs diverged from those of mammals. The segmented primary amino acid structure of the ER family, with two highly conserved regions, led to the hypothesis that these regions might represent distinct domains correlated with receptor function.

FUNCTION

The hormone binding domain. Steroid hormone receptors might be considered as proteins which exhibit (at least) three basic functional characteristics: they bind their cognate ligands, they interact with hormone responsive elements (HREs), usually located in the upstream region of target genes, and they activate transcription. One interpretation of the high degree of conservation of segments of the ERs was that these might correspond to functional domains, notably a hormone-binding domain, and/or a DNA-binding domain that triggers transcriptional activation. In order to test this working hypothesis, a series of deletion mutants (6) and the full-length estrogen receptor (2) was constructed and transiently expressed in HeLa-cells using the SV40-based eukaryotic expression vector pKCR2 (7). In order to define the hormone-binding domain, cytosolic

```
hER    1  MTMTLHTKASGMALLHQIQGNELEPLNRPQLKIPLERPLGEVYLDSSKPAVYNYPEGAAYEFNAAAA-----ANAQVYGQTGLPYGPGSEAAAFGSNGLG
rER    1                          M M  A    V N    F              AAAAG S P    SSIT           A S            A·B
cER    1           VT     T T S   S SDM VE N TG F      T D ---------GTT P   S TSAT  --S   SS A
xER    1         P PN TT VTF   SS  T T P  S   MTVENNRTGIF     TT D A     --------P  SSAS S AAS  --T   SS T

hER   96  GFPPLNSVSPSPLMLLHPPPQLSPFLQPHGQQVPYYLENEPSGYTVREAGPPAFYRPNSDNRRQGGRERLASTNDKGSMAMESAKETRYCAVCNDYASGY
rER  101  A Q                      HV   H  H          A A DT     S        N    S SSE N I                       C
cER   90  HS N P   VVF QTA   IHH S        QGSFGM  A    S     HSI  MS E  LS              S
xER   91  LHT N P  VVF AKL   IHH          S QGTFA   A T   SSS       S    MS A   PPSM T           S

hER  196  HYGVWSCEGCKAFFKRSIQGHNDYMCPATNQCTIDKNRRKSCQACRLRKCYEVGMMKGGIRKDRRGGRMLKHKRQRDDGEGRGEVGSAGDMRAANLWPSP
rER  201                                                                            L   N M TS                  D
cER  190                                                                   E M Q    EEQDS NGEASSTEL  PT  T
xER  191                                                                  L         KEEQ QKND DPSEIRT  SITVN-

hER  296  LMIKRSKKNSLALSLTADQMVSALLDAEPPILYSEYDPTRPFSEASMMGLLTNLADRELVHMINWAKRVPGFVDLTLHDQVHLLECAWLEILMIGLVWRS
rER  301  V HT    P                        LI    S                          G N                                E
cER  290  VV HN    P      E        E     V       N N     T
xER  291  SV--K MKL PV     E LI    ME A V  H SKL        T                                                V I

hER  396  MEHPVKLLFAPNLLLDRNQGKCVEGMVEIFDMLLATSSRFRMMNLQGEEFVCLKSIILLNSGVYTFLSSTLKSLEEKDHIHRVLDKITDTLIHLMAKAGL
rER  401  G                                                                                      N              E
cER  390  G                                AA                                     R Y                        S
xER  388  V  G S        R   L   VT AT   R R                                       E  DTL II   I   V F  S

hER  496  TLQQQHQRLAQLLLILSHIRHMSNKGMEHLYSMKCKNVVPLYDLLLEMLDAHRLHAPSRGGASVEETDQSHLATAGSTSSHSLQKYYI-TGEAEGFPATV  595
rER  501      R               N                       A  M VPP  PS Q TS   A    T  -PP        N I  600       F
cER  490  S   R               N                      AA SA PM  ENRNQ T  -PA     SF  NSK E SMQN I  589
xER  488  S   QR                                     I T KDKTTT-Q  DSRSPPT TVNGA PC  P  T-DT EVSLQS  586
```

Fig. 1. Comparison of the human (hER), rat (rER), chicken (cER) and Xenopus (xER) estrogen receptor amino acid sequences. Gaps (−) were introduced into the sequence to obtain maximal alignment of identical amino acids. The numbers on the left-hand side refer to the amino acid sequence. The sequence was divided into six regions (A–F) based on sequence homology between the four receptors. The three most highly conserved regions, A, C and E, are boxed.

extracts were prepared and analyzed for specific estradiol binding. It is apparent from Figure 2 that while regions A, B, C and F are dispensable for hormone binding, mutant HE14 contains all the sequences which are required for specific, high-affinity interaction with the steroidal ligand. Thus, it was concluded that region E comprises the estradiol-binding domain (6).

DNA binding. In the absence of steroid hormones, receptors are usually located in the cell nucleus and, upon homogenization, they can be recovered from the cytosolic fraction. After exposure to hormone in vivo, the receptor becomes tightly associated with nuclear structures and is isolated from nuclear preparations only by extraction with high concentrations of salt, e.g., with 400 mM KCl. To determine the region(s) responsible for tight nuclear binding, HeLa cells, after transient transfection with ER mutants deleted in the regions A, B, C and F, were exposed to radioactively labeled estradiol, and the radioactivity in the nuclear fraction was determined. The results clearly identified region C as being indispensable for the tight nuclear association of the steroid hormone receptor complex (Fig. 3, reference 6).

In vivo, steroid binding is the prerequisite for the hormone receptor complex to specifically bind to the hormone responsive enhancer element(s) of target genes. Having defined region C as indispensable for tight binding to the nucleus, the next question was whether this domain contained all the elements for the recognition of a HRE. In this respect, it was important to consider specific structural peculiarities of the 66 amino acid long core of region C which contains cysteine residues in a configuration reminiscent of the Xenopus 5S RNA transcription factor TFIIIA (13; for review, see reference 1 and references therein; see also below). To test the hypothesis that this region defined target gene specificity, a chimeric receptor was constructed which was basically an estrogen receptor but having the core of region C exchanged with the human

Region E is the hormone-binding domain

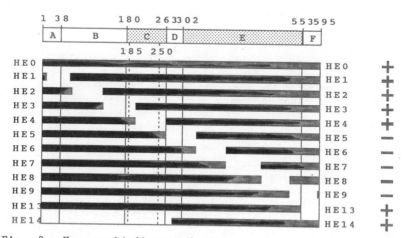

Fig. 2. Hormone-binding analysis of human estrogen receptor mutants. HE0 represents the wild type receptor, gaps indicate deletions. The division of the estrogen receptor into the six regions A-F is shown on the top (see Figure 1), numbers refer to amino acid positions. Plus (+) indicates the presence, minus (-) the absence of estradiol binding in cytoplasmic extracts of HeLa cells transiently transfected with the mutant receptors.

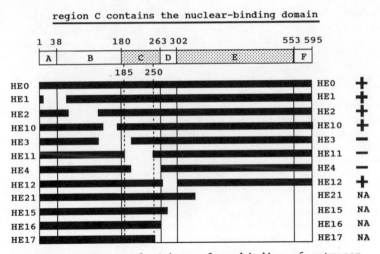

Fig. 3. Analysis of tight nuclear binding of estrogen receptor mutants. For description of the graphic presentation, see Figure 2; for details of the analysis, see text and reference 6.

glucocorticoid receptor (HGR) (8). This chimeric ER/GR was then analyzed for activation of the reporter genes vit-tk-Cat and MMTV-Cat which contain estrogen (ERE) and glucocorticoid (GRE) responsive elements, respectively. As is shown in Figure 4 (for further details, the reader is referred to references 1 and 8), it is now possible to activate the MMTV-GRE by the chimeric receptor ER-GR˙CAS under the control of estrogen. As expected, the ER-GR˙CAS is no longer able to activate the ERE of the vit-tk-Cat construct (Fig. 4). A reverse chimera has been constructed which results in a glucocorticoid receptor capable of activating the ERE of vit-tk-Cat by glucocorticoids due to the presence of an "ER-cassette" in the C region (9). These data indicate that the 66 amino acid long core of region C contains all the information necessary for the recognition of a target gene.

Further evidence supporting this conclusion came from "competition" experiments performed with C-terminally truncated mutants. HE0 and vit-tk-Cat were introduced into HeLa cells and the effect of cotransfected mutants (Fig. 5) on the activation of the vit-ERE was measured after estrogen treatment. All the mutants that are depicted in Figure 5 have either low (≤5% of HE0) or no capacity for activating transcription themselves (see also below). It is obvious from the comparison of mutants HE21 and HE36 that it is the core of region C which is apparently responsible for the inability of HE36 to compete with HE0 for binding to the vit-ERE. That HE16 and HE17 are not able to affect the HE0-induced transcription suggests that these particular truncations, close to or within region C, weaken the affinity for the ERE.

A superfamily of molecular receptor genes. A comparison of the primary amino acid sequences of all steroid and thyroid hormone receptors available to date (for review and references, see reference 1; see also references 10 and 11) reveals a strikingly similar structural organization (12). Regions which are homologous to the two highly conserved regions C and E of the estrogen receptor as described above can be found at corresponding positions in the progesterone, glucocorticoid, mineralocorticoid and vitamin D receptors and also in the c-erb A gene products. The DNA-binding domain containing region C (see above) is the region of

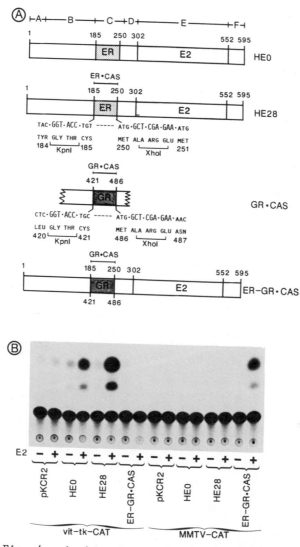

Fig. 4. A chimeric estrogen receptor (ER) containing the 66 amino acid core region of the glucocorticoid receptor (GR) transactivates transcription from the MMTV-LTR-GRE under the control of estrogen (E2). For details, see text and reference 8.

highest homology between all of these receptors, which differ from each other in size mainly due to the different lengths of the nonconserved regions A/B and D. Its most striking characteristics are the perfect conservation of the two motifs $Cys-X_2-Cys-X_{13}-Cys-X_2-Cys$ and $Cys-X_4-Cys-X_9-Cys-X_2-Cys-X_4-Cys$ (Fig. 6) which, interestingly, correspond to different exons of the chicken PR gene. The N-terminal cysteine motif is reminiscent of the DNA-binding region of a class of eukaryotic transcription factors that contain similar cysteine and histidine arrangements (for further details and references, see reference 1). In the Xenopus 5S RNA transcription factor TFIIIA (13), such a motif is repeated 9 times. Each repeat is believed to fold into DNA-binding "fingers" with the invariant cysteine and histidine pairs chelating Zn^{++} ions and that specific DNA

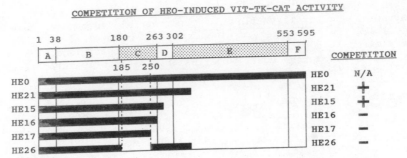

COMPETITION EXPERIMENTS SUGGEST THAT THE NUCLEAR BINDING
DOMAIN (REGION C), BUT NOT THE HORMONE BINDING DOMAIN
(REGION E), IS REQUIRED FOR RECOGNITION OF A TARGET GENE ERE.

COMPETITION OF HE0-INDUCED VIT-TK-CAT ACTIVITY

Fig. 5. Estrogen receptors containing an intact region
C are able to compete with wild type receptor (HE0) for
the activation of the vitellogenin estrogen responsive
element. For details, see text and reference 9.

contacts are made by some of the other amino acids. Assuming that cysteine and histidine are functionally equivalent with respect to the
chelation of Zn^{++} or other metal ions, the DNA-binding domain C of
steroid/thyroid hormone receptors might fold into similar structures.

Activation of transcription. An extensive panel of mutants was used
in order to define the region(s) which is (are) responsible for the
activation of transcription. The analysis was performed by CAT-assay and
by quantitative S1 mapping, using two different sets of constructs containing the vit-ERE and the PS2-ERE (Fig. 7, reference 9). As expected,
region C is indispensable for transcriptional activation. Since this
region contains the DNA-binding domain (see above), this is not a surprising result. Interestingly, however, all deletions affecting the
integrity of the hormone-binding domain E generate ER mutants (HE5 to HE9)
which are no longer able to transactivate transcription from the vit- or
PS2-ERE containing reporter genes (Fig. 7). Deletions in the N-terminal
region A/B of the estrogen receptor had different effects on the two
reporter genes. Whereas vit-tk constructs were insensitive to any deletion in this region, the pS2 construct showed a significant drop in the
ability to transactivate transcription from the pS2-ERE. Deletion of most
or of all of region A/B resulted in a five- to tenfold reduced transcriptional activity (mutants HE18 and HE19) when compared with HE0. Thus, it
appears that the presence of region A/B is not absolutely required for
stimulation of transcription, but it may be necessary so as to obtain
maximal stimulation with some estrogen responsive genes.

To further define the effects of C-terminal deletions on transcription, the set of mutants shown in Figure 8 was analyzed by quantitative S1
mapping. Whereas HE13 (deletion of region F) is fully active, HE21 and
HE15 are reduced in their potential to activate transcription from the
vit- or pS2-ERE by a factor of ~ 20. HE16 and HE17 do not activate
transcription, presumably due to a decrease in affinity to the EREs.

Mutant analysis of the cloned chicken progesterone receptor (cPR)
reveals structure-function characteristics similar to the estrogen receptor. Cloning (14) and sequencing (15) of the cPR demonstrated a structural organization characteristic for the steroid/thyroid hormone receptor

```
hER      185  CAVNDYASGYHYGVWSCEGCKAFFKRSIQG--HNDYMCPATNQCTIDKNRRKSCQACRLRKCYEVGM
hPR      567  CLICGDEASGCHYGVLTCGSCKVFFKRAMEGQ-HN-YLCAGRNDCIVDKIRRKNCPACRLRKCCQAGM
hGR      421  CLVCSDEASGCHYGVLTCGSCKVFFKRAVEGQ-HN-YLCAGRNDCIIDKIRRKNCPACRYRKCLQAGM
cVitD3    35  CGVQGDRAIGFHFNAMTCEGCKGFFRRSMKR--KAMFTCPFNGDCKITKDNRRHCQACRLKRCVDIGM
hc-erbA  102  CVVCGDKAIGYHYRCITCEGCKGFFRRTIQKNLHPSYSCKYEGKCVIDKVTRNQCQHCRFKKCIYVGM

GAL4      11  CDICRLKKLKCSKEKPKCAKCLKNNWEC
PPRI      34  CKRCRLKKIKCDQEFPSCKRCAKLEVPC
ARGII     21  CWTCRGRKVKCDLRHPHCQRCEKSNLPC

TFIIIA        C .DGCDKRFTKK..LK*RH..*.H
consenus

ADRI      98  CEVCTRAFARQEHLK*RHYR*SH
Repeat 1
```

Fig. 6. Alignment of receptor DNA-binding domains. Shown are the human estrogen (hER), the human progesterone (hPR), the human glucocorticoid (hGR), and the chicken vitamin D$_3$ (cVitD3) receptors together with human c-erb-A (hc-erb-A) gene product. Boxed areas indicate complete amino acid identity between all the sequences, and dashes (-) indicate amino acid gaps for optimal alignment. Conserved cysteines are shaded. The Cys-(X)$_2$-Cys-(X)$_{13}$-Cys-(X)$_2$-Cys motif present in the putative DNA-binding domain of the GAL4, PPR1 and ARGII yeast regulatory proteins is aligned with the corresponding motif of the steroid hormone receptors and erbA gene product. The consensus motif of the Xenopus transcription factor TFIIIA and the corresponding repeat 1 of the yeast regulatory proteins ADR1 are also shown. The pairs of cysteine and histidine residues dictating the postulated "finger" structures are boxed. Asterisks indicate positions where amino acid insertions may occur, and dots in the consensus sequence indicate variable residues. Numbers indicate the position of amino acid residues in each sequence. For review and references, see reference 1.

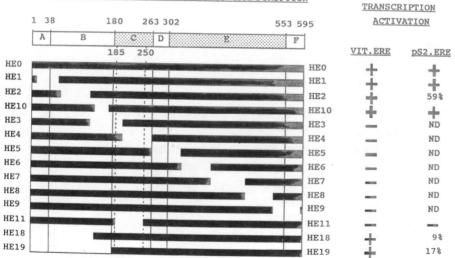

Fig. 7. Activation of transcription from the vitellogenin (vit) and pS2 estrogen responsive elements (EREs) by cotransfection of estrogen receptor mutants; for details see text and reference 9.

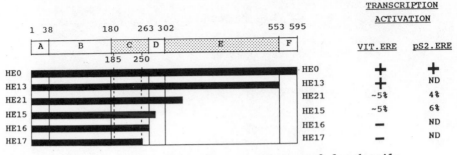

Fig. 8. As for Figure 7, see reference 9 for details.

supergene family described above. In an amino acid sequence comparison between the cPR and its rabbit (16) and human (17) homologues, the structural segmentation of the cPR shown in Figure 9 was defined (15 and see above) using the terminology of Krust et al. (3). As expected, the domains responsible for tight nuclear binding ("Nucl" in Figure 9) and progestin binding ("Cytopl." in Figure 9) could be correlated with regions C and E, respectively (15).

Quantitative S1 mapping and CAT-assays were used to define the PR regions which are indispensable for efficient transcriptional activation. Activation was monitored by interaction of the cPR with the hormone responsive element of the mouse mammary tumor virus (MMTV) long terminal repeat (LTR) which has the characteristics of a progesterone responsive element (PRE) (18). By comparison with a cloned human glucocorticoid receptor (19) inserted into the pKCR2 (7) eukaryotic expression vector (HG1 in Figure 10 and reference 9), it was found that the cPR had a fivefold higher potential to activate the MMTV-LTR-HRE (cPR0 in Figure 10). Deletion of the entire region A/B resulted in a 100 x lower transcriptional activity (cPR3) which was similar to deletions of the C-terminal hormone-binding domain E (cPR4 and cPR5). Mutant cPR5 exhibited constitutive activity as shown in the CAT-assay of Figure 10A. No trans-

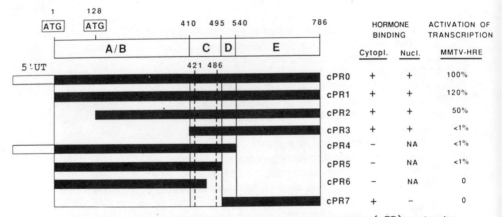

Fig. 9. Analysis of chicken progesterone receptor (cPR) mutants for hormone binding (Cytopl.), tight nuclear binding (Nucl.) and transactivation of the MMTV-LTR hormone responsive element (HRE). For details, see reference 15.

activation of transcription was observed for cPR mutants where the C-terminal deletion extended into region C (see cPR6 in Figure 10A). In conclusion, we find that in a fashion similar to that found with the estrogen receptor, the regions A/B and the hormone-binding domain are required in addition to the DNA-binding domain to efficiently activate transcription.

THERE ARE TWO TISSUE-SPECIFIC MECHANISMS WHICH MIGHT BE RESPONSIBLE FOR THE APPEARANCE OF THE CHICK OVIDUCT PROGESTERONE RECEPTOR FORMS A AND B

The chick oviduct PR [and the human T47D PR] differs from the other members of the steroid receptor family in that two forms A (79 kDa) and B (109 kDa) have been described and that different functional characteristics have been attributed to these forms (for review, see 20). Recent work has shown, however, that both forms are structurally and immunologically closely related (21, 22 for review, see 23). The cloning of the cPR cDNA (14,15) and gene (our unpublished results) excludes that forms A and B are the products of different genes. Furthermore, no evidence has been found that form A could be translated from an mRNA that is processed differently from that of form B. Since both forms bind the hormone and since the hormone-binding domain is located in the C-terminus, it is most probable that the difference between A and B is a consequence of different

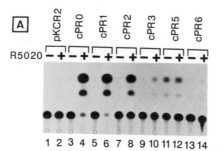

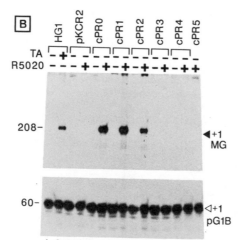

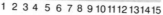

Fig. 10. Activation of transcription from the MMTV-LTR-HRE by cotransfection of chicken progesterone receptor (cPR) mutants. (A) Cat assay; (B) quantitative S1 mapping analysis. For details, see reference 15.

lengths of the N-terminal region. Thus, the two possibilities which have to be considered are (i) initiation of translation at an internal AUG; or, (ii) proteolysis in the N-terminus. As there is only one AUG (position 128) between the first AUG and the region C, this was the only candidate for internal initiation of translation. Using oligonucleotides complementary to the RNA sequences around AUG 1 or AUG128, it was shown that in vitro internal initiation can occur at AUG128 (15). This initiation was, however, less pronounced than initiation at other internal AUGs present in region E during in vitro translation. Expression of a protein initiating at AUG 128 in COS-1 cells (Fig. 11, lane 4) yielded a protein with a MW indistinguishable from that of natural chick oviduct PR from A (lane 1, 79 kDa form A). As expected, the protein expressed from the expression vector cPR0 or cPR1, containing the entire open reading frame of the PR, yielded a protein indistinguishable from oviduct form B (compare lanes 2 and 3 with lane 1 for the 109 kDa form B). Only in some cases (lane 2) on overexposed autoradiographs, a band corresponding in size to form A was noticed among other proteolytic fragments of the cPR form B. Thus, it was concluded that the appearance of form A is a chick oviduct cell-specific characteristic, presumably generated by either N-terminal proteolysis of form B close to, and/or internal initiation from, AUG 128.

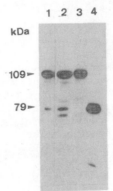

Fig. 11. Western blot of cytoplasmic extracts of Cos cells transiently transfected with cPR0 (lane 2), cPR1 (lane 3) and cPR2 (lane 4). A Western blot of a partially purified chick oviduct progesterone receptor form B preparation, run on the same gel, is shown for comparison (lane 1). The position of form B (109 kDa) and form A (79 kDa), still present in the form B preparation, are indicated.

REFERENCES

1. Gronemeyer H, Green S, Kumar V, Jeltsch JM, Chambon P. In: Sheridan, Blum, Trachtenberg, eds. Steroid receptors and disorders: cancer, bone and circulatory disorders. New York: Marcel Dekker Inc., 1987 (in press).
2. Green S, Walter P, Kumar V, et al. Human oestrogen cDNA: sequence, expression and homology to v-erb-A. Nature 1986; 320:134-9.
3. Krust A, Green S, Argos P, et al. The chicken oestrogen receptor sequence: homology with v-erbA and the human oestrogen and glucocorticoid receptors. EMBO J 1986; 5:891-7.
4. Koike S, Sakai M, Muramatsu M. Molecular cloning and characterization of rat estrogen receptor cDNA. Nucleic Acids Res 1987; 15:2499-

513.

5. Weiler IJ, Lew D, Shapiro DJ. The Xenopus laevis estrogen receptor: sequence homology with human and avian receptors and identification of multiple estrogen receptor messenger ribonucleic acids. Molecular Endocrinology 1987 (in press).

6. Kumar V, Green S, Staub A, Chambon P. Localisation of the oestradiol-binding and putative DNA-binding domains of the human oestrogen receptor. EMBO J 1986; 5:2231-6.

7. Breathnach R, Harris BA. Plasmids for the cloning and expression of full-length double-stranded cDNAs under control of the SV40 early or late gene promoter. Nucleic Acids Res 1983; 1111:7119-36.

8. Green S, Chambon P. Oestradiol induction of a glucocorticoid-responsive gene by a chimaeric receptor. Nature 1987; 325:75-8.

9. Kumar V, Green S, Stack G, Berry M, Jin JR, Chambon P. Functional domains of the human estrogen receptor. Cell 1987 (in press).

10. Arriza JL, Weinberger C, Cerelli G, et al. Cloning of human mineral-corticoid receptor complementary DNA: structural and functional kinship with the glucocorticoid receptor. Science 1987; 237:268-74.

11. Thompson CC, Weinberger C, Lebo R, Evans RM. Identification of a novel thyroid hormone receptor expressed in the mammalian central nervous system. Science 1987; 237:1610-4.

12. Green S, Chambon P. A superfamily of potentially oncogenic hormone receptors. Nature 1986; 324:615-7.

13. Miller J, McLachlan AD, Klug A. Repetitive zinc-binding domains in the protein transcription factor IIIA from Xenopus oocytes. EMBO J 1985; 4:1609-14.

14. Jeltsch JM, Krozowski Z, Quirin-Stricker C, et al. Cloning of the chicken progesterone receptor. Proc Natl Acad Sci USA 1986; 183:5424-8.

15. Gronemeyer H, Turcotte B, Quirin-Stricker C, et al. The chicken progesterone receptor: sequence, expression and functional analysis. EMBO J 1987 (in press).

16. Loosfelt H, Atger M, Misrahi M, et al. Cloning and sequence analysis of rabbit progesterone-receptor complementary DNA. Proc Natl Acad Sci USA 1986; 83:9045-9.

17. Mirashi M, Atger M, d'Auriol L, et al. Complete amino acid sequence of the human progesterone receptor deduced from cloned cDNA. Biochem Biophys Res Commun 1987; 143:740-8.

18. Cato ACB, Miksicek R, Schutz G, Arnamann J, Beato M. The hormone regulatory element of mouse mammary tumour virus mediates progesterone induction. EMBO J 1986; 5:2237-40.

19. Govindan MV, Devic M, Green S, Gronemeyer H, Chambon P. Cloning of the human glucocorticoid receptor. Nucleic Acids Res 1985; 13:8293-304.

20. Schrader WT, Birnbaumer ME, Hughes MR, Weigel NL, Grody WW, O'Malley BW. Studies on the structure and function of the chicken progesterone receptor. Recent Prog Horm Res 1980; 37:583-633.

21. Gronemeyer H, Harry P, Chambon P. Evidence for two structurally related progesterone receptors in chick oviduct cytosol. FEBS Lett 1983; 156:287-92.

22. Gronemeyer H, Govindan MV, Chambon P. Immunological similarity between the chick oviduct progesterone receptor forms A and B. J Biol Chem 1985; 260:6916-25.

23. Gronemeyer H, Govindan MV. Affinity labelling of steroid hormone receptors. Mol Cell Endocrinol 1986; 46:1-19.

12

MOLECULAR DETERMINANTS OF POSITIVE AND NEGATIVE REGULATION BY LIGAND-REGULATED TRANSCRIPTION FACTORS

Michael G. Rosenfeld, Christopher K. Glass, Rodrigo Franco, Stuart Adler, Marian L. Waterman, and Xi He

HHMI, Eukaryotic Regulatory Biology Program
University of California, School of Medicine
La Jolla, California 92093 USA

INTRODUCTION

The cloning of the glucocorticoid and estrogen receptors (1-5) permitted identification of a super-family of ligand-regulated transcription factors (e.g., 6-12), including the c-erb A gene products, which bound thyroid hormone (9,11). Knowledge of the structure of these transcription factors has permitted initial exploration of the functional domains. In the case of the glucocorticoid receptor, the DNA binding domain has been identified and appears to be sufficient for stimulation of transcription (13-17). In this manuscript, we review data regarding the regulation of rat prolactin and growth hormone gene expression by the estrogen and thyroid hormone receptors, respectively. The cis-active elements and the molecular determinants of positive and negative regulation of the prolactin gene by estrogen are defined. The T3 regulatory element in the rat growth hormone gene is defined, using an avidin/biotin complex DNA (ABCD) binding assay, and demonstrated to bind the c-erb A gene product.

DETERMINANTS OF ESTROGEN REGULATION OF THE RAT PROLACTIN GENE

Steroid hormone receptors are members of a family of ligand-activated intracellular receptors which increase transcription of regulated genes as a consequence of binding to specific DNA elements (2). Because the primary amino acid sequences have been deduced by analysis of cDNA clones of the receptor mRNAs and the DNA control elements responsible for induction are also known (1-12, 18-22), these transacting factors present a unique opportunity to study the mechanisms of regulation of transcription.

The primary sequence of the glucocorticoid receptor predicted three functional protein domains: a central DNA binding domain, a carboxy-terminal ligand-binding domain, and an amino-terminal domain (1,3,12). Site-directed mutagenesis of the glucocorticoid receptor cDNA provided experimental documentation of the putative domains, and demonstrated that the DNA binding domain was itself sufficient for activation of gene transcription (13-17). The subsequent cloning of the estrogen receptor revealed regions of high amino acid sequence homology to the glucocorticoid receptor (4,5); with highest conservation in the DNA binding (61.5%

homology) and steroid hormone binding domains (30% homology) (23). In vitro hormone binding and nuclear localization assays have confirmed the importance of these regions for DNA sequence recognition and estrogen binding (24,25).

In order to study the interaction of estrogen receptor with its DNA transcriptional element, we have utilized the rat prolactin (rPRL) gene because 17-beta-estradiol (E2) stimulates prolactin synthesis both in vitro and in cultured pituitary cells due to an accumulation of prolactin mRNA (26-31). Maurer reported a rapid increase in rPRL gene transcription after in vivo injections of E2 (32). Further evidence that estrogen directly increases prolactin gene transcription has been provided by transcription run-on assays using nuclei from rat GH4 pituitary cells (Fig. 1A). Based on the immediate 4.5-fold stimulation of the transcription rate, it was reasonable to suggest that the estrogen receptor directly interacted with a DNA element(s) near or within the prolactin gene.

Mapping of the ERE and Transfer of Regulation to a Heterologous Promoter

Deletion mapping of the 5' flanking sequences of the rat prolactin gene, using phenol red and serum-free media (33) localized the sequence conferring estrogen responsivity to a 235 bp fragment also containing a tissue-specific enhancer for the prolactin gene (34). Fragments containing the entire enhancer region transferred both enhancing activity and estrogen responsivity to the Herpes virus thymidine kinase (tk) promoter. Correct transcription start site usage in the absence and presence of estrogen were confirmed using primer extension to determine the cap site.

A 53 base pair oligonucleotide (PER-53) centering around a 15 bp (-1582-1568) sequence homologous to a glucocorticoid receptor consensus binding sequence (18,19) transferred estrogen responsivity to both the prolactin and tk promoters (Fig. 1B), consistent with the presence of a functional estrogen regulatory element (ERE) within this sequence. Transfer of this 53 base pair region itself conferred a threefold enhancement of both prolactin and tk promoters even in the absence of estrogen; this is consistent with the presence of an adjacent but separate tissue-specific enhancer element within this 53 base pair region (34).

Estrogen Receptor Binding to the ERE

The Avidin-Biotin-Conjugated DNA binding (ABCD) assay (35) was utilized to define the minimal ERE. An ^{35}S-methionine-labeled, in vitro translation product of the human estrogen receptor was incubated with the double stranded ERE oligonucleotide PER-53, containing biotin-11-dUMP at various positions as shown in Fig. 2B. Following the binding reaction, protein-DNA complexes were precipitated using streptavidin-conjugated to agarose beads. Precipitation of ^{35}S-methionine labeled receptor was dependent on specific rPRL sequences. An unrelated biotinylated probe derived from the rat prolactin gene (Fig. 2B) failed to precipitate significant levels of receptor (Fig. 2A). Estrogen receptor also bound to truncated rPRL ERE sequences containing 26 base pairs or 23 base pairs (PER-26 and PER-23 respectively, Fig. 2A, 2B). An element which transfers estrogen responsivity to the Xenopus vitellogenin A[2] gene (22) contains a 15 bp palindromic sequence with close homology to the prolactin ERE (Fig. 2D). To further delimit the nucleotides in the prolactin genomic element responsible for binding of the estrogen receptor, a biotinylated probe was prepared. Human estrogen receptor recognized and bound efficiently to an oligonucleotide containing 26 base pairs of Xenopus vitellogenin A2 5' flanking sequence centered around this sequence VER-26, reflecting a

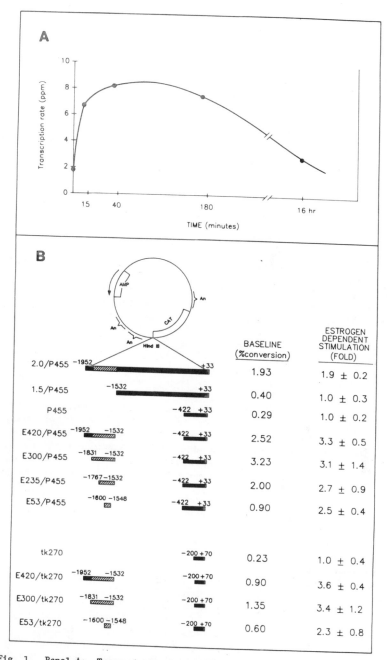

Fig. 1. _Panel A:_ Transcriptional analysis of the endogenous rPRL gene. Transcription of the prolactin gene was quantitated by a nuclear run-off assay following addition of 17-beta-estradiol. Values represent the average of triplicate hybridizations (each with 10^7 cpm input labeled RNA) in parts/million/kb probe size. _Panel B:_ Mapping the rPRL ERE. Fragments of the 5'-flanking region of the rPRL gene were placed 5' of the bacterial CAT gene and plasmids transfected in GC2 cells. 17-beta-estradiol (10^{-8} M) was added 24 h after transfection and cells harvested 48 hours posttransfection. Estrogen-dependent fold stimulation represents the increase in CAT activity with 17-beta-estradiol treatment of duplicate plates and are the average of 2-8 experiments. The hatched region represents the upstream enhancer for the rPRL gene.

preference for this palindromic sequence (Fig. 2B). Because the only sequence in common between the vitellogenin and prolactin 26 bp EREs is the central 15 base pairs, we have proposed the minimal binding site shown in Figure 2D (36). Introduction of a mutation in this region of the prolactin enhancer such that 11 base pairs (approximately one helix turn of DNA) abolished estrogen regulation (Fig. 2C). Removal of these 11 base pairs lowers baseline expression approximately 25% when compared to activity of the wild-type construction even in the absence of estrogen (Fig. 2, panel C). Although it is possible that a lower baseline reflects the loss of basal activation by the unoccupied estrogen receptor, an effect on the adjacent tissue-specific enhancer element is suggested to be a more likely explanation.

Estrogen Receptor Mutations: Regulation and DNA Binding

The rPRL ERE was utilized for functional analysis of estrogen receptor mutations. In order to investigate the functional consequences of removing the amino-terminal region, and the carboxy-terminal steroid binding domain, amino acids 40-144 were removed, and truncations beyond the DNA binding domain were constructed by introducing stop codons after amino acids 251, 264, and 318 (Fig. 3A). Point mutations were introduced within the DNA binding domain to convert two conserved cysteines at amino acids 185 and 221, to serine and glycine (S-185 and G-221), respectively. Each of these two amino acids is the first cysteine of two sequential amino acid motifs that resemble the zinc coordinated "finger" first described for transcription factor TFIIIA, and which is thought to be important for DNA binding (37). In addition, each of the putative fingers was removed by loop-out mutagenesis.

Estrogen receptor cDNA carrying site-specific mutations or deleted portions of the estrogen receptor molecule were placed into a plasmid such that the altered receptor coding regions could be transcribed in vitro with T3 RNA polymerase and subsequently translated in vitro in reticulocyte lysates. In vitro Translation products of T3 RNA polymerase-catalyzed transcripts of each cDNA were confirmed to exhibit the predicted size of the mutant proteins.

The estrogen receptor cDNAs were each fused 3' of the Rous Sarcoma Virus Long Terminal Repeat (RSV LTR) and co-transfected with rat prolactin, tk luciferase reporter genes to evaluate regulated expression. Co-transfection of wild type receptor cDNA and the ERE-containing reporter fusion gene into an estrogen receptor-negative breast carcinoma cell line (MB231N cells) followed by estrogen treatment 24 h later, resulted in a three- to sevenfold stimulation of luciferase activity. Estrogen receptor dependence was established by co-transfection with a control plasmid in which the cDNA for the neomycin resistance gene replaced the estrogen receptor cDNA which exhibited no hormone-dependent stimulation of luciferase activity above baseline (Fig. 3B). N-terminal deletion of the estrogen receptor resulted in retention of a small but significant estrogen-dependent stimulation; while DNA binding domain mutants including mutation of cysteine residues or deletion of either metal coordinated finger exhibited no significant estrogen dependent transcriptional activation (Fig. 3B). Mutations of the DNA binding domain are also abolished in DNA binding (Fig. 2A). Our results are consistent with the proposed importance of a coordinated finger structure for DNA recognition.

In the case of the glucocorticoid receptor, removal of the steroid-binding domain results in a constitutively activated transcription factor, implying that neither this domain nor the steroid hormone is itself required for transcriptional activation (14-17). This observation raises the question whether all members of this gene family would exhibit similar constitutive activation with removal of their respective ligand binding domain. Truncation of the estrogen receptor at amino acid 251 causes the receptor to become completely inactive, while mutations with truncations at amino acid 264 or 318 exhibited full, constitutive activity (Fig. 3B). The constitutively active receptor exhibited normal DNA binding activity (Fig. 2A).

These analyses provide an initial molecular identification of receptor domains conferring estrogen regulation upon the prolactin gene. Analysis of the C-terminal truncated estrogen receptor, in concert with similar data for the glucocorticoid receptor, suggests that the C-terminal ligand-binding domain of the steroid receptor gene family exerts a regulatory function and is itself not required for transcriptional activation. These studies, analogous to studies of the glucocorticoid receptor (20-24), indicate that the properties of DNA binding and transcriptional activation reside within the estrogen receptor region containing basic amino acids and the conserved cysteines and histidines. The carboxy-terminal boundary of this critical DNA binding and transcriptional domain appears to reside between amino acid 249 and 263.

The ERE we have identified in the rPRL gene lies >1.5 kb upstream from the PRL transcriptional start site. This ERE is adjacent to a binding site for a tissue-specific enhancer protein, which we refer to as Pit-1. Potential interaction between this tissue-specific factor and estrogen receptor is indicated in Figure 2C; baseline tissue specific expression in the absence of estrogen is decreased when the ERE is removed. The ERE identified for the rPRL gene is similar but not identical to the previously identified ERE sequence for Xenopus vitellogenin A2. There is no information regarding potential binding sites of other transcription factors adjacent to the vitellogenin ERE. Also, unlike the rPRL ERE, the vitellogenin ERE is a palindrome, and binds the estrogen receptor very efficiently in vitro (Fig. 2A). It is suggested that the higher affinity of binding may indicate an axis of symmetry in the active receptor, perhaps the consequence of dimerization.

Negative Regulation of the Rat Prolactin Gene by Steroid Hormones

The rat prolactin gene is under negative regulation by glucocorticoids and by high levels of estrogen receptor following removal of the ERE. At least four separate 5'-flanking regions confer this negative regulation, none of which contain a consensus ERE or GRE, but all of which contain a Pit-1 binding site. Further, based on a series of experiments, the DNA binding domain of the estrogen receptor is not required for the negative effect, but a sequence of hormone-binding domain is 63 amino acids between the DNA-binding and hormone-binding domains is obligatory for this inhibition of prolactin gene expression. These data suggest that two different domains are responsible for positive and negative regulation of prolactin gene transcription, respectively.

Regulation of Growth Hormone by T3

1,3,3-Triiodothyronine (T_3) stimulates growth hormone (GH) gene transcription in rat pituitary tumor cells (37-40), presumably the consequence of binding of nuclear T_3 receptors to regulatory elements which have been functionally identified 5' to the transcriptional start site (41-43). The study of the molecular mechanisms by which thyroid hormone activates gene transcription has been limited by the failure to purify nuclear T_3 receptors due to their low abundance and by the absence of defined T_3 receptor-DNA binding sites conferring T_3 regulation. Recently, human and avian c erb A gene products have been demonstrated to bind thyroid hormone with high affinity (9,10) and to exhibit molecular weight

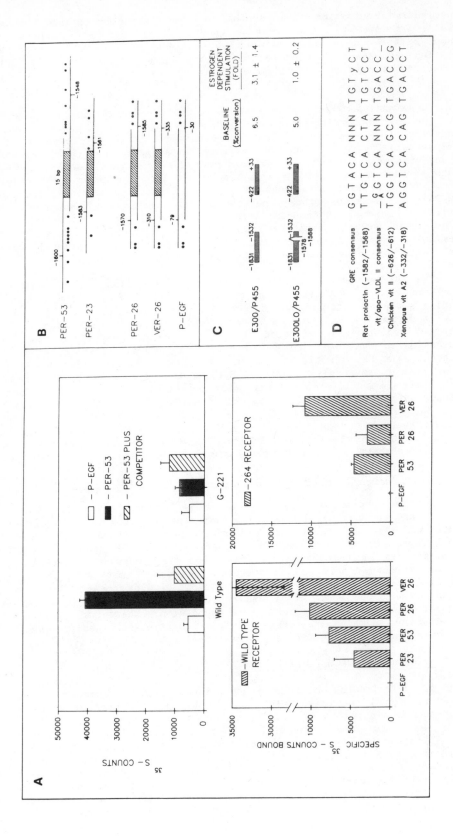

and nuclear association characteristic of the thyroid hormone receptor. We have developed an avidin-biotin complex DNA-binding (ABCD) assay which has permitted elucidation of the specific, high affinity binding of rat pituitary cell T_3 receptors.

Initial experiments identified the cis-active element in the growth hormone 5' flanking genomic sequence necessary for T_3' regulation (Fig. 4). An assay to detect specific binding was devised[3] which we term the ABCD (avidin-biotin complex DNA-binding) assay. Double stranded oligonucleotides containing the 5' flanking region of the GH gene necessary for T_3 regulation were prepared containing biotin-11-dUTP at various positions as shown in Figure 2A. As shown in Figure 5B, probe G209-146 resulted in specific precipitation of ^{125}I-T_3 activity over background; representing the binding of approximately 3.2 fmol of T_3 receptor, approximately 40% of the total T_3 receptor present in the binding reaction. Addition of a one hundredfold molar excess of unlabeled T_3 reduced the precipitated ^{125}I-T_3 to background levels (Fig. 2B), indicating that the T_3 binding protein that was being precipitated by the probe was present in limited quantities. The equilibrium binding constant for the T_3 receptor-DNA complex was estimated to be 1.4×10^{-9} M (35). The precipitation of ^{125}I-T_3 by G209-146 is dependent on the rat GH sequence contained within that probe (Fig. 5B).

Attempts to localize a T_3 receptor binding site by conventional DNase 1 footprinting techniques were successful using buffer conditions optimal for the ABCD binding assay, identifying a 16 bp protected region in the antisense strand between nucleotides -179 and -164 (Fig. 6). This

←

Fig. 2 (opposite page). Panel A: Avidin-Biotin-Conjugated-DNA binding of estrogen receptor mutants. Estrogen receptor was translated in the presence of 20 µM $ZnCl_2$ in rabbit reticulocyte lysates primed with capped RNA synthesized by T3 RNA polymerase using standard techniques. Oligonucleotide binding of in vitro translated wild type and G-221 receptor (Fig. 3A). Reactions with competitor used fiftyfold molar excess of restriction fragment containing rPRL nucleotides -1833 to -1532. Results shown are average and standard deviation of total counts from duplicate reactions. Lower left panel: Estrogen receptor binding to oligonucleotides containing the 15 bp ERE. Lower right panel: Binding of constitutive estrogen receptor to EREs. 25 µl reactions containing 10 µl (80,000 cpm, approximately 70 fmol) of 264 receptor (Fig. 3A). Specific counts shown are average and standard deviation of duplicate reactions minus nonspecific precipitated counts. Panel B: Schematic representation of the oligonucleotide probes used to assay estrogen receptor binding. PER-53, PER-23, PER-26, and P-EGF contain rPRL sequences with the illustrated 5' and 3' boundaries, flanked by identical restriction sites. VER-26 contains sequences from the Xenopus vitellogenin A2 gene. The hatched region depicts the 15 base pair homology common to four of the probes. P-EGF lacks this apparent homology. Asterisks indicate the positions of biotin-11-dUMP incorporation. Panel C: Site-directed mutagenesis of the ERE. Plasmid E300L0/P455 contains a deletion of 11 base pairs of the 15 base pair homology. Panel D: Sequence of the rPRL ERE and comparison with the GRE consensus and EREs of other genes.

sequence, which in the sense strand corresponds to 5' CAGGGACGTGACCGCA 3', is contained in the oligonucleotide probe demonstrated to specifically bind T₃ receptors and corresponds in location to a previously identified T₃-dependent DNase I hypersensitive site (15). A clear footprint could

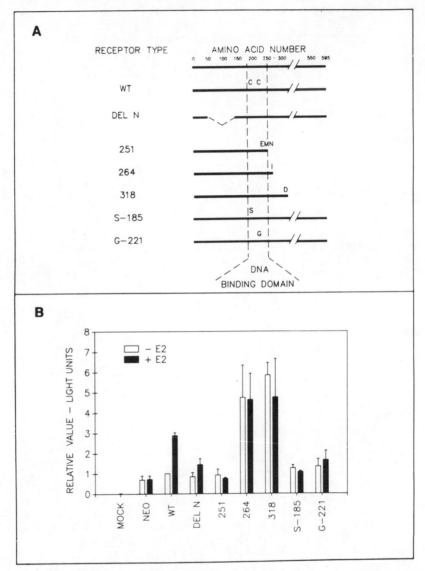

Fig. 3. Panel A: Mutant human estrogen receptors are represented by length and key amino acid changes. The DNA binding domain, amino acids 185-250, contains the two cysteine finger motifs. DEL N, (deletes amino acids 40-144 and includes a G-145->E); 251, (carboxy terminal deletion after amino acid 251); 264, (carboxy terminal deletion after amino acid 264); 318, (carboxy terminal deletion after 318); S-185, (amino acid C185->S); G-221, (amino acid C-221->G). Panel B: Transfectional analysis of estrogen receptor mutations. MB231N cells were co-transfected with estrogen receptor mutants and luciferase reporter plasmids under estrogen free conditions and hormone treated (10⁻⁸ M E2).

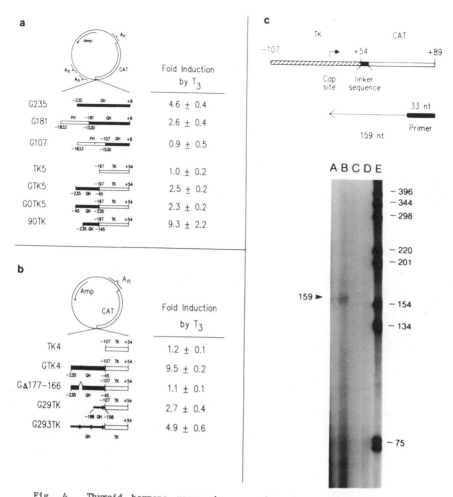

Fig. 4. Thyroid hormone responsiveness of various gene fusions containing rat GH 5' flanking sequences in GC cells. (a) Responsiveness of 5' and 3' deletions of the rat GH gene. The illustrated 3' deleted fragments were fused to a TK promoter fragment extending from -197 to +54 bp of the CAP site and placed proximal to the CAT gene in the same vector. (b) Functional analysis of the putative T_3 receptor binding site. Mutant G delta 177/166 contains a deletion of 11 bases of the T_3 receptor binding site from -177 to -166 base pairs from the CAP site. Plasmids G29TK and G293TK contain the 28 base pair region of the rat GH gene that binds the T_3 receptor in one and three copies, respectively. (c) Messenger RNA transcription initiation site analysis using a 33-nucleotide primer complimentary to nucleotides 67 to 89 of the CAT coding sequence used to determine the CAP site of transcripts of plasmids containing the TK promoter. Primer extension analysis was performed on 50 µg of total RNA. Lanes A and B represent the extension product from cells transfected with a plasmid containing the GH fragment from -235 to -45 fused to the TK promoter. Lanes C and D represent the extension product from cells transfected with a plasmid containing the TK promoter alone. No extension products were observed. The products shown in lanes A and C were from cells incubated in the absence of T_3 while those in lanes 2 and 4 were from cells treated with T3 at a concentration of 10^{-9} M. Lane E represents the products of a HindIII digest of pBR322 which are used as markers (in nucleotides).

not be detected in the sense strand itself, primarily due to inefficient digestion by DNase I in this G-rich region.

Removal of the putative T_3 receptor binding region identified by oligonucleotide and DNase I binding assays abolished the ability of the GH enhancer to confer T_3 regulation to the TK promoter (Fig. 4B), and a short oligonucleotide containing this sequence transferred T_3 regulation (Fig. 4B).

The short oligonucleotide used for transfer of T_3 regulation to the TK promoter (G186-158) also specifically bound nuclear T_3 receptors (Fig. 4), although significantly less efficiently than oligonucleotide G209-146. The possibility that this difference was due to the presence of an additional T_3 receptor binding site in G209-146 was ruled out using an oligo-

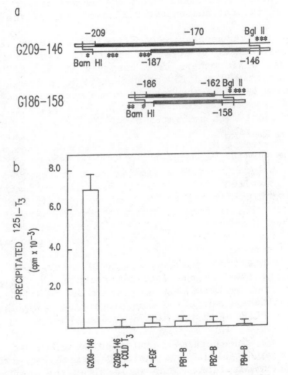

Fig. 5. Binding of T_3 receptors to oligonucleotide probes containing biotin-11-dUTP. (a) Schematic representation of two oligonucleotide probes used to assay T_3 receptor binding to GH 5' flanking sequences. Heavy lines indicate synthesized oligonucleotides with complementary 3' ends. (b) Precipitation of ^{125}I-T_3 labeled T_3 receptors from GC2 nuclear extracts by various oligonucleotide probes containing biotin-11-dUTP. P-EGF, PB1-B, PB2-B, and PB4-B are oligonucleotides of 68, 53, 55 and 58 base pairs containing 10, 11, 10 and 10 biotin-11-dUTPs respectively, representing rat prolactin genomic 5' flanking that lack apparent homology to the rat GH T_3 regulatory sequence. Precipitations were performed using 100 femtomole of each probe.

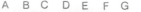

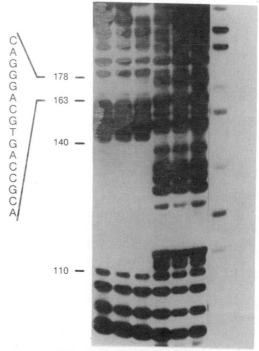

Fig. 6. DNase I footprinting of the rat GH enhancer element by GC2 nuclear extracts. A 16 bp protected region in the antisense strand is shown. A second footprint extending from -110 to -140 bp from the CAP site is also evident. Lanes A-C: Digestion of labeled GH enhancer following incubation with GC2 nuclear extract using 24, 12 and 4 µg of DNase I, respectively. Lanes D-F: Digestion of labeled GH enhancer with 24, 12 and 4 µg of DNase I in the absence of GC2 nuclear extract. Lane G: Molecular weight markers.

nucleotide containing the rat GH sequence from -177 to -235. This oligonucleotide failed to bind measurable amounts of T_3 receptors (data not shown). Competition experiments were also performed in which non-biotinylated G209-146 and G186-159 were used to compete for the binding of T_3 receptors with biotinylated G209-146. These experiments indicated that the relative affinity of T_3 receptors for G209-146 was two- to threefold higher than G186-159 (data not shown). A sequence extending from -209 to -146 bound T_3 receptor much better than a shorter sequence extending from -186 to -158. GC2 nuclear extracts may contain additional factors that stabilize the binding of T_3 receptors to the longer probe.

To test whether hc erb A also binds to this element, an ^{35}S-methionine-labeled in vitro translation which migrated as a doublet of approximate MW of 48 and 52 K_D on SDS gel electrophoresis and bound T_3 with a k_d of 5 x 10[-11] was tested for function. The hc erb A in vitro translation product bound to both the long and short probes bound the in vitro translation product significantly above background, while probes lacking homology to the T_3 receptor binding site of the GH gene, such as P-EGF, did not (Fig. 7). The hc erb A in vitro translation product was bound

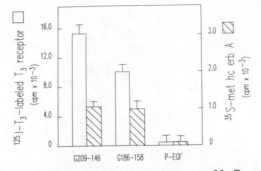

Fig. 7. Binding of rat pituitary cell T_3 receptors and an in vitro translation product of hc erb A to oligonucleotides containing 64 (-209 to -146) and 29 (-186 to -158) base pairs of 5' flanking GH sequence. Twenty-five μl of GC2 nuclear extract were labeled with ^{125}I-T_3, or four microliters of hc erb A in vitro translation product labeled with ^{35}S-methionine were assayed for binding to these oligonucleotides in an identical manner in the presence of 10 nM T_3.

equivalently by long and short T_3 regulatory regions. These results indicate that the hc erb A gene product specifically binds to the identical T_3 regulatory sequence that is bound by T_3 receptors from GC2 nuclear extracts and provide further evidence that the c erb A gene product functions to mediate the transcriptional effects of T_3.

The finding that the erb A in vitro translation product binds equivalently to short and long T_3 regulatory regions is consistent with the possibility that crude GC2 nuclear extracts contain an additional factor(s) that binds to the sequence between -210 and -181 and stabilizes the binding of the T_3 receptor to its cognate binding site. The T_3 regulatory element is highly homologous to the glucocorticoid or estrogen regulatory element if one could permit a difference in spacing between critical nucleotides. The operation of such a possibility is under investigation.

ACKNOWLEDGMENTS

CKG is a recipient of a Lucille P. Markey Scholarship for Biochemical Sciences, SA, an NIH Postdoctoral Fellowship. The studies presented in this manuscript were performed under HEMI and NIH support.

REFERENCES

1. Hollenberg SM, Weinberger C, Ong ES, et al. Primary structure and expression of a functional human glucocorticoid receptor cDNA. Nature 1985; 318:635-41.
2. Green S, Chambon P. A superfamily of potentially oncogenic hormone receptors. Nature 1986; 324:615-7.
3. Miesfeld R, Rusconi S, Godowski PJ, et al. Genetic complementation of a glucocorticoid receptor deficiency by expression of cloned receptor cDNA. Cell 1986; 47:389-99.
4. Greene GL, Gilna P, Waterfield M, Baker A, Hort Y, Shine J. Sequence and expression of human estrogen receptor complementary DNA. Science 1986; 231:1150-4.

5. Green S, Walter P, Kumar V, Krust A, Bornert J-M, Argos P, Chambon P. Human oestrogen receptor cDNA: sequence, expression and homology to v-erb-A. Nature 1986; 320:134-9.

6. Jeltsch JM, Krozowski Z, Quirin-Stricher C, et al. Cloning of the chicken progesterone receptor. Proc Natl Acad Sci USA 83:5424-8.

7. Loosfelt H, Atger M, Misrahi M, et al. Cloning and sequence analysis of rabbit progesterone-receptor complementary DNA. Proc Natl Acad Sci USA 1986; 83:9045-9.

8 Arriza, JL, Weinberger C, Cerelli G, Glaser TM, Handelin BL, Housman DE, Evans RM. Cloning of human mineralocorticoid receptor complementary DNA: structural and functional kinship with the glucocorticoid receptor. Science 1987; 237:268-75.

9. Sap J, Munoz A, Damm Y, et al. The c-erb-A protein is a high affinity receptor for thyroid hormone. Nature 1986; 324;635-40.

10. Weinberger C, Thompson CC, Ong ES, Lebo R, Gruol DJ, Evans RM. The c-erb-A gene encodes a thyroid hormone receptor. Nature 1986; 324:641-6.

11. McDonnell DP, Mangelsdorf DJ, Pike JW, Haussler MR, O'Malley BW. Molecular cloning of complementary DNA encoding the avian receptor for vitamin D. Science 1987; 235:1214-7.

12. Danielsen M, Northrop JP, Ringold GM. The mouse glucocorticoid receptor: mapping of functional domains by cloning, sequencing, and expression of wild type and mutant receptor proteins. EMBO J 1986; 5:2513-22.

13. Giguere V, Hollenberg SM, Rosenfeld MG, Evans RM. Functional domains of the human glucocorticoid receptor. Cell 1986; 46:645-52.

14. Hollenberg SM, Giguere V, Segui P, Evans RM. Colocalization of DNA-binding and transcriptional activation functions in the human glucocorticoid receptor. Cell 1987; 49:39-46.

15. Godowski PJ, Rusconi S, Miesfeld R, Yamamoto KR. Glucocorticoid receptor mutants that are constitutive activators of transcriptional enhancement. Nature 1987; 325:365-8.

16. Rusconi S, Yamamoto KR. Functional dissection of the hormone and DNA binding activities of the glucocorticoid receptor. EMBO J 1987; 6:1309-15.

17. Miesfeld R, Godowski PJ, Maler BA, Yamamoto KR. Glucocorticoid receptor mutants that define a small region sufficient for enhancer activation. Science 1987; 236:423-7.

18. Jantzen H-M, Strahle U, Gloss B, et al. Cooperativity of glucocorticoid response elements located far upstream of the tyrosine amino-transferase gene. Cell 1987; 49:29-38.

19. Scheidereit C, Westphal HM, Carlson C, Bosshard H, Beato M. Molecular model of the interaction between the glucocorticoid receptor and regulatory elements of inducible genes. DNA 1986; 5:383-91.

20. Walker P, Germond J-E, Brown-Luedi M, Givel F, Wahli W. Sequence homologies in the region preceding the transcription initiation site of the liver estrogen-responsive vitellogenin and apo-VLDLII genes. Nucleic Acids Res 1984; 12:8611-26.

21. Jost J-P, Seldran M, Geiser M. Preferential binding of estrogen-receptor complex to a region containing the estrogen-dependent hypomethylation site preceding the chicken vitellogenin II gene. Proc Natl Acad Sci USA 1984; 81:429-33.

22. Klein-Hitpass L, Schorpp M, Wagner U, Ryffel GU. An estrogen-responsive element derived from the 5' flanking region of the Xenopus vitellogenin A2 gene functions in transfected human cell. Cell 1986; 46:1053-61.

23. Krust A, Green S, Argos P, Kumar V, Walter P, Bornert J-M, Chambon P. The chicken oestrogen receptor sequence: homology with v-erb-A and the human oestrogen and glucocorticoid receptors. EMBO J 1986; 5:891-7.

24. Kumar V, Green S, Staub A, Chambon P. Localization of the oestradi-

ol-binding and putative DNA-binding domains of the human oestrogen receptor. EMBO J 1986; 5:2231-6.

25. Green S, Chambon P. Oestradiol induction of a glucocorticoid-responsive gene by a chimaeric receptor. Nature 1987; 325:75-8.

26. Maurer RA, Gorski J. Effects of estradiol-17-beta and pimozide on prolactin synthesis in male rats and female rats. Endocrinology 1977; 101:76-84.

27. Haug E, Gautvik KM. Effects of sex steroids on prolactin secreting rat pituitary cells in culture. Endocrinology 1976; 99:1482-9.

28. Lieberman ME, Maurer RA, Gorski J. Estrogen control of prolactin synthesis in vitro. Proc Natl Acad Sci USA 1978; 75:5946-9.

29. Stone RT, Maurer RA, Gorski J. Effect of estradiol-17-beta on preprolactin messenger ribonucleic acid activity in the rat pituitary gland. Biochemistry 1977; 16:4915-21.

30. Ryan R, Shupnik MA, Gorski J. Effect of estrogen on preprolactin messenger ribonucleic acid sequences. Biochemistry 1979; 18:2044-8.

31. Seo H, Refetoff S, Vassart G, Brocas H. Comparison of primary and secondary stimulation of male rats by estradiol in terms of prolactin synthesis and mRNA accumulation in the pituitary. Proc Natl Acad Sci USA 1979: 76;824-8.

32. Maurer RA. Estradiol regulates the transcription of the prolactin gene. J Biol Chem 1982; 257;2133-6.

33. Berthois Y, Katzenellenbogen JA, Katzenellenbogen BS. Phenol red in tissue culture media is a weak estrogen: implications concerning the study of estrogen-responsive cells in culture. Proc Natl Acad Sci USA 1986; 83:2496-500.

34. Nelson C, Crenshaw EB III, Franco R, Lira SA, Albert VR, Evans RM, Rosenfeld MG. Discrete cis-active genomic sequences dictate the pituitary cell type-specific expression of rat prolactin and growth hormone genes. Nature 1986; 322:557-62.

35. Glass CK, Franco R, Weinberger C, Albert V, Evans RM, Rosenfeld MG. A c-erbA binding site in the rat growth hormone gene mediates transactivation by thyroid hormone. Nature 1987 (in press).

36. Waterman ML, Adler S, Nelson C, Greene GL, Evans RM, Rosenfeld MG. A single domain of the estrogen receptor confers DNA binding and transcriptional activation of the rat prolactin gene. Mol Endocrinol 1987 (in press).

37. Evans RM, Birnberg NS, Rosenfeld MG. Glucocorticoid and thyroid hormones transcriptionally regulate growth hormone gene expression. Proc Natl Acad Sci USA 1982; 79:7659-63.

38. Diamond DJ, Goodman HM. Regulation of growth hormone messenger RNA synthesis by dexamethasone and triiodothyronine: transcriptional rate and mRNA stability changes in pituitary tumor cells. J Mol Biol 1985; 181:41-62.

39. Spindler SR, Mellon SH, Baxter JD. Growth hormone gene transcription is regulated by thyroid and glucocorticoid hormones in cultured rat pituitary tumor cells. J Biol Chem 1982; 257:11627-32.

40. Yaffee BM, Samuels HH. Hormonal regulation of the growth hormone gene relationship of the rate of transcription to the level of nuclear thyroid hormone-receptor complexes. J Biol Chem 1984; 259:6284-91.

41. Larsen PR, Harney JW, Moore DD. Sequences required for cell-type specific thyroid hormone regulation of rat growth hormone promoter activity. J Biol Chem 1986; 261:14373-6.

42. Flug F, Copp RP, Casanova J, Horowitz ZD, Janocko B, Plotnick M, Samuels HH. Cis-acting elements of the rat growth hormone gene which mediate basal and regulated expression by thyroid hormone. J Biol Chem 1987; 262:6373-82.

43. Casanova J, Copp RP, Janocko L, Samuels HH. 5' flanking DNA of the rat growth hormone gene mediates regulated expression by thyroid hormone. J Biol Chem 1985; 260:11744-8.

13

THE MAMMALIAN PROGESTERONE RECEPTOR: CLONING, IMMUNOLOCALIZATION AND MECHANISM OF INTERACTION WITH DNA

Jean-Francois Savouret, Hugues Loosfelt, Micheline Misrahi, Michel Atger, Alain Bailly, Martine Perrot-Applanat, Anne Guiochon-Mantel, Michel Rauch, and Edwin Milgrom

Hormones et Reproduction (INSERM U. 135), Faculte de Medecine Paris-Sud, 94275 Le Kremlin-Bicetre Cedex, France

Steroid hormone receptors have two essential functions: hormone binding, then DNA binding and transcription modulation. Although these two properties have been thoroughly characterized (review in 1), their structural basis has been only recently unraveled. The obtention of monoclonal antibodies against purified receptor and the subsequent cloning of receptor cDNA has been the key to the recent progress in the case of the progesterone receptor (2) as well as other steroid receptors (3-5).

STRUCTURE OF THE PROGESTERONE RECEPTOR (PR)

Rabbit PR

Poly A^+ RNA from rabbit uterus has been used to prepare cDNAs, which have been inserted in a λgt11 expression library, that was screened with monoclonal and polyclonal antibodies against PR (6). Positive clones were cross-controlled in several ways: antibody binding to fusion proteins was inhibited by purified receptor; conversely, fusion proteins blocked monoclonal antibody binding to the receptor.

The positive clones were used as probes in Northern blot analysis of mRNAs in various rabbit tissues. As expected, they hybridized with a mRNA species of 5900 nt present in the uterus, where it was induced by estrogen treatment, and in the vagina. Nontarget tissue mRNAs yielded no detectable signal (liver, spleen, kidney and gut). In a second step, the screening of a λgt10 cDNA library produced several cross-hybridizing clones that gave the complete sequence of the PR cDNA (Fig. 1). It consists of 930 amino acids and contains a central basic, cysteine-rich region (residues 568-645) bearing extensive homology to the glucocorticoid and estrogen receptors and the c-erbA oncogene. This segment defines two lateral regions. The C-terminal part is the steroid-binding domain and shows a strong homology to the glucocorticoid receptor and significant homology to the estradiol receptor. The N-terminal part, on the contrary, is extremely variable in the three receptors and c-erbA. No homology can be found, and its length variation accounts entirely for the size differences between these proteins. It has a high content in proline, a feature which associated to the central basic region has prompted some authors to compare these receptors to homeotic proteins (7). These comparative data remain hypothetical at the present time. cDNA clones for the chicken PR have also been isolated (8,9), but the sequence of this receptor has not been published.

Human PR

We have used the rabbit PR cDNA in the detection of its human counterpart in the breast cancer cell line T47D (10). Four overlapping clones were used to establish the full cDNA sequence shown in Figure 2.

The cDNA contains an open reading frame for 933 amino acids (930 in rabbit cDNA). The overall homology is 88.3% which is in agreement with the cross-hybridization of sequences and the cross-reaction of monoclonal antibodies between the two receptors (2).

Homology rises to 100% in the cysteine-rich basic segment, showing the selective pressure characteristic of a functionally important domain. This region is, in fact, responsible for the interaction of steroid receptors with DNA as will be discussed in section III (7,11). The C-terminal, steroid-binding region is also highly conserved which is in agreement with the similarities in hormonal specificities of both receptors. The N-terminal proline-rich region has somewhat lower homologies (82%) with its rabbit counterpart although 2 clusters of higher score (89% and 96%) may reveal functionally important segments that could be involved in interactions with the transcriptional machinery.

Northern blot analysis of mRNAs from T47D cells, MCF7 cells and normal uterine tissues revealed four major species (5100, 4300, 3700 and 2900 nt) and a minor one (5900 nt). The concentrations of PR mRNA in various cell lines and the uterus match their respective receptor content. The availability of this probe will be of interest in the search for mutated or abnormally expressed genes in cancer biopsies, as well as in the study of receptor expression in the genital tract and nervous system. Chromosome mapping studies have been performed in collaboration with M. F. Rousseau-Merck (INSERM U. 301) (12). The human PR gene was localized to 11q22-q23 and not to 11q13 as previously reported by Law et al. (13). These authors speculated about the presence in the same band 11q13 of c-int-2, a proto-oncogene that has been implicated in mouse mammary tumors. The 11q22-q23 localization has no relation with breast cancer-related oncogenes. The c-ets proto-oncogene has been mapped to 11q23-q24 by de Taisne et al. (14).

IMMUNOLOCALIZATION

Initial immunocytochemical studies using monoclonal antibodies confirmed the exclusive nuclear localization of PR even in the absence of hormone (15) as already reported by King and Green for the estradiol receptor (16). No staining could be detected in nontarget organs.

A strong heterogeneity in staining was observed among cells of a same type in several target tissues, suggesting the existence of differences or desynchronization in the hormonal sensitivity of sister cells.

Subcellular localization was further analyzed in uterine stromal cells using an immunogold method (17). Most of PR was localized in the nucleus where it was randomly associated with condensed chromatin in the absence of hormone. A very small amount of staining was also associated with the rough endoplasmic reticulum. This can be interpreted either as newly synthesized receptor or as an indication of a posttranscriptional function of the receptor. Upon hormone administration, the chromatin underwent extensive rearrangement while the receptor was displaced towards the borders of condensed chromatin and also the dispersed chromatin, both regions being the most active sites of transcription. These techniques have been applied to breast cancer biopsies, where immunolocalization of PR in the nucleus of breast cancer cells was in agreement with quantitative data from steroid-binding assays on tumor extracts. These studies revealed again a marked heterogeneity in staining between cells of a same lineage (18).

INTERACTION OF PR WITH GENOMIC DNA

High affinity interactions of hormone-receptor complexes with chromatin have been studied for a long time (19). Unfortunately, the complexity of the model has precluded the obtention of clearly interpretable results. The recent purification of receptors has, however, made possible the analysis of their interaction in vitro with naked DNA (20). These studies have revealed that purified receptors bind with high affinity to distinct portions of DNA mainly upstream and also within structural genes (21).

The portions of upstream sequence that bind hormone-receptor complexes have been linked to nonregulated promoters directing the transcription of their own genes or heterologous genes such as Chloramphenicol Acetyl Transferase. These constructions were used in transfection experiments on receptor-containing cell lines, where they displayed hormone-dependent transcription levels. Since these DNA sequences conferred hormone responsiveness, they were dubbed "hormone responsive elements" (HRE) (review in 22). These experiments have been performed with several HREs such as the vitellogenine gene estradiol HREs (23), the MMTV glucocorticoid and progesterone HREs (24), the lysozyme estradiol HREs (25) among others.

The mechanism of action of receptors seemed quite straightforward at that time. Upon hormone binding, receptors interact with HREs, considered as hormone-dependent enhancers, and induce chromatin modifications leading to the onset of RNA polymerase activity. However, only the advent of monoclonal antibodies allowed us to prepare ligand-free purified receptors to study the role of hormone agonists and antagonists on DNA binding. It came as a surprise that the hormone dependency of receptor binding to DNA or chromatin is observed in vivo and in crude cellular extracts, but not in vitro with purified receptor. The progesterone HREs in the uteroglobin gene have been mapped by filter-binding assay and DNAse footprinting. High affinity sites were found far upstream (-2700 to -2500) from the transcription start and within the first intron. These sites were occupied by the receptor in similar conditions whether it was ligand free, hormone bound or antagonist bound (RU 38486). In all cases, identical footprints were observed. These results led to the putative conclusion that in situ, the free receptor is stabilized away from the DNA by interacting with some nuclear component(s) that prevent its activation. The nature of this factor is unknown; a possible candidate is the 90 K protein (26). The purified receptor, liberated from that interaction might then readily activate and bind DNA. Other noteworthy data is the fact that hormone-dependent phosphorylation and antagonist binding do not modify the DNA receptor interaction (27). Thus, the biological significance of these two situations has to be searched elsewhere in the course of hormone-regulated gene expression.

As reported in the first section, the central cysteine-rich region of the receptors (C-region) is responsible for DNA binding as shown by

```
(-125) CGGGTCCAGcCAAACCCCACACCCATTTTCTCCTCCCTCTGcCCTATATCCCGGCACCCCTCCTCTC TAGCCTTTCCCTCCTCCCGAGAGACGGGGGAGGGAGAGAAAAGGGGAGTTCAGGTCGAC   -1
                                            10                  20                  30

        MetThrGluLeuLysAlaLysGluProArgAlaProHisValAlaLeuGlyGlyAlaProLeuLeuArgLeuArgProAspArgProGlyProPheGlnLeuGlySerGlnThrSer
        AtGACTGAGCTGGAGAAGGCAAAGGAACCTCGGGCTCCCCACGTGGCATTGGGTGGTGCTCCCCTACTCCGGCTGCGGCCGGACCGTCCTGGCCCTTCCAGGGGAGCCAGACCTCA 129
              40                  50                  60                  70                  80

        GluAlaSerSerValValSerAlaIleProIleSerAlaIleProProAspGlyLeuLeuProPheProArgProCysGlnLysGlnLeuAsnProProSerLeuSerAspValGluGly
        GAGGCCTCGTCTAGTCTCGTAGTCCCCATCCCCATCTCCCTGGACGGGTTGCTCTTCCCCGGCGTTGCAGGGGCAGAACCCCCACACCGTCGTTGTCAGcGTGGAGGGC 258
           90                  100                 110                 120

        AlaPhePheProGlyValGlyValGluAlaGlyAlaAspSerSerSerArgProProGluLysProGlyLeuLeuAspSerArgValLeuAlaAspThrLeuLeuAlaProSerGlyGlnSerHis
        GCATTTCCTGGAGTGGAAGTCCCCGGAGGGGCAGGAGCACGCAGCTCCAGAAAAGGACAGCGGGTGTCCTCGACGcTCGTcGGCCTCGGGTCCCGGCAGAGCCAC 387
        130                 140                 150                 160                 170

        AlaSerProAlaAlaThrCysGluAlaIleIleSerProTrpCysLeuProGluGlyProGluAspProArgAlaAlaAlaProAlaAlaAlaThrLysGlyValValAlaProLeuMetSerArgProGluAspLys
        GCCAGCCCTGCCACCTGCGAGGCCATCAGCCCGTGGTGCCTGCCTTGGGGGGACCTTCCCGAAGAcCCCCGGCTGCCCGCTGCCGCCACTAAAGGGTGTTGGCCCCGGTCATGAGCCGCCCGGAGGACAAG 516
                  180                 190                 200                 210

        AlaGlyAspSerSerGlyThrAlaAlaAlaHisLysValValProLeuPheSerProArgArgGlnLeuLeuLeuLeuLeuProSerGlySerGlyProHisIleTrpProAlaAlaValValProSerProGlnPro
        GCAGGCGGACAGCTCTGGGACGGCAGCGGCCCACAGGTGCTGCCCAGGCAGCTGCTCCCTCTCTGGAGAGCCCTCACTGGCCGCAGTGAAGGCCATCCCCGAGCCC 645
                  220                 230                 240                 250

        AlaAlaValGlnValGlnAspGluAspSerGluGlyLlyThrArgValGlyGlnThrAlaLeuGluGlyLyGlyThrAlaAlaAlaGlyGlyValAlaAlaProValAlaAlaSerGly
        GCTGCCGGTGCAGGTAGACGAGGAGACAGCTCCGAATCCGGGGCACCGTGGGCCGGCCAACCTGGGCACTGGGAGGCACGGGAGACCGGGCCGGGAGAGCTGCCCCCGTCGCTGGA 774
                  260                 270                 280                 290                 300

        AlaAlaAlaAlaGlyLlyValAlaLeuValProLysGlyAspProSerProArgAlaAlaProGluPheSerArgAlaLeuProGlyValArgSerLeuValAlaGluValSerAlaProGlyProGlyValAlaProGlyProGlnProTrpThrHisArgLeuGlyThrArgSerProLeuAlaProGlyArgGlySerProLeuAlaAlaThrSerValValAsp
        GCGGCCCAGGAGGCGTGCCCTTGTCCCCAAGGAAGATTCTCGCTTCTGGCGCGCCCAGGGTCTCTTGGCGGAGAAGACGCGCCGGTGGGCGTCCCGGTGGCGCTGGCCACCTCGGTGGTGGAT 903
                  310                 320                 330                 340

        PheIleHisValProIleLeuProLeuAsnHisAlaPheLeuAlaLlrThrArgThrArgLeuGluGlyThrGlnLeuLeuValLeuGlyLeuGlyLyValAlaAlaAlaAlaAlaAlaSerProPheValProGlnArgGlySer
        TTCATCCACGTGCCCATCCTGCCTCTCAACCAGCTTTCCAACCACAGCTTCCGACCGACCAGCTACGACGGCGGGCGCCGGGCCCTTCGTCCCCAGCGGGGCTCC 1032
                  350                 360                 370                 380

        ProSerAlaSerSerThrProValAlaAlaGlyGlyValGlyLeuProLysSerAspAspAspAlaPheProLeuTyrGlyAspPheGlnProProAlaLeuLeuLysIleLeuLys
        CCCTCTGCCTCGTCCACCCCTGTGGCGGGCGGCAGTTCCCCGACGTTCCCCTCTCACGGCGACCCGCCGCCCGGCCCCTCAAGATAAAG 1161
                  390                 400                 410                 420                 430

        GluGluLeuGluLaAlaGlyLluAlaIleAlaAlaAlaAlaAlaAlaAsnProAlaLeuAlaGlyAlaAlaAsnProAlaLeuAlaProAspPheGlnLeuLeuAlaAlaProAlaProAlaAlaProGlnGlnSerLeuProAspPheGlnLeuLeuAlaProAlaProAlaAlaProPheGlnLeuLeuAlaAlaAlaProValProAlaAlaProSerLeuProProGlnArgProProSerLeuProProPheGlnLeuLeuValAla
        GAGGAGGAAAAGCCGGCGGCGGCGGCATTCCCCGGACTTCCAGCTTGCAGAGCCGCGCGCCACCCTCGCTGCCGCCTCCGAGTG 1290
                                           440                 450                 460                 470

        ProSerSerArgProGlyGluValAlaValAlaAlaSerProGlySerAlaSerValSerSerSerSerGlySerThrLeuGluCysIleLeuLeuTyrLysAlaGluGluAlaProGlnGln
        CCCTCTCCAGACCCGGGAGCCGGCGGGTGGCGGCCTCCGTCCCTGTCCTGCGTCTGTCGGGGTGCACTCTGTACAAGGCAGAAGGCGGCCGGCCCCAGCAG 1419
                  480                 490                 500                 510

        GlyProPheAlaProLeuProGlyValAlaGlyValAlaGlyLysProProGlyGluValAlaIleLeuProArgAspPheGlyLeuLeuProSerThrSerGlyAlaSerAlaGlyAlaAlaGlyLyValAlaAlaAlaLeuAlaProAlaLeuGluTyrProThrLeu
        GGCCCCTTCGGCGCGCTGCCCTGCAAGCCTCCGGGGCGGCCCCTGCCCTCCACCTCGGCGACGGCCCTCGCCTCTGCCGCGCTC 1548
                  520                 530                 540                 550
```

GlyLeuAsnGlyLeuProGlnLeuGlyTyrGlnAlaAlaAlaValLeuLysGluGlyLeuProGlnValTyrThrProTyrLeuAsnTyrLeuArgProAspSerGluAlaSerGlnSerProGlnTyrSer
GGCCTCAACGGACTCCCGCAGCTGGGCTACCAGGCGGCCGCTGCTCAAGGAGGGCCTGCCGCAGGTCTACACGCCCTATCTCAACTACCTCAGGCCGGATTCAGAAGCCAGTCAGAGCCCACAGTACAGC 1677
560   570   580   590   600

PheGluLeuProGlnLysLysCysGlyLeuIleCysGlyHisAlaSerGluAlaSerGlyAlaSerHisTyrGlyLysLysTyrGlyValPheLeuValLeuLeuThrCysGlySerLysLysTyrGlnHisHisTyr
TTCGAGTCACTACCTCAGAAGATTGTTTGATCTGTGGGATGAAGCATCAGCTGTCATTATGGTGTCCTCACCTGTGGGAGCTGTAAGGCTCTTTTTAAAGGCGCAGCATAACTAT 1806
610   620   630   640

LeuCysAlaGlyIleArgAlaAsnAspCysIleLeuValAspLysIleArgArgLysAsnCysProAlaCysArgLeuArgLysCysCysGlnAlaGlyMetValLeuGlyGlyArgLysPheLysLysPheAsnLys
TTATGTGCTGGAAGAAATGACTGCATTGTTGATAAAATCCGGAGGAAAAACTGCCCAGCGTGTCGCCTTAGAAAGTGCTGCCAGGCATGGTCCTTGGAGGCGAAAGTTTAAAAAGTTCAATAAA 1935
650   660   670   680

ValArgValMetArgAlaLeuAspAlaValAlaLeuProGlnProValGlyIleProAsnGluSerGlnAlaLeuSerGlnArgPheThrPheSerProGlySerGlnIleThrIleGluAsnLeuLeu
GTCAGAGTCATGAGAGCACTCGATGCTGTTGCTCTCCCACAGCCAGTGGGCATTCCAAATGAAAGCCAAGGCACTCTCTCAACTGTTAATCAACCTGTTA 2064
690   700   710   720   730

MetSerIleGluProAspValIleTyrAlaGlyHisAspAsnThrLysProAspThrSerSerLeuLeuThrSerLeuAsnGlnLeuGlyGluArgGlnLeuLeuSerValValLysTrpSerLys
ATGAGCATTGAACCAGATGTGATCTATGCAGGACATGACAACACAAAGCCTGATACCTCCAGTTCTTTGCTGACGAGTCTTAATCAACTAGGCGAGCGGCAACTTCTTTCAGTGGTAAAATGGTCCAAA 2193
740   750   760   770

SerLeuProGlyPheArgAsnLeuHisIleAspAspGlnIleThrLeuIleGlnTyrSerTrpMetSerLeuMetValPheGlyLeuGlyTrpArgSerTyrLysHisValSerGlyGlnMetLeuTyr
TCTCTTCCAGGTTTTCGAAACTTACATATTGATGACCAGATAACTCTCATCCAGTATTCTTGGATGAGTTTAATGGTATTTGGACTAGGATGGAGATCCTACAAACATGTCAGTGGGCAGATGCTGTAT 2322
780   790   800   810

PheAlaProAspLeuIleLeuAsnGluGlnArgMetLysGluSerSerPheTyrSerLeuCysLeuThrMetTrpGlnIleProGlnGluPheValLysLeuGlnValSerGlnGluGluPheLeuCys
TTTGCACCTGATCTCATAATATTAAATGAACAGCGGATGAAAGAATCATCATTCTATTCACTATGCCTTACAATGTGGCAGAATACCGCAGGAGTTTGTCAAGCTTCAAGTTAGCCAAGAAGAGTTCCTCTGC 2451
820   830   840   850   860

MetLysValLeuLeuLeuLeuAsnThrIleProLeuGluGlyLeuArgSerGlnThrGlnPheGluGluMetArgSerSerTyrIleArgGluLeuIleLysAlaIleGlyLeuArgGlnLysGlyValVal
ATGAAAGTATTACTACTTCTTAATACAATTCCTTTGGAAGGACTAAGAAGTCAAAGCCAGTTTGAAGAGATGAGATCCAGCTACATTAGAGAGCTCATCAAGGCAATTGGTTTGAGGCAAAAAGGAGTT 2580
870   880   890   900

ValSerSerSerGlnArgPheTyrGlnLeuThrLysLeuLeuAspAsnLeuHisAspLeuValLysGlnLeuHisLeuTyrCysLeuAsnThrPheIleGlnSerArgAlaLeuSerValGluPhePro
GTTTCCAGCTCACAGCGTTTCTATCAGCTCACAAAACTTCTTGATAACTTGCATGATCTTGTCAAACAACTTCACCTGTACTGCCTGAATACATTTATCCAGTCCCGGGCGCTGAGTGTTGAATTCCA 2709
910   920   930

GluMetMetSerGluValIleLeuAlaAlaGlnMetValLysProLeuLeuPheHisLysLys
GAAATGATGTCTGAAGTTATTGCTGCAGGTTACCCAAGATATTGGCAGGGATGGTGAAACCACTTCTTCTTTCATAAAAGTGAATATTTTTCAAAGAATTAAGTGTTGTGGTATGTCTTTTC 2838

Fig. 1. Nucleotide sequence of the complete coding region of rabbit progesterone receptor cDNA and predicted amino acid sequence of the deduced protein. The cysteine-rich basic region is underlined. Stop codons and initiator codon defining the beginning and the end of the open reading frames are also underlined.

```
(-175) CTGACCAGCGCCGCCTCCCCGCCCCGACCCAGGAGGTGGAGATCCTCCGGT                              -121

CCAGCCACATTCAACACCCACTTTCTCCTCCTGCCCCTATATTCCGAAACCCCTCCTTCCTTTTCCCTTGGAGAGGGGAGGAGAAAAGGGAGTCCAGTCGTC   -1

     1                                  10                                  20                                  30
ATG ACT GCC CCA GCC GCT GTG CTC CCC CAC GCT ACC TCG CTG CAG ACC TTC CTG GAC GTT CTG ATC CCT GAG GTC TCC GTC CTG TGT CGC      90
MET THR ALA PRO ALA ALA VAL LEU PRO HIS ALA THR SER LEU GLN THR PHE LEU ASP VAL LEU ILE PRO GLU VAL SER VAL LEU CYS ARG
                                        40                                  50                                  60
GCA AAG CCG TTC CGG GCC GAC TCG GGA AGC GGT CAG CGG CCC GCC ACC CAG CGG CCC GTT TGC GAC GTG GAC CTG TAT CCT TCC AGA CGC     180
ALA LYS PRO PHE ARG ALA ASP SER GLY SER GLY GLN ARG PRO ALA THR GLN ARG PRO VAL CYS ASP VAL ASP LEU TYR SER PRO SER ARG
                                        70                                  80                                  90
CCT CGG CCC TGC GGA GAC AGC AGC CAA CCC CCA GTT TCC ATG CGG CTC AGC CCG GTC TTG GTC GAC AGT GAC CTG GAC AGT CTT CCC GAT     270
PRO ARG PRO CYS GLY ASP SER SER GLN PRO PRO VAL SER MET ARG LEU SER PRO VAL LEU VAL ASP SER ASP LEU ASP SER LEU PRO ASP
                                       100                                 110                                 120
GAA GCT ACA AGG CCC GGG CAG CAA CCC GGG GAA AAG GTC ACC AGC CGG TCC GAG GTG GAC CTG CTG GAC GAT CTT AGC AGC GGA GCT GCA     360
GLU ALA THR ARG PRO GLY GLN GLN PRO GLY GLU LYS VAL THR SER ARG SER GLU VAL ASP LEU LEU ASP ASP LEU SER SER GLY ALA ALA
                                       130                                 140                                 150
CCC TCA GGT GGC GGG GCC ACC CCC GCC GTT TCC CCG GTT GGG GTG GTC TTT GGC CCC CTT CCC GAA GAT GTC TTG GAC ACT CTG GAC GAT     450
PRO SER GLY GLY GLY ALA THR PRO ALA VAL SER PRO VAL GLY VAL VAL PHE GLY PRO LEU PRO GLU ASP VAL LEU ASP THR LEU ASP ASP
                                       160                                 170                                 180
CCA CCG GCT CGG GCC AGC CAG CGG CGG AGC ATG CTC CCG TCC CTG GAC GAC TGG TGG TGC CTG TGG CCC GAA GGG GTC TCC CCC ACG GCA     540
PRO PRO ALA ARG ALA SER GLN ARG ARG SER MET LEU PRO SER LEU ASP ASP TRP TRP CYS LEU TRP PRO GLU GLY VAL SER PRO THR ALA
                                       190                                 200                                 210
CCA CAT AAA CGG GTG CTG TCA CCA GTT CTC AGC TCC CTG GGG TGC AAG GTT GTT AGC GCC CCA GCC GCA TCC GGG GCC GCG ACG GCA GCT     630
PRO HIS LYS ARG VAL LEU SER PRO VAL LEU SER SER LEU GLY CYS LYS VAL VAL SER ALA PRO ALA ALA SER GLY ALA ALA THR ALA ALA
                                       220                                 230                                 240
GCC CAT GTG TCT CCG GCG GCT GGC GGT GAG GTT GGA GAG TCT GGC GCA GCA GCC CTC CTG GGG TCT CTG GGG GCC AGC TGG TCC GGT GGC     720
ALA HIS VAL SER PRO ALA ALA GLY GLY GLU VAL GLY GLU SER GLY ALA ALA ALA LEU LEU GLY SER LEU GLY ALA SER TRP SER GLY GLY
                                       250                                 260                                 270
AAG CCG TCT CGG CAG CCC GCT GCA GGA GGA GGA GGT GTC GTC GTC AGC GCC CCG CTC CCC CTG GCC ACC GTG AAG CTC CCC CTG GTC CCG     810
LYS PRO SER ARG GLN PRO ALA ALA GLY GLY GLY GLY VAL VAL VAL SER ALA PRO LEU PRO LEU ALA THR VAL LYS LEU PRO LEU VAL PRO
                                       280                                 290                                 300
CCT CGG GCT TCA GCG TTC GCC GGC GCG GCG GCC CTG GTC GTG GGG GCC GCG ATG GCG GCA GCC ACC GGC GCC ACC ACG ACG GTG AAG GTG     900
PRO ARG ALA SER ALA PHE ALA GLY ALA ALA ALA LEU VAL VAL GLY ALA ALA MET ALA ALA ALA THR GLY ALA THR THR THR VAL LYS VAL
                                       310                                 320                                 330
GGC GAT GTC TCA CAC GTG CTG ATC GCC CTG CTC AAT CTC TTG GCA GCC ACT CGG CTG GAA GAC AGT TAC GTA GGC TTC GAC GAC TAC GAC     990
GLY ASP VAL SER HIS VAL LEU ILE ALA LEU LEU ASN LEU LEU ALA ALA THR ARG LEU GLU ASP SER TYR VAL GLY PHE ASP ASP TYR ASP
                                       340                                 350                                 360
GGC GGG GCC GGG TTT GCC GCC ACC GCC CCG CCG CCC TCA GCC GCG CCC TCC GCC CCG GTC GCC CTG GCC GTC TTC GGC GAC TTC CCC GAC    1080
GLY GLY ALA GLY PHE ALA ALA THR ALA PRO PRO PRO SER ALA ALA PRO SER ALA PRO VAL ALA LEU ALA VAL PHE GLY ASP PHE PRO ASP
                                       370                                 380                                 390
TGC GCG TAC GCC GAC GCC GAC GAG GCC GCC CCT CTC TAC GGT GTG GTA GCC GCT CTA AAG ATA AAG GAG GAG GAG GAG GCC TTC CCG GAT    1170
CYS ALA TYR ALA ASP ALA ASP GLU ALA ALA PRO LEU TYR GLY VAL VAL ALA ALA LEU LYS ILE LYS GLU GLU GLU GLU ALA PHE PRO ASP
                                       400                                 410                                 420
GAG GAA GGC GGC GAG TCC TCC CGT CGC TAC CGT CCG GGT GCC GGT GCG GCC GGT GAT TTC CCG GAT GAC CCG GGG GGA GAG GAG GAG TTG    1260
GLU GLU GLY GLY GLU SER SER ARG ARG TYR ARG PRO GLY ALA GLY ALA ALA GLY ASP PHE PRO ASP ASP PRO GLY GLY GLU GLU GLU LEU
                                       430                                 440                                 450
CCA CCG CCG CCG CCG CTG CCG CCG AGA GCG ACC TCC AGA AGC CGA ATC GCC GTG GCG ACG GCC GCC GCA TCA CGC TCG GTC TCA TCT TCG    1350
PRO PRO PRO PRO PRO LEU PRO PRO ARG ALA THR SER ARG SER ARG ILE ALA VAL ALA THR ALA ALA ALA SER ARG SER VAL SER SER SER
                                       460                                 470                                 480
GCG TCC TCC TCG GAG TGC TGC ATC CTG TAC AAA CTG ATC CTG TAC CTG AGC CCC CAG GCC CCC CAG GGC CCC CCC CGG CCG TTC CCG CCC TGC   1440
ALA SER SER SER GLU CYS CYS ILE LEU TYR LYS LEU ILE LEU TYR LEU SER PRO GLN ALA PRO GLN GLY PRO PRO ARG PRO PHE PRO PRO CYS
```

Fig. 2. Nucleotide sequence of the complete coding region of human progesterone receptor cDNA and amino acid sequence of the deduced protein. Stop codons and initiator codon defining the beginning and the end of the open reading frame are underlined.

```
                              490                    500                      510
AAG  GCG  CCG  GGC  AGC  TGC  CTG  CTC  CCG  CGG  GAC  GGC  GGC  CTG  CCG  CCC  TCC  ACC  TCT  GCC  GCC  GCC  GGG  GCC  CCC  GCG
LYS  ALA  PRO  GLY  SER  CYS  LEU  LEU  PRO  ARG  ASP  GLY  GLY  LEU  PRO  PRO  SER  THR  SER  ALA  ALA  ALA  GLY  ALA  PRO  ALA        1530

                              520                    530                      540
CTC  TAC  CCT  GCA  CTC  GGC  CTC  AAC  TAC  CTG  CCG  CTC  CCG  CAG  CCG  CTC  TAC  GGC  CAG  GTC  CTG  CCG  TAC  CCG
LEU  TYR  PRO  ALA  LEU  GLY  LEU  ASN  TYR  LEU  PRO  LEU  PRO  GLN  PRO  LEU  TYR  GLY  GLN  VAL  LEU  PRO  TYR  PRO                    1620

                              550                    560                      570
TAT  CTC  AAC  TAC  CTG  CTG  CCG  GAC  CTG  CTC  CAG  GTC  TTA  CCT  TCA  AGC  TTC  TAC  ATC  TGT  TTA  ATC  TGT
TYR  LEU  ASN  TYR  LEU  LEU  PRO  ASP  LEU  LEU  GLN  VAL  SER  PHE  SER  PHE  LEU  TYR  ILE  CYS  LEU  ILE  CYS                        1710

                              580                    590                      600
GGG  GAT  GAA  GCA  GCA  GAG  GAT  GTT  GGT  GGG  AGC  GTC  ACC  AGC  TTC  AGC  GTC  AAG  GTC  GCA  ATG  GAA  GGG  CAG  CAC  AAC
GLY  ASP  GLU  ALA  ALA  GLU  ASP  VAL  GLY  GLY  SER  VAL  THR  SER  PHE  SER  VAL  LYS  VAL  ALA  MET  GLU  GLY  GLN  HIS  ASN        1800

                              610                    620                      630
TAC  TTA  TGT  GCT  GGA  AGA  AAT  GAC  TGC  ATC  GTT  GAT  AAA  ATC  CGC  CGC  AAA  AAC  TGT  CCG  GCT  GCT  AGA  AAG  TGC  GCT
TYR  LEU  CYS  ALA  GLY  ARG  ASN  ASP  CYS  ILE  VAL  ASP  LYS  ILE  ARG  ARG  LYS  ASN  CYS  PRO  ALA  ALA  ARG  LYS  CYS  ALA        1890

                              640                    650                      660
GGC  ATG  GTC  CTT  GGA  GGT  GGC  AAA  TTT  AGA  TTC  GTG  AGA  GCA  CTG  GAT  GCT  GTT  GCT  CTC  CCA  CAG  CCA  CCA  GTG
GLY  MET  VAL  LEU  GLY  GLY  GLY  LYS  PHE  ARG  PHE  VAL  ARG  ALA  LEU  ASP  ALA  VAL  ALA  LEU  PRO  GLN  PRO  PRO  VAL            1980

                              670                    680                      690
GGC  GTT  CCA  AAT  GAA  AGC  CTA  GCC  GTT  TCA  ACT  TTT  TCA  CCA  AGA  TTC  TTC  CCA  ATA  TTG  CTG  ATC  CTG  AAC  CTG
GLY  VAL  PRO  ASN  GLU  SER  LEU  ALA  VAL  SER  THR  PHE  SER  PRO  ARG  PHE  PHE  PRO  ILE  LEU  LEU  ILE  LEU  ASN  LEU            2070

                              700                    710                      720
TTA  ATG  AGC  ATT  GAA  ATT  GGT  ATC  GAT  GTG  CCA  GGA  CAT  GAC  AGT  TCT  TTG  ACA  AGT  CTT  AAT  CAA
LEU  MET  SER  ILE  GLU  ILE  GLY  ILE  ASP  VAL  PRO  GLY  HIS  ASP  SER  SER  LEU  THR  SER  LEU  ASN  GLN                            2160

                              730                    740                      750
CTA  GGC  GAG  AGG  CAA  CTT  TCA  GTA  GTC  AAG  TCT  TGG  AGA  AAC  TTG  CCA  GGT  GTT  AAC  TCC  AGT  CAG  ATA  CTC
LEU  GLY  GLU  ARG  GLN  LEU  SER  VAL  VAL  LYS  SER  TRP  ARG  ASN  LEU  PRO  GLY  VAL  ASN  SER  SER  GLN  ILE  LEU                    2250

                              760                    770                      780
ATT  CAG  TAT  TCT  TGG  ATG  AGC  TTA  ATG  GTG  TTT  GGT  CTA  GGA  TGG  AGA  TCC  TAC  GTC  AGT  CAG  ATG  CTG  TAT  TTT  GCA
ILE  GLN  TYR  SER  TRP  MET  SER  LEU  MET  VAL  PHE  GLY  LEU  GLY  TRP  ARG  SER  TYR  VAL  SER  GLN  MET  LEU  TYR  PHE  ALA        2340

                              790                    800                      810
GAT  CTA  ATA  CTA  AAT  GAA  CAA  CGG  ATG  CAG  GAG  TCA  ACC  ATG  TAC  TGC  TTA  TTA  TCA  CCA  ATC  CCA  CAG  GAG  TTT  GTC
ASP  LEU  ILE  LEU  ASN  GLU  GLN  ARG  MET  GLN  GLU  SER  THR  MET  TYR  CYS  LEU  LEU  SER  PRO  ILE  PRO  GLN  GLU  PHE  VAL        2430

                              820                    830                      840
CTT  CAA  GTT  AGC  CAA  GAA  GAG  TTC  CTC  TGT  ATG  AAA  GTA  TTG  CTT  CTT  CTT  AAT  ACA  ATT  CCT  TTG  GAA  GGG  CTA  CGA
LEU  GLN  VAL  SER  GLN  GLU  GLU  PHE  LEU  CYS  MET  LYS  VAL  LEU  LEU  LEU  LEU  ASN  THR  ILE  PRO  LEU  GLU  GLY  LEU  ARG        2520

                              850                    860                      870
TTT  GAG  GAG  ATG  TCA  GGG  ATT  GCA  AAG  GCA  ATT  GGT  TTG  AGG  CAA  AAA  GGA  GTT  GTG  TCG  AGC  TCA  CAG  CGT  TTC
PHE  GLU  GLU  MET  SER  GLY  ILE  ALA  LYS  ALA  ILE  GLY  LEU  ARG  GLN  LYS  GLY  VAL  VAL  SER  SER  SER  GLN  ARG  PHE            2610

                              880                    890                      900
TAT  CAA  CTT  ACA  AAA  CTT  CTT  GAT  AAC  CTA  CAG  GAG  CTT  GTC  AAG  CTC  CAT  CAG  TCG  TAC  AGT  ATT  CAG  AAA  CCC  GCA
TYR  GLN  LEU  THR  LYS  LEU  LEU  ASP  ASN  LEU  GLN  GLU  LEU  VAL  LYS  LEU  HIS  GLN  SER  TYR  SER  ILE  GLN  LYS  PRO  ALA        2700

                              910                    920                      930
CTG  AGT  GTT  GAA  TTT  CCA  GAA  ATG  ATG  TCT  GAA  GTT  ATT  GCT  GCA  ATA  TTG  GCA  GGG  ATA  TTG  CCC  CTT  CTC  TTT
LEU  SER  VAL  GLU  PHE  PRO  GLU  MET  MET  SER  GLU  VAL  ILE  ALA  ALA  ILE  LEU  ALA  GLY  ILE  LEU  PRO  LEU  LEU  PHE            2790

CAT  AAA  AAG  TGAATGTCATCTTTTCTTTAAGAATTAAATTTGTGG
HIS  LYS  LYS                                                                                                                            2839
```

deletion experiments (11). Steroid and DNA-binding domains can be dissociated and recombined in a heterologous manner between different receptors, indicating their relative independence (28). Conversely, DNA binding and transcription regulation activities cannot be dissociated. Deletion studies show that the removal of the steroid-binding domain elicits a constitutive unregulated induction of transcription by the deleted receptor (29). These results can be explained either by the loss of attachment sites to the stabilizing factor or by unmasking of preexistent DNA-binding sites. We have addressed this problem by electron microscopy studies, performed in collaboration with B. Theveny and E. Delain (CNRS UA 147). Receptor oligomers bind to the HREs of the MMTV LTR promoter and the uteroglobin promoter. Native DNA molecules, where HREs are present in doublets separated by spacer DNA as in the case of the uteroglobin gene, interact with purified receptors to form loops.

The size of proteins bridging the loops is roughly twice the size of the proteins involved in single site interaction, suggesting the loops are formed by protein-protein interactions between two DNA-bound receptor oligomers. The promoter of the MMTV LTR has two adjacent HREs. Progesterone receptors bound at both positions. Since these sites were close one to the other, it was difficult to decide if the receptors were interacting or just apposed. However, tight protein-protein interactions appear more likely than simple side-by-side apposition since no receptor molecule was ever observed in a "trans" position, and receptor oligomers were able to bridge independent DNA fragments when incubated with a molar excess of DNA (30). The existence of cooperative processes in these interactions is currently under study in our laboratory. Similar interactions have been described in prokaryotic systems such as the bacteriophage lambda (31).

A function for this receptor-receptor association upon binding to the HREs could be to induce a further protein-protein interaction with a transcription factor and/or RNA polymerase to activate transcription. This interaction may take place at a distance since the intervening DNA could then loop out.

The loop formation might explain why almost all steroid regulated genes have several HREs (22) and the activity of the HREs at distance of the start sites for transcription upstream or downstream from these sites. Experimental support to this hypothesis is also given by transfection experiments which show that deletion of one HRE of a native pair lowers considerably the efficiency of hormone induction of transcription (32). Cordingley et al. have recently shown that glucocorticoid receptor binding to the HREs in MMTV occurs simultaneously with the binding of Nuclear Factor 1 (NF1) (33). Mutagenesis experiments on receptors will certainly shed light on the role and the nature of these receptor-receptor interactions at a finer level and help to define their correlation with biological activity.

REFERENCES

1. Eriksson H, Gustafsson JA. Steroid hormone receptors: structure and function. Nobel Symposium n°57. Amsterdam: Elsevier Science Publishers, 1983.
2. Logeat F, Vu Hai MT, Fournier A, Legrain P, Buttin G, Milgrom E. Monoclonal antibodies to rabbit progesterone receptor: crossreaction with other mammalian progesterone receptors. Proc Natl Acad Sci USA 1983; 80:6456-9.
3. Okret S, Wikstrom AC, Wrange O, Anderson B, Gustafsson JA. Monoclonal antibodies against the rat liver glucocorticoid receptor. Proc Natl Acad Sci USA 1984; 81:1609-13.

4. Westphal HM, Moldenhauer G, Beato M. Monoclonal antibodies to the rat liver glucocorticoid receptor. EMBO J 1982; 11:1467-71.
5. Greene GL, Nolan C, Engler JP, Jensen E. Monoclonal antibodies to human estrogen receptor. Proc Natl Acad Sci USA 1980; 77:5115-9.
6. Loosfelt H, Atger M, Misrahi M, et al. Cloning and sequence analysis of rabbit progesterone-receptor complementary DNA. Proc Natl Acad Sci USA 1986; 83:9045-9.
7. Weinberger C, Hollenberg SM, Rosenfeld MG, Evans RE. Domain structure of human glucocorticoid receptor and its relationship to the v-erb-A oncogene product. Nature 1985; 318:670-2.
8. Conneely OM, Sullivan WP, Toft DO, et al. Molecular cloning of the chicken progesterone receptor. Science 1986; 233:767-70.
9. Jeltsch JM, Krozowski Z, Quirin-Stricker C, et al. Cloning of the chicken progesterone receptor. Proc Natl Acad Sci USA 1986; 83: 5424-8.
10. Misrahi M, Atger M, d'Auriol L, et al. Complete amino acid sequence of the human progesterone receptor deduced from cloned cDNA. Biochem Biophys Res Commun 1987; 143:740-8.
11. Kumar V, Green S, Staub A, Chambon P. Localisation of the oestradiol-binding and putative DNA-binding domains of the human oestrogen receptor. EMBO J 1986; 5:2231-6.
12. Rousseau-Merck MF, Misrahi M, Loosfelt H, Milgrom E, Berger R. Localization of the human progesterone receptor gene to chromosome 11q22-11q23. Hum Genet 1987 (in press).
13. Law ML, Kao FT, Wei Q, et al. The progesterone receptor gene maps to human chromosome band 11q13, the site of the mammary oncogene int-2. Proc Natl Acad Sci USA 1987; 84:2877-81.
14. de Taisne C, Gegonne A, Stehelin D, Bernheim A, Berger R. Chromosomal localization of the human proto-oncogene c-ets. Nature 1984; 310:581-3.
15. Perrot-Applanat M, Logeat F, Groyer-Picard MT, Milgrom E. Immunocytochemical study of mammalian progesterone receptor using monoclonal antibodies. Endocrinology 1985; 116:1473-84.
16. King WJ, Greene GL. Monoclonal antibodies localize oestrogen receptor in the nuclei of target cells. Nature 1984; 307:745-7.
17. Perrot-Applanat M, Groyer-Picard MT, Logeat F, Milgrom E. Ultrastructural localization of the progesterone receptor by an immunogold method: effect of hormone administration. J Cell Biol 1986; 102: 1191-9.
18. Perrot-Applanat M, Groyer MT, Lorenzo F, et al. Immunocytochemical study with monoclonal antibodies to progesterone receptor in human breast tumors. Cancer Res 1987; 47:2652-61.
19. Barrack ER, Coffey DS. The role of nuclear structure in hormone action: the nuclear matrix. In: Eriksson H, Gustafsson JA, eds. Steroid hormone receptors: structure and function. Nobel Symposium n°57. Amsterdam: Elsevier Science Publishers, 1983:221-31.
20. Payvar F, Wrange O, Carlstedt-Duke J, Okret S, Gustafsson JA, Yamamoto KR. Purified glucocorticoid receptors bind selectively in vitro to a cloned DNA fragment whose transcription is regulated by glucocorticoid in vitro. Proc Natl Acad Sci USA 1981; 78:6628-32.
21. Payvar F, De Franco D, Firestone GL, et al. Sequence-specific binding of glucocorticoid receptor to MMTV DNA at sites within and upstream of the transcribed region. Cell 1983; 35:381-92.
22. Yamamoto KR. Steroid receptor regulated transcription of specific genes and gene networks. Annu Rev Genet 1985; 19:209-52.
23. Klein-Hitpab L, Schorpp M, Wagner U, Ryffel GU. An estrogen-responsive element derived from the 5'flanking region of the Xenopus vitellogenin A2 gene functions in transfected human cells. Cell 1986; 46:1053-61.
24. Cato ACB, Miksicek R, Schutz G, Arnemann J, Beato M. The hormone

regulatory element of mouse mammary tumor virus mediates progesterone induction. EMBO J 1984; 5:2237–40.

25. Renkawitz R, Schutz G, von der Ahe D, Beato M. Sequences in the promoter region of the chicken lysozyme gene required for steroid regulation and receptor binding. Cell 1984; 37:503–10.

26. Catelli MG, Binart N, Jung-Testas I, et al. The common 90-kd protein component of non-transformed "8S" steroid receptors is a heat-shock protein. EMBO J 1985; 4:3131–5.

27. Bailly A, Le Page C, Rauch M, Milgrom E. Sequence-specific DNA binding of the progesterone receptor to the uteroglobin gene: effects of hormone, antihormone and receptor phosphorylation. EMBO J 1986; 5:3235–41.

28. Green S, Chambon P. Oestradiol induction of a glucocorticoid-responsive gene by a chimaeric receptor. Nature 1987; 325:75–8.

29. Godowski PJ, Rusconi S, Miesfeld R, Yamamoto KR. Glucocorticoid receptor mutants that are constitutive activators of transcriptional enhancement. Nature 1987; 325:365–8.

30. Theveny B, Bailly A, Rauch C, Rauch M, Delain E, Milgrom E. Association of DNA-bound progesterone receptors. Nature 1987; 329:79–81.

31. Ptashne M. DNA-binding proteins. Nature 1984; 308:753–4.

32. Kuhnel B, Buetti E, Diggelmann H. Functional analysis of the glucocorticoid regulatory elements present in the mouse mammary tumor virus long terminal repeat. A synthetic distal binding site can replace the proximal binding domain. J Mol Biol 1986; 190:367–78.

33. Cordingley MG, Riegel AT, Hager GL. Steroid-dependent interaction of transcription factors with the inducible promoter of mouse mammary tumor virus in vivo. Cell 1987; 48:261–70.

14

ISOLATION AND SEQUENCE OF THE HUMAN GLUCOCORTICOID RECEPTOR GENE PROMOTER. CLONING OF THE HUMAN ANDROGEN RECEPTOR cDNA

Manjapra V. Govindan, Marco Burelle, Celine Cantin,
Martine Devic,[2] Claude Labrie, Fernand Labrie,
Yves Lachance, Gilles Leblanc, Claude Lefebvre,
Pravin Patel,* Jacques Simard, and Udo Stropp[2]

MRC Group in Molecular Endocrinology, Laval
University Medical Center, Quebec G1V 4G2;
*Department of Microbiology, Faculty of Medicine,
Laval University, Quebec, G1K 7P4, Canada;
[2]L.G.M.E., C.N.R.S., U-184, INSERM Institut de
Biochimie Biologique, 27085 Strasbourg, France

We have isolated the promoter region of the human glucocorticoid receptor (hGR) gene from the λEMBL-3 human genomic library using synthetic oligonucleotides corresponding to the 5' end of hGR cDNA. The clone was fine mapped by restriction digestion, hybridization with hGR cDNA probes and by DNA sequence analysis and found to contain an open reading frame corresponding to the hGR cDNA from amino acids 1-131 separated by a large intron from the 5' noncoding sequences. The promoter region of the hGR has been identified by primer extension, nuclease S_1 mapping using hGR mRNA from human prostatic carcinoma cells (LNCaP) and human breast tumor cells (MCF-7), by in vitro transcription using hGR-DNA fragments as template and by DNA sequence analysis. The sequence of the hGR promoter reveals that it contains neither a "TATA box" nor a "CAAT box" and has an extremely high "G+C" content. Gene transfer studies with hGR-CAT chimeric plasmids into COS-cells showed that the hormonal regulatory sequences of hGR is contained within a 4 kb EcoRl-XbaI fragment.

In order to define the functional domains of the human androgen receptor (hAR) involved in gene regulation by androgens, complementary DNA (cDNA) clones encoding the human androgen receptor has been isolated from a human testis λgt-11 cDNA library using synthetic oligonucleotides homologous to the human glucocorticoid, estradiol, progesterone and aldosterone receptors as probes. The cDNA clones were characterized after their insertion into a bacterial expression vector in the proper orientation and in vitro transcription using T7-RNA polymerase and in vitro translation of the mRNA in rabbit reticulocyte lysate followed by incubation with tritium-labeled DHT (dihydrotestosterone) in the presence and absence of various steroid hormones. The clones giving rise to proteins which bound [³H]-DHT with high affinity and specificity were chosen for further studies. Northern hybridization results, obtained by using the AR cDNA as probe, detected the presence of multiple mRNA species in human MCF-7 cells, human LNCaP cells and rat ventral prostate. Using a similar approach, human mineralocorticoid receptor (hMR) cDNA from the human testis cDNA library was also isolated.

INTRODUCTION

Steroid hormone receptors are a family of regulatory proteins, which control the gene expression through their dependency of binding to their respective ligand. Activation or inhibition of transcription of selected genes results from the specific interaction of the hormone-receptor complex with the promoter elements (1). The ability of the purified glucocorticoid receptor (GR) to interact with specific sequences in different regulated genes has been well documented (2-10). The studies of steroid hormone receptors is of paramount interest not only for elucidating how the receptor interacts specifically with its ligand, but also for understanding the mechanism leading to the regulation of transcription through specific DNA-protein interactions. To investigate the regulation of the expression of the human GR gene (hGR) at the molecular level, we identified and characterized the 5' flanking region of this gene.

Steroid hormones interact with specific receptors to regulate gene expression in target cells (1,11-14). Critical to the understanding of the molecular mechanism of androgen action is the determination of the structure and function of its receptor (15).

The characterization of the androgen receptors (AR) has been severely hampered by the low levels of AR found in target tissues. The isolation and expression of AR cDNA should permit further insight into AR structure and function as well as its regulation at the molecular level. Based upon our current knowledge of the mechanism of steroid hormone action, androgen AR complexes play a major role in the growth of prostate cancer in man (16-18). It has also been demonstrated that a deficient or qualitatively abnormal AR is responsible for the unresponsiveness found in the testicular feminization syndrome (Tfm) in which genotypic males develop female secondary sex characteristics (19-22). A better understanding of androgen action would lead to improved treatments for androgen-dependent diseases.

Various investigators have reported the monomeric form of AR to range from 3 to 4.5S and 42 to 61Å, indicating a molecular weight ranging from 60,000 to 120,000 (23-26). AR purified from steer seminal vesicle was shown to consist of two polypeptides of 60,000 and 70,000 Da (5) while rat prostate AR weighed 86,000 Da (6) and demonstrated specific activity. AR purified from rat Dunning R3327 tumor showed a band of 120,000 Da (19).

The recent cloning of the human estradiol (27), glucocorticoid (28,29), progesterone (30), mineralocorticoid (31) and androgen receptor (32) have demonstrated a high degree of structural homology between these transcriptional regulatory proteins. The putative DNA-binding of these receptors is a highly conserved 66-amino-acid region which have the potential to adopt a conformation analogous to the two DNA-binding fingers proposed for the Xenopus 5S genes encoding the transcriptional factor III A, but involving two pairs of cysteines instead of pairs of cysteines and histidines (33). Significant homology is also found in the hormone-binding region located in the C-terminal half of each of the receptors. We describe here the isolation and characterization of cDNA clones corresponding to the human AR mRNA.

MATERIALS AND METHODS

DNA analysis and sequencing were performed as described (34). Poly A+ RNA was isolated from human prostatic carcinoma cells (LNCaP), human breast tumor cells (MCF-7) and prostates of intact, castrated and DHT-treated castrated DHT (5α-dihydrotestosterone) rats (35). Primers were synthesized in a Biosearch DNA synthesizer and primer extension was performed as described (36). Nuclease S_1 mapping was done according to a modification of procedures described in "Basic Methods in Molecular Biology" (37). In vitro transcription using the Hela cell extracts were performed according to the manufacturer's instruction (Gibco-BRL, Eukaryotic in vitro transcription system) and the transcripts were purified as described by Weingartner and Keller (38). Nuclease S_1 mapping of the transcripts were done as described (37).

The Probes for Screening the cDNA Library

Oligonucleotides corresponding to homologous regions of the putative DNA and hormone-binding domains of hGR in open reading frame (orf) were synthesized in a Biosearch DNA synthesizer and purified by high pressure liquid chromatography (HPLC). Oligonucleotides 358, 359 and 361 encoded amino acids 435 to 448, 468 to 477 and 616 to 626, respectively. The 3 oligonucleotides were [^{32}P]5' end-labeled separately and an equimolar mixture was used for screening (2 x 10^6 Cherenkow counts per filter).

cDNA Library, Screening and Characterization

A human testis cDNA library in λgt-11 (Clonetech Laboratories, USA) containing double-stranded cDNA prepared from poly A+ RNA of high molecular weight was used. The library was retitrated and found to contain 85.3% recombinants. The library was plated at a density of 25,000 recombinants on 85 mm agar plates made in NZCYM medium using 4 ml of 0.7% top agarose in the same medium. A total of 2.5 x 10^6 recombinants were screened. The positive plaques were purified by a second cycle of screening and the λgt-11 recombinants were prepared by phage lysate using Y1088 as host. The insert size was determined by EcoR1 digestion, separation of the DNA fragments on 1% agarose gel by electrophoresis followed by staining with ethidium bromide and photography. The agarose gels were then transferred onto Hybond N membranes (39).

The filters were hybridized subsequently with 358, 359, 361, hGR$_{orf}$, and hER$_{orf}$ and hPRcDNA, respectively. The clones other than hGR ^{orf} and larger than 1 kb were subcloned into pBR 322 and analyzed by restriction digestion and electrophoresis. The clones were classified into different groups based on their cross-hybridization to one another and intensity of cross-hybridization. The largest cDNA clones from each batch were subcloned into an expression vector BlueScribe M13 (BSM13) (Stratagene, Palo Alto, USA). Clones were selected in both orientation and large-scale plasmids were prepared.

Expression of the Protein and Hormone Binding Assay

The plasmids in BSM13 were digested with BamHI or HindIII restriction enzymes to linearize the cDNA. 0.5 µg of the linearized cDNAs were transcribed in vitro using the T7-RNA polymerase and the mRNAs were dissolved in 1 µl water and translated in vitro using rabbit reticulocyte lysate N90 from Amersham and labeling with 2 µCi of [^{35}S]-methionine in a final volume of 10 µl. The in vitro translation products were analyzed by SDS-PAGE and fluorography (40).

Hormone Binding Assay

50 µg of the plasmids containing the cDNAs inserted in the proper orientation were linearized with BamHI or HindIII, and in vitro transcription was performed on a large scale to produce 40 µg of mRNA. 20 µg of

the RNAs were translated in vitro (final volume, 250 μl) and after the translation, diluted to 500 μl with binding buffer (20 mM Tris-HCl, pH 7.4, 50 mM NaCl, 2 mM EDTA, 5 mM β-mercaptoethanol, 0.2 mM PMSF and 10% glycerol). 100 μl of the diluted translation products were incubated in duplicate with 5 nM [^{3}H]-DHT in the presence and absence of 500 nM cold R1881, 5 nM [^{3}H]-aldosterone in the presence and absence of 500 nM cold aldosterone and 25 nM [^{3}H]-dexamethasone in the presence and absence of 2.5 μM cold dexamethasone overnight at 4°C.

The contents of each tube were further diluted to 200 μl and an equal amount of hydroxylapatite (1:1 suspension in phosphate buffer) was added and incubated at 0°C for 1 h with occasional mixing. After centrifugation and washing the hydroxylapatite 5 times with 1 ml phosphate buffer, the protein bound radioactivity was released by incubating with 1 ml ethanol for 1 h with occasional mixing. The ethanol supernatant was separated by centrifugation and the radioactivity was determined by scintillation counting. The ER$_{orf}$ served as controls during these experiments.

Northern Blot Analysis

To determine the size and nature of AR mRNA, poly A+ RNA from LNCaP cells and MCF-7 cells as well as poly A+ RNA from intact prostates of castrated (3 days) and DHT-treated castrated rats were isolated and size separated on a 1% formaldehyde-agarose gel (39). The RNAs were transferred onto Zeta probe-membrane (BioRad, Canada) and hybridized with nick-translated hAR-cDNA probe.

Southern Blot Hybridization

20 μg of human DNA prepared from MCF-7 were digested with ECOR1, HindIII and PstI restriction enzymes to completion and separated on a 1% agarose gel. After Southern transfer (41) onto Zeta probe membrane, the blot was hybridized under high stringency conditions with a nick-translated hAR probe.

RESULTS AND DISCUSSION

Southern Analysis

The genomic organization of the hGR gene was analyzed by digestion of human MCF-7 DNA with several restriction enzymes followed by Southern analysis (Fig. 1 A and B). The same blot was hybridized with nick-translated hGR cDNA sequences from 1-1630 (panel A) and 1-2850 (panel B). cDNA sequences 1-1630 contained the complete amino-terminus until the end of v-erbA homology region. 1-2850 contained the complete hGR$_{orf}$. The hGR cDNA has been mapped to human chromosome No. 5 and evidences are found that similar sequences may be present elsewhere (28). These results suggest the complexity of the hGR gene and also that it may be between 20-30 kb.

Isolation of 5'-Specific hGR Genomic Clones

Genomic clones containing the 5' end of the hGR gene were isolated from a human λEMBL-3 genomic library (42) by screening with [^{32}P]-end labeled 5'ATC TCC CCT CTC CTG AGC AAG CAC ACT GCT 3' corresponding to the anti-mRNA strand coding for amino acids 16-25 of hGR. The first exon of hGR gene was detected with a synthetic oligonucleotide "338" corresponding to the anti-mRNA strand of hGR "5' TCCGCAGTTCCCGCCGCG3' from the 5' nontranslated region. One of the positive clones isolated contained 3 EcoR1 fragments of 4.5, 3.5 and 0.8 kb, respectively. The 3.5 kb EcoR1-

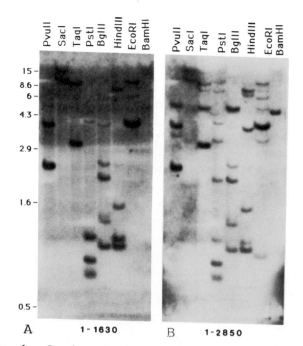

Fig. 1. Southern analysis: Human genomic DNA (30 µg) was digested with one of the following enzymes: PVUII, SacI, TaqI, PstI, BglII, HindIII, EcoRl or BamHI, and electrophoresed on a 1.5% agarose gel. The DNA was transferred to diazo-benzyloxymethyl (DMB) paper and hybridized with the nick-translated hGR 1-1630 and hGR 1-2850 cDNA probes. The position of the DNA size markers are indicated in kilobases.

EcoRl genomic subclone contained the possible codons of the amino acids at the amino terminus of the hGR (1-131), including 14 nucleotides of the 5' noncoding region. The 4.5 kb EcoRl-EcoRl genomic subclone contained 1600 bp SmaI-SmaI fragments which hybridized to the oligo "338" and found to contain the nucleotides -88 to -45 from the 5'-untranslated region of the hGR cDNA. Sequence analysis of the SmaI-SmaI subclone of the 4.5 kb EcoRl-EcoRl genomic clone revealed that one exon is located within this fragment. This exon contains the 5'-untranslated region (-88 to -45) and ends at CG and the adjacent intron begins with the sequence GT. The sequence between the beginning of hGR$_{orf}$ and the first exon was not found in the SmaI-SmaI fragment. These 27 nucleotides may be present in a separate exon.

Primer Extension

To identify the 5' boundary of the hGR RNA, 5' end [^{32}P]-labeled oligonucleotide "338" (-45 to -62) corresponding to the anticoding strand was prepared and hybridized to LNCaP and MCF-7 poly A + RNA. The primer was extended with murine reverse transcriptase and the sizes of the resulting products were determined by gel electrophoresis under dena-turing conditions, followed by autoradiography. The most abundant extension product has a length of 88 bases (Fig. 2, indicated by an arrow) from both LNCaP and MCF-7 mRNAs (Fig. 3, lane 6 and 8, respectively). Minor extension products of 163, 136, 132, 120, 110 and 39 bases in length were observed in which the 136 bases long product appears to be more predominant in LNCaP than in MCF-7 cells mRNA. This may suggest that the hGR gene transcription may be heterogenous. At least two of these start sites, 136 and 39 bases which are unique to LNCaP cells, suggest that amplified and rearranged hGR genes are present in LNCaP cells. The predominant extended product in both MCF-7 and LNCaP is of 88 bases long, indicating the major hGR population is transcribed from the same gene and transcription is occurring at the same start site in both cell types.

Nuclease S₁ Mapping

The SmaI-SmaI (1.6 kb) genomic subfragment (Fig. 2) inserted into the BSM13 [BS(SmaI-SmaI 1.6] at the 3' to 5' orientation to the T7-RNA pol-

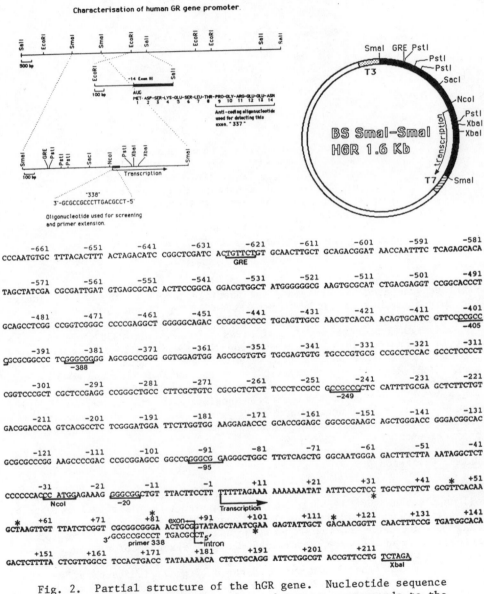

Fig. 2. Partial structure of the hGR gene. Nucleotide sequence of the 5' portion of hGR gene where the arrow corresponds to the transcription initiation site.

ymerase, linearized with NcoI (31 bp 5' to the transcription initiation mapped) was used in synthesizing a uniformly [^{32}P]-CTP labeled anti-mRNA probe (Fig. 2). When this probe was hybridized with 2 μg each of LNCaP and MCF-7 poly A+ RNA and digested with nuclease S_1, multiple protected fragments were detected. The major fragments had lengths of 88, 81 and 80 bases (Fig. 3). The largest of these protected fragments co-migrated with the major primer extension product demonstrating that the 5' end of the primer is at the 3' end of the exon. There are no other protected larger

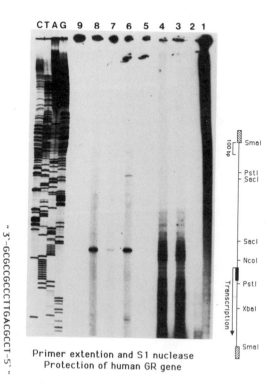

Primer extension and S1 nuclease
Protection of human GR gene

Fig. 3. Mapping of the hGR mRNA capsite. The SmaI-SmaI fragment of the hGR gene (Fig. 2) was subcloned into M13mp18 and BSM13-. The sequencing of the M13mp18 clone with oligonucleotide 5'TCCGCAGTTCCCGCCGCG3' "338" as primer is shown on the right side (GATC). The BS plasmid containing the insert in the 5' to 3' orientation with regard to T3-RNA promoter was linearized at the NcoI site and a uniformly [^{32}P]-CTP labeled anti-mRNA probe was synthesized using T7-RNA polymerase. 2 μg of each poly (A)+ RNA from LNCaP (lane 3) and MCF-7 (lane 4) were hybridized with the anti-mRNA probe, digested with S_1 nuclease, the protected fragments were separated on 7M Urea/6% polyacrylamide sequencing gel. Lane 1 contained the labeled probe alone, Lane 2 contained the probe hybridized to tRNA and S1 digested. Primer extension mapping was performed using [^{32}P]-end labeled primer "338," reverse transcriptase and poly (A)+ RNA from LNCaP (1 μg, Lane 5; 2 μg, Lane 6) and MCF-7 (1 μg, lane 7, 2 μg, lane 8) cells. The primer was extended in the presence and absence (Lane 9) of RNA without treatment with S_1 nuclease. The arrow shows the position of the 5' end of the hGR mRNA as defined by either primer extension or S1 mapping.

193

fragments visible, indicating the presence of a major strong transcription
start site in the hGR gene promoter.

The primer extension, nuclease S_1 mapping and sequencing data (Figs.
2 and 3) together suggest that the hGR cDNAs isolated from MCF-7 cDNA
library extend to the extreme 5' end of the hGR gene. Weinberger et al.
(28) isolated hGR cDNA clone which contained identical 5'-untranslated
cDNA sequences.

Sequence Around the hGR Promoter is G+C Rich

The nucleotide sequence upstream of the hGR RNA start site contains
neither a "TATA box" nor a "CAAT box" (Fig. 2). Most other characterized
eukaryotic genes have these two sequence elements approximately 30 and
80 bp, respectively, upstream of the RNA initiation site (43). Since in
vitro transcription studies have shown that the "TATA box" serves to fix
start site of transcription (44), it is surprising that hGR gene without a
"TATA box" has a unique transcriptional start site (Fig. 3). It has been
demonstrated that EGF receptor gene possessing similar structural features
as hGR gene has numerous transcriptional initiation sites (45) contain
neither a "TATA box" nor a "CAAT box." The sequence between -661 and -1
(Fig. 2) contains the putative promoter and part of 5' untranslated
region, has a G+C content of 72.5%. Further analysis of hGR gene 5'
flanking region shows similar to the EGF receptor that a specific sequence
"CCGCCC" and its inverted repeats "GGGCGG" are repeated many times (see
Figure 2) in the putative promoter region. The element "CCGCCC" is the
same sequence that is repeated 6 times within the simian virus 40 (SV40)
early promoter (44). The 5' flanking region of the hGR gene, therefore,
differs from the corresponding regions of most other eukaryotic genes
analyzed to date but resembles the SV40 early promoter, the EGF receptor
promoter, the mouse metallothionein promoter and the hydroxy methylglu-
taryl-CoA reductase (HMG-CoA reductase) promoter (45,51).

The SV40 early promoter has a G+C region, about 80 bp upstream of the
RNA start site, which is essential for transcription (44,46-49) and
contains 6 copies of the sequence "CCGCCC" (45,51). The gene HMG-CoA
reductase does not possess a typical "TATA box," has 5 transcriptional
start sites (50) and contains 3 repeats of the sequence "CCGCCC" at the 5'
flanking region. The c-myc proto-oncogene promoter also contains the
"CCGCCC" sequence and is G+C rich (Fig. 6). The 5' flanking region of the
EGF receptor gene is G+C rich and contains 5 "CCGCC" repeats. The mouse
metallothionein-1 gene promoters appear to include two "CCGCCC" elements
present in an inverted configuration (51). Like the corresponding regions
of these genes, the 5' flanking region of the hGR gene is G+C rich.
Within this area, there are two repeats of "CCGCCC" sequence and three of
the inverted elements "GGGCGG"; however, the sequence of the hGR gene is
found to contain in addition at -621 bp a putative GR-binding site
"TGTTCT." A recent report demonstrates that the human Hela transcription
factor Spl that stimulates in vitro transcription of the SV40 early
promoter binds to specific SV40 early promoter region containing CCGCCC
sequences (52). Because Spl-binding protein is found in uninfected cells,
it seems likely that it plays a role in the expression of cellular as well
as viral genes (53). An attractive hypothesis is that some "growth
control" genes like hGR gene that contain the repeat "CCGCCC" in the
promoter region are regulated by binding of the Spl protein.

In Vitro Transcription of the hGR Gene

To determine whether the cloned genomic DNA containing the 5' flanking region of the hGR gene is active in initiating transcription (Fig.
4), we performed an in vitro transcription assay using extracts from Hela

cells (Gibco-BRL). The plasmid containing the 4.5 kb EcoR1-EcoR1 genomic subfragment was linearized with XbaI, downstream from the initiation start site and then used as template (Fig. 2). The XbaI cuts at a site 211 bp downstream of the putative RNA start site mapped by primer extension and nuclease S_1 mapping. Transcription products were purified on CsCl gradient, hybridized to uniformly [^{32}P]CTP-labeled anti-mRNA probe synthesized from the NcoI linearized (BS SmaI-SmaI 1.6) template and digested with nuclease S_1. The protected fragments were fractionated under denaturing conditions on a 7M urea/6% polyacrylamide gel. A major protected fragment of 211 bp was observed (Fig. 4). This demonstrates that in vitro

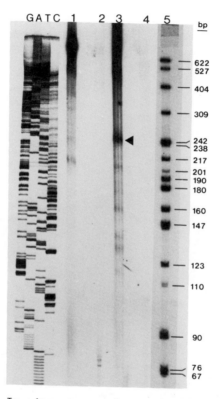

Fig. 4. In vitro transcription of the hGR gene. The plasmid containing the 4.5 kb EcoR1-EcoR1 genomic fragment, linearized with XbaI (see Figure 2) was used as template for in vitro transcription. RNAs were synthesized using the Hela cell in vitro transcription kit (BRL). RNAs were purified on CsCl gradient as described by Weingartener and Keller (38). The transcripts were hybridized with the anti-mRNA probe (Fig. 3), digested with S_1 nuclease and the protected fragments were analyzed on sequencing gels as described (Fig. 3). Lane 1, probe alone. Lane 2, probe hybridized to tRNA and S_1 nuclease treated. In vitro transcribed RNA in the absence (Lane 3) and in the presence (Lane 4) of α-amanitin, hybridized with the probe and treated with S_1 nuclease. Lane 5 contains the labeled pBR322 digested with MspI. The arrow indicates the major protected transcription product.

as well as in vivo transcription initiation occurs precisely at the same site, corroborating the results obtained above by primer extension and nuclease S_1 mapping (Fig. 3).

Regulation of the hGR Gene Studied With hGR-CAT Chimeric Plasmids

GR is known to be down-regulated by glucocorticoids and extensive studies on the level of mRNA are reported using rat GR cDNA probes (54). It has been also shown that a putative GR-binding site is present in the 3'-untranslated region of rat GR cDNA (54). It is postulated that the binding of GR at this site is involved in the down-regulation of GR by glucocorticoid. To study the regulation of hGR at the molecular level, the hGR gene promoter containing plasmids inserted with bacterial chloramphenicol acetyl transferase (CAT) gene was constructed (Fig. 5). As a control for hormonal regulation, MMTV-LTR-CAT plasmids were used (Fig. 5). The hGR-CAT as well as MMTV-CAT were transfected into COS-1 cells by calcium phosphate precipitation (55). After transfection, the cells were grown in hormone depleted medium for 48 h and separated into two batches. The first batch was used as nontreated controls and the second batch of plates were treated for 12 h with 1 μM dexamethasone. The cells were collected and cell extracts were prepared. The CAT activity was determined using ^{14}C-chloramphenicol and the acetylated products were separated by thin-layer chromatography followed by autoradiography.

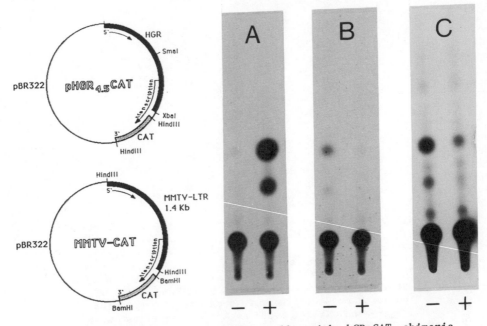

Fig. 5. Transfection of COS-1 cells with hGR-CAT chimeric plasmids. Semi-confluent COS-1 cells were transfected with constructs containing MMTV-CAT (panel A) and hGR-CAT (panels B and C). The cells were grown in hormone-depleted medium for 48 h. Twelve h before harvesting, dexamethasone (1 μM) was added to duplicate culture plates. Extracts were prepared and CAT activity was determined using the procedure described by Gorman et al. (25). Minus (-) indicates absence of hormone, plus (+) indicates presence of 1 μM dexamethasone. Panels B and C show autoradiograms obtained after exposure for 1 and 5 days, respectively.

As it has been demonstrated (56), the cells transfected with MMTV-CAT showed a glucocorticoid-dependent stimulation of the CAT activity. There was a basal level of CAT activity observed in the nontreated MMTV-CAT transfected cells, whereas the CAT activity increased manyfold in hormone-treated cells (Fig. 5A). However, the contrary results are observed in the hGR-CAT transfected cells (Fig. 5 B and C). The CAT activity was at least 5 times higher in the nonhormone-treated hGR-CAT transfected cells than the hormone-treated hGR-CAT transfected cells. This is the first demonstration of the regulation of a regulatory protein gene, such as hGR, by a glucocorticoid ligand. These experiments define that the sequences required for the feedback regulation of hGR are contained within a 4 kb EcoRl-XbaI fragment, which contains the transcription start site, 5' flanking region containing two "CCGCCC," three "GGGCGG" elements and a putative GR-binding site "TGTTCT" approximately 620 bp upstream of the transcription start site. These findings support the hypothesis that some "growth control" genes such as hGR containing the repeat CCGCCC in the promoter region are regulated by binding the Sp1 protein (52). The hGR gene may be induced by the Sp1 protein interaction in the absence of steroidal ligand for GR. The interaction of GR with its ligand follows binding of GR hormone complex to the hGR gene promoter at the putative GR binding site. We postulate that the interaction of occupied GR binding site "TGTTCT" by GR complex as well as the interaction of Sp1 protein at the "CCGCCC" and "GGGCGG" result in steric hindrance through protein-protein interactions. These steric hindrances in turn interfere with the transcription machinery resulting in the "switching off" of the transcription of the GR. The specific features of the 5' flanking region of hGR gene may prove to be important to our understanding of the regulation of regulatory protein expression.

HUMAN ANDROGEN RECEPTOR cDNA CLONING

Screening the cDNA Library

We have chosen the homologous amino acid sequences between 438-447, 468-477 and 617-625 of hGR_{orf} to synthesize oligonucleotides as probes for screening the cDNA library (Fig. 6). Optimal conditions for hybridization and washings were determined by varying the formamide (10-40%) concentration of the hybridization solution and by testing different washing temperatures (30-42°C). Hybridization at 42°C in 20% formamide followed by washes at 37°C in 2X SSC/0.1% SDS gave the best signals with minimal background (Fig. 7). A total of 214 positive clones were purified by a second screening and the λgt-11 recombinant phage DNA was prepared from all of them. The λgt-11 clones were analyzed by dot plaque hybridization technique parallely. The plaques were blotted onto 5 nitrocellulose filter discs and hybridized with nick-translated hGR_{orf}, hER_{orf} and a human PR cDNA probe isolated from a breast tumor cell cDNA library$_{orf}$ using the same oligonucleotides as probes (Govindan MV and Lachance Y, unpublished results) to eliminate their respective clones present in the 214 testis cDNA clones. Restriction fragmentation and hybridization showed that 194 out of 214 cDNA clones were coding for the glucocorticoid receptor mRNA. None of them hybridized to the hPR cDNA or hER_{orf} nick-translated probes. From the remaining 20 cDNA clones, 14 were not characterized further because they were smaller than 1 kb in length. The remaining six were subcloned into pBR 322 and mapped by restriction digestion. Two groups of cDNA clones were found. In the first group, 4 cross-hybridizing cDNA clones contained internal EcoRl sites with the longest insert being 2.4 kb (clone 2). The second group consisted of 2 cDNA clones which hybridized with one another (clones 77 and 94) (Fig. 8). The clone 77 is approximately 1.9 kb long and the clone 94 of size approximately 2.6 kb. The largest cDNA clones (2, 77 and 94) were subcloned

DNA binding ■358 ■359

```
rPR   568  CLICGDEASGCHYGVLTCGSCKVFFKRAMEGQ-HN-YLCAGRNDCIVDKIRRKNCPACRLRKCCQAGM
cPR        CLICGDEASGCHYGVLTCGSCKVFFKRAMEGQ-HN-YLCAGRNDCIYDKIRRKNCPACRLRKCCQAGM
cER   179  CAVCNDYASGYHYGVWSCEGCKAFFKRSIQG---HNDYMCPATNQCTIDKNRRKSCQACRLRKCYEVGM
hER   185  CAVCNDYASGYHYGVWSCEGCKAFFKRSIQG---HNDYMCPATNQCTIDKNRRKSCQACRLRKCYEVGM
hGR   421  CLVCSDEASGCHYGVLTCGSCKVFFKRAVEGQ-HN-YLCAGRNDCIIDKIRRKNCPACRYRKCLQAGM
erbA   37  CVVCGDKATGYHYRCITCEGCKSFFRRTIQKNLHPTYSCTYDGCCVIDHITRNQCQLCRFKKCISVGM
```

Hormone binding

```
rPR   684  LINLLMSIEPDVIYAGMENTKPDTSSSLLTSLNQLGERQLLSVVKWSKSLPGFRNLMIDDQ
hER   309  MVSALLEAEPPIVYSEYDPNRPFNEASMMTLLTNLADRELVHMINWAKRVPGFVDLTLHDQ
hER   315  MVSALLDAEPPILYSEYDPTRPFSEASMMGLLTNLADRELVHMINWAKRVPGFVDLTLHDQ
hGR   532  LVSLLEVIEPEVLYAGYDSSVPDSTWRIMTTLNMLGGHQVIAAVKWAKAIPGFRNLHDDDQ
erbA  173  RKFLLEDIGQSPMASMLDGDKVDLEA---FSEFTKIITPAITRVVDFAKNLPMFSELPCEDQ
```

■361

```
rPR   745  ITLIQYSWMSLMVFGLGWRSY-KMVSGQMLYFAPDLILNEQRMKESSKYSLCLTMWQIPQE
cER   370  VHLLECAWLEILMIGLVWRSM-EHQGKLL-FAPNLLLDRNQGKCVEGMVEIFDMLLATAAR
hER   376  VHLLECAWLEILMIGLVWRSM-EHPVKLL-FAPNLLLDRNQGKCVEGMVEIFDMLLATSSR
hGR   593  MTLLQYSWMFLMAFALGWRSYRQSSANLLCFAPDLIIN-EQRMTLPCMYDQCKHMLYVSSE
erbA  232  IILLKGCCMEIMSLRAAVR-YDPESETLT-LSGEMAVKREQLKN-GGLGVVSDAIFDLGKS
```

Fig. 6. Homologous regions corresponding to the DNA-binding and hormone-binding domains of steroid receptors. Darkly shaded areas represent the amino acid sequences encoded by the three oligonucleotide probes (358, 359, 361) derived from hGR.

into an expression vector, and large scale plasmids were prepared. The first group of cDNA clones contained an internal XbaI site and BamHI site which were used for subcloning and joining the EcoRl fragments together using the BSM13 (Statagene) vector.

Expression of the Protein and Hormone Binding

The plasmids in BSM13 were digested with BamHI or HindIII restriction enzymes to linearize the cDNA. The transcription products of these linearized cDNAs with T7-RNA polymerase followed by in vitro translation were analyzed by SDS-PAGE and fluorography. The cDNAs 77 and 94 gave

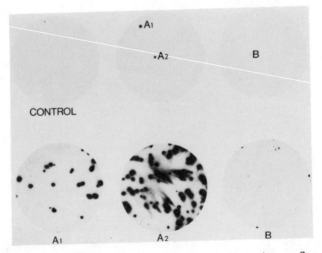

Fig. 7. Example of filters from screening. Control: Filters without any signal. A1 and A2: Filter containing two signals of hGR cDNA. B: filter containing the clone hAR 94. Lower panel: Purification of A1, A2 and B by second screening.

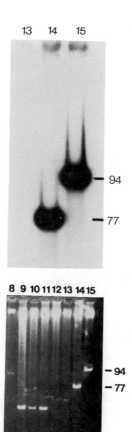

Fig. 8. Cross-hybridization λgt-11 clones 77 and 94: λgt-11 DNAs were digested with EcoR1, size fractionated on 1% agarose, stained with ethidium bromide and photographed (lower panel), Lane 14 contained DNA from clone 77 and lane 75 contained DNA from clone 94. The gel was Southern transferred onto Hybond N and hybridized with nick-translated insert of clone 77 (upper panel).

translation products of 38,000 and 85,000 Da respectively (Fig. 9). The clone No. 2 contained a translatable mRNA for a polypeptide of 45,000 Da (not shown).

Large-scale in vitro transcription was performed to produce suffi-cient mRNAs from clones 2, 77 and 94. The in vitro translation of these mRNAs in rabbit reticulocyte lysate was used to synthesize these polypep-tides encoded by the cDNA clones. The hormone-binding experiments were initially performed with the polypeptides synthesized by all the three clones to determine the specificity following the incubation with [^{3}H]-DHT in the absence and presence of one hundredfold excess of competitor. Polypeptides synthesized by the mRNA transcribed by clones 77 and 94 were found to bind with DHT specifically. The polypeptide expressed by clone 2 did not bind [^{3}H]-DHT and was not analyzed further for the hormone-binding experiments.

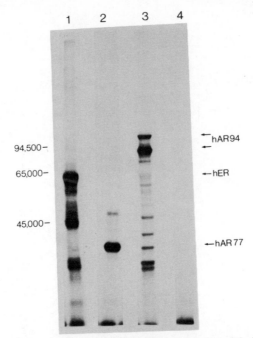

Fig. 9. Expression of the protein binding specifically to [^{3}H]-DHT. The in vitro translation products were analyzed by 7.5% SDS-polyacrylamide gel electrophoresis. Lane 1 hER$_{orf}$,(64,000 Da) cloned in BSM13 served as control. Lane 2 clone 77; lane 3 clone 94; lane 4 control (without added RNA).

Since clone 77 and 94 contained identical restriction pattern and both produced translation products which interacted specifically with [^{3}H]-DHT, they contain coding information for the human androgen receptor. These cDNAs did not correspond to hGR, hER hPR or hMR as found by cross-hybridization and restriction fragmentation.

Clones 77 and 94 encoded homologous regions present in all the steroid receptor cDNAs cloned so far. Even though clone 77 encodes only a polypeptide of 38,000 Da, this polypeptide bound [^{3}H]-DHT specifically. The translation of clone 94 yielded two major polypeptides, one with 100,000 Da and a predominant 85,000 Da protein.

To determine the specificity and selectivity of hormone interaction with the translation product of clone 77, this protein was incubated with 5 nM [^{3}H]-DHT in the presence of 10^{-5}-10^{-10} M competitor DHT, 5 nM [^{3}H]-R1881 in the presence and absence of 10^{-5}-10^{-10} M cold R1881, 5 nM [^{3}H]-DHT in the absence and presence of one hundredfold excess estradiol hydroxyflutamide, R5020 and cortisol (Fig. 10). These data demonstrate that the protein synthesized interact with [^{3}H]-DHT with the same affinity and specificity as the cellular counterpart (26,57,58). As expected at these high concentrations (26,57) hydroxyflutamide, the active metabolite of the pure antiandrogen flutamide, displaced competitively [^{3}H]DHT from the in vitro translated androgen receptor. Partial competition was also observed with estradiol and R5020 but no competition was found with cortisol and aldosterone. This demonstrates that the hAR synthesized in vitro has similar, if not identical, specificity and affinity towards [^{3}H]-DHT as

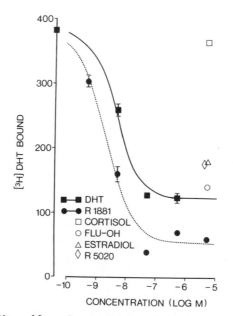

Fig. 10. Competition with in vitro synthesized receptor.

the receptor found in target tissues and cells. As the clone 94 gave two translation products and clone 77 behaved similar in hormone-binding experiments, clone 77 was chosen for further screening of overlapping cDNA clones and hybridization experiments.

Northern Analysis

The nick-translated hAR77 probe was hybridized to poly A+ RNA (Fig. 11) from human LNCaP and MCF-7 cells, as well as from prostates of intact castrated (3 days) and DHT-treated castrated rats. Multiple mRNA species were observed. It should be mentioned that this probe contained the conserved region of erbA homology and hormone-binding carboxy terminal. Cross-reactivity using such probes under low stringency condition is observed with GR and PR. Hybridization of the human northern blot was performed at 42°C and the blot-containing rat prostate RNA at 37°C. The washing of human northern blot was performed at 64°C in 0.2X SSC/0.1% SDS and the rat prostate at 2X SSC/0.1% SDS at 42°C. In both cases, the largest mRNA is of 6.5 kb and a major band has a size of 4.5 kb. The latter mRNA appeared to be induced in castrated rat prostates in contrast to the 6.5 kb mRNA species which is slightly increased in the DHT-treated castrated rat prostates. These preliminary data have to be confirmed by additional experiments to understand the regulation of human and rat androgen receptors.

Southern Analysis

The genomic organization of the human AR gene was analyzed by digestion of human (T47D) DNA with several restriction enzymes followed by Southern analysis (Fig. 12). For each digest hAR-77 hybridized to 2-4 bands, suggesting that the hAR gene may be present as single copy gene. Hybridization of hAR-77 with genomic blots of human-mouse hybrid cell lines have localized the human AR gene to the human X chromosome.

CONCLUSION

Cloning and expression of hAR cDNA will provide new insight and should stimulate new interest into the molecular mechanism underlying the complexity of androgen action. The isolation of the hAR cDNA should allow the elucidation of the pharmacologic and physiologic function of the hAR and allow investigation of the role of hAR in a number of disease states, among them testicular feminization syndrome and prostate cancer, where the study of the heterogeneity in androgen sensitivity from one cell to

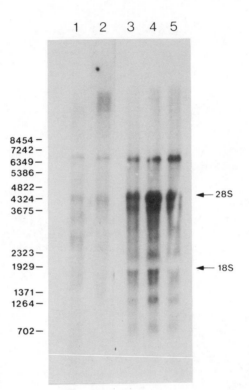

Fig. 11. Northern blot of poly A+ RNA: Lane 1: LNCaP; lane 2: MCF-7; lane 3: intact; lane 4: castrated; and, lane 5: DHT-treated castrated.

another as well as antiandrogen AR interaction may lead to an improvement in therapeutical regimens for such androgen-dependent diseases. Expression of full length hAR cDNA in eukaryotic and prokaryotic cells and overproduction of this rare receptor protein will provide additional tools to study the molecular aspects of androgen action. Primary structure of the androgen receptor deduced from the cDNA sequences will delineate its relationship to other steroid receptors and shed light on its uniqueness. Further DNA sequencing revealed clone 2 to be identical to the human mineralocorticoid receptor cDNA sequence published recently (31).

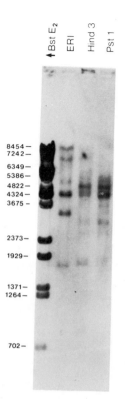

Fig. 12.   Southern blot analysis (see
Materials and Methods).

ACKNOWLEDGMENTS

We thank Prof. P. Chambon for his encouragement and interest in this
project. This project is supported by MRC Group grant for MRC Group in
Molecular Endocrinology, National Cancer Institute grant (M.V.G.).

REFERENCES

1. Yamamoto KR. Steroid receptor regulated transcription of specific
    genes and gene networks. Annu Rev Genet 1985; 19:209-52.
2. Payvar F, Wrange O, Carlstedt-Duke J, et al. Purified glucocorticoid
    receptors bind selectively in vitro to a cloned DNA fragment whose
    transcription is regulated by glucocorticoids in vivo. Proc Natl
    Acad Sci USA 1981; 78:6628-32.
3. Govindan MV, Spiess E, Majors J. Purified glucocorticoid receptor-
    hormone complex from rat liver cytosol binds specifically to cloned
    mouse mammary tumor virus long-terminal repeats in vitro. Proc Natl
    Acad USA 1982; 17:5157-61.
4. Geisse S, Scheidereit C, Westphal HM, et al. Glucocorticoid recep-
    tors recognize DNA sequences in and around murine mammary tumour
    virus DNA. EMBO J 1982; 1:1613-9.
5. Pfahl M. Specific binding of the glucocorticoid-receptor complex to
    the mouse mammary tumor proviral promoter region. Cell 1982; 31:
    475-82.
6. Scheidereit C, Geisse S, Westphal HM, et al. The glucocorticoid
    receptor binds to defined nucleotide sequences near the promoter of

mouse mammary tumour virus. Nature 1983; 749–52.

7. Payvar F, De Franco D, Firestone GL, et al. Sequence-specific binding of glucocorticoid receptor to MTV DNA at sites within and upstream of the transcribed region. Cell 198; 35:381–92.

8. Scheidereit C, Beato M. Contacts between hormone receptor and DNA double helix within a glucocorticoid regulatory element of mouse mammary tumor virus. Proc Natl Acad Sci USA 1984; 81:3029–33.

9. Karin M, Haslinger A, Holtgreve H, et al. Characterization of DNA sequences through which cadmium and glucocorticoid hormones induce human metallothionein-IIA gene. Nature 1984; 308:513–9.

10. Renhawitz R, Schutz G, von der Ahe D, et al. Sequences in the promoter region of the chicken lysozyme gene required for steroid regulation and receptor binding. Cell 1984; 37:503–10.

11. Liao S. Cellular receptors and mechanisms of action of steroid hormones. Int Rev Cytol 1975; 41:87–172.

12. Mooradian AD, Morley JE, Korenman L. Biological actions of androgens. Endocr Rev 1987; 1–28.

13. Smith RG, Nag A, Syms AJ, Norris JS. II. Steroid receptor, gene structure and molecular biology: steroid regulation of receptor concentration and oncogene expression. J Steroid Biochem 1986; 24:51–5.

14. Tindall DJ, Chang CH, Lobl TJ, Cunningham GR. Androgen antagonists in androgen target tissues. Pharmacol Ther 1984; 24:367–400.

15. Rowley DR, Tindall DJ. Androgen receptor protein: purification and molecular properties. In: Litwack G, ed. Biochemical actions of hormones; vol XIII. New York: Academic Press, 1984.

16. Labrie F, Dupont A, Belanger A, et al. Treatment of prostate cancer with gonadotropin-releasing hormone agonists. Endocr Rev 1986; 7:67–74.

17. Labrie F, Luthy I, Veilleux R, Simard J, Belanger A, Dupont A. New concepts on the androgen sensitivity of prostate cancer. In: Murphy GP, Khoury S, Kuss R, Chatelain C, Denis L, eds. New York: Alan R. Liss, Inc., 1987:145–52.

18. Labrie F, Dupont A, Giguere M, et al. Advantages of the combination therapy in previously untreated and treated patients with advanced prostate cancer. J Steroid Biochem 1986; 25:877–83.

19. Bardin CW, Catterall JF. Testosterone: a major determinant of extragenital sexual dimorphism. Science 1981; 211:1285–94.

20. Keenan BS, Meyer WJ, Hadjian AJ, Jones HW, Migeon CJ. Syndrome of androgen insensitivity in man: absence of 5-alpha-dihydrotestosterone-binding protein in skin fibroblasts. J Clin Endocrinol Metab 1974; 38:1143–6.

21. Meyer WJ, Migeon BR, Migeon CJ. Locus of human X chromosome for dihydrotestosterone receptor and androgen insensitivity. Proc Natl Acad Sci USA 1975; 72:1469–72.

22. Wilson JD, George FW, Griffin JE. The hormonal control of sexual development. Science 1981; 211:1278–84.

23. Chang CM, Rowley DR, Lobl TJ, Tindall DJ. Purification and characterization of androgen receptor from steer seminal vesicle. Biochemistry 1982; 4102–9.

24. Chang CM, Tindall DJ. Physiochemical characterization of the androgen receptor in rat uterine cytosol. Endocrinology 1983; 113:1486–93.

25. Rowley DR, Chang CM, Tindall DJ. Effects of sodium molybdate on the androgen receptor from the R3327 prostatic tumor. Endocrinology 1984; 114:1776–83.

26. Asselin J, Melancon R, Moachon G, Belanger A. Characteristics of binding to estrogen, androgen, progestin and glucocorticoid receptors in 7,12-dimethylbenz(a)anthracene-induced mammary tumors and their hormonal control. Cancer Res 1980; 40:1612–22.

27. Barnert JM, Jeltsch JM, Staub A, Jensen E, Scrace G, Waterfield M,

Chambon P. Cloning of the human estrogen receptor cDNA. Proc Natl Acad Sci USA 1985; 82:7889–93.

28. Hollenberg SM, Weinberger C, Ong ES, et al. Primary structure and expression of a functional human glucocorticoid receptor cDNA. Nature 1985; 318:635–41.

29. Govindan MV, Devic M, Green S, Gonemeyer H, Chambon P. Cloning of the human glucocorticoid receptor cDNA. Nucleic Acids Res 1985; 13:8293–304.

30. Misrahi M, Atger M, D'Auriol L, et al. Complete amino acid sequence of the human progesterone receptor deduced from cloned cDNA. Biochem Biophys Res Commun 1987; 143:740–8.

31. Arriza JL, Weinberg C, Cerelli G, et al. Cloning of human mineralo-corticoid receptor complementary DNA: structural and functional kinship with the glucocorticoid receptor. Science 1987; 237:268–75.

32. Govindan MV, Burelle M, Cantin C, et al. Cloning of human androgen receptor cDNA. Proc of the Int Conf on Hormones and Cancer, Hamburg, 1987.

33. Miller J, McLachlan AD, Klug A. Repetitive zinc-binding domains in the protein transcription factor III-A from Xenopus oocytes. EMBO J 1985; 41:1609–14.

34. Sanger F, Nicklen S, Coulson AR. DNA sequencing with chain terminating inhibitors. Proc Natl Acad Sci USA; 74:5463–7.

35. Lemeure M, Glandville N, Mandel JL, Gerlinger P, Palmiter R, Chambon P. The ovalbumin gene family: hormonal control of X and Y gene transcription and mRNA accumulation. Cell 1981: 23:561–71.

36. Nelsen C, Crenshaw EB III, Franco R, Lira SA, Alber VR, Evans RM, Rosenfeld MV. Discrete cis-active genomic sequences dictate the pituitary cell type-specific expression of rate prolactin and growth hormone genes. Nature 1986; 322:557–62.

37. Davis GL, Dibner MD, Battey JF. Basic methods in molecular biology. New York: Elsevier, 1986.

38. Weingartener B, Keller W. Transcription and processing of adenoviral RNA by extracts from Hela cells. Proc Natl Acad Sci USA 1981; 78:4092–6.

39. Maniatis T, Fritsch EF, Sambrook J. Molecular cloning. Cold Spring Harbor Laboratory.

40. Laemmli UK. Cleavage of structural proteins during the assembly of the head of the bacteriophage T4. Nature; 227:680.

41. Southern E. Detection of specific sequences among DNA fragments separated by gel electrophoresis. J Mol Biol 1975; 98:503.

42. Frischauf AM, et al. Lambda replacement vectors carrying polylinker sequences. J Mol Biol 1983; 170:827–42.

43. Breathnach R, Chambon P. Organization and expression of eucaryotic split genes coding for proteins. Annu Rev Biochem 1981; 50:349–83.

44. Fromm M, Berg P. Deletion mapping of DNA regions required for SV40 early region promoter function in vivo. J Mol Appl Genet 1982; 1:457–81.

45. Ishii S, Xu Y-H, Stratton RH, et al. Characterization and sequence of the promoter region of the human epidermal growth factor receptor gene. Proc Natl Acad Sci USA 1985; 82:4920–4.

46. Benoist C, Chambon P. In vivo sequence requirement of the SV40 early promoter region. Nature 1981; 290:304–10.

47. Hansen U, Sharp PA. Sequences controlling in vitro transcription of SV40 promoters. EMBO J 1983; 2:2293–303.

48. Wasylyk B, Chambon P. Potentiator effect of the SV40 72-bp repeat on initiation of transcription from heterologous promoter elements. Cold Spring Harbor Symposium. Quant Biol; 47:921–34.

49. Tjian R. T antigen binding and the control of SV40 gene expression. Cell 1981; 26:1–2.

50. Reynolds GA, Basu SK, Osborne TH, et al. HMG CoA reductase: a negatively regulated gene with unusual promoter and 5'-untranslated regions. Cell 1984; 38:275–85.

51. Serfling E, Jasin M, Shaffner W. Enhancers and eukaryotic gene transcription. Trends in genetics. August 1985, 224-30.

52. Gidoni D, Dynan WS, Tjian R. Multiple specific contacts between a mammalian transcription factor and its cognate promoters. Nature 1984; 312:409-13.

53. Dynan WS, Tjian R. Isolation of transcription factors that discriminate between different promoters recognized by RNA polymerase II. Cell 1983; 32:669-80.

54. Okret S, Poellinger L, Dong Y, Gustafsson JA. Down-regulation of glucocorticoid receptor mRNA by glucocorticoid hormones and recognition by the receptor of a specific binding sequence within a receptor cDNA clone. Proc Natl Acad Sci USA 1986; 83:5899-903.

55. Gorman MC, Moffat FL, Howard BH. Recombinant genomes which express chloramphenicol acetyltransferase in mammalian cells. Mol Cell Biol 1982; (Sep):1044-51.

56. Miefsfeld R, Ruscini S, Godowski PJ, et al. Genetic complementation of a glucocorticoid receptor deficiency by expression of cloned receptor cDNA. Cell 1986; 46:389-99.

57. Asselin J, Labrie F, Gourdeau Y, Bonne C, Raynaud JP. Binding of [^{3}H]methyltrienolone (R1881) in rat prostate and human benign prostatic hypertrophy (BPH). Steroids 1976; 28:449-59.

58. Simard J, Luthy I, Guay J, Belanger A, Labrie F. Characteristics of interaction of the antiandrogen flutamide with androgen receptor in various target tissues. Mol Cell Endocrinol 1986; 44:261-70.

V. BIOCHEMICAL ACTIONS AND ANTIHORMONES

15

ESTROGEN AND ANTIESTROGEN REGULATION OF PROLIFERATION AND PROTEIN SYNTHESIS OF HUMAN BREAST CANCER CELLS

Benita S. Katzenellenbogen, Yhun Yhong Sheen,
Catherine E. Snider, and Yolande Berthois

Department of Physiology and Biophysics
University of Illinois, Urbana, Illinois 61801

INTRODUCTION

Estrogenic hormones are known to stimulate a variety of biosynthetic processes in hormone-responsive target cells, such as those of the breast and uterus, and nonsteroidal antiestrogens have been shown to antagonize many of the actions of estrogens (1-3). Indeed, antiestrogens have proven to be effective in controlling the growth of estrogen-responsive breast cancers (4). The actions of estrogens appear to be mediated via inter-action with an intracellular receptor protein (5-7). Ligand-free estrogen receptors are weakly associated with nuclear components. Following ligand binding, receptor complexes become tightly associated with specific nuclear components, and this association presumably alters gene expression (8-10). Antiestrogens also bind directly to the estrogen receptor, and the resulting antiestrogen-receptor complexes also become associated with chromatin, but presumably block the events which promote cell growth (11,12).

Estrogen responsive breast cancer cell lines, and most notably the MCF-7 human breast cancer cell line, have been used extensively in studies aimed at analyzing the mechanisms by which hormones affect cell prolif-eration and protein synthesis, and the use of in vitro cell culture systems has enabled responses to be studied under carefully controlled conditions of hormone exposure (3,13-16).

In the MCF-7 human breast cancer cell line, which contains functional estrogen receptors, estrogen stimulates cell proliferation, pS2 mRNA levels, plasminogen activator activity, thymidine incorporation and DNA synthesis, and progesterone receptor levels (11). Estrogen treatment of MCF-7 cells also results in the stimulation of two specific secreted proteins (MW 160,000 and MW 52,000) and a cytoplasmic protein (MW 24,000) (16-18).

In order to gain further insight into how estrogens and antiestrogens modulate cell function, we have examined the effects of estrogen and antiestrogen on cell proliferation and on the synthesis of specific secreted proteins by breast cancer cells. We have also directly studied the interactions of radiolabeled antiestrogens with the estrogen receptor system and have provided considerable evidence suggesting that the effects of antiestrogens on protein synthesis and cell proliferation are mediated via the estrogen receptor and not via additional estrogen–noncompetable binding sites (reviewed in 11 and 19; see also 20,21). The reader is directed to these review articles for references to the work of this laboratory and others regarding evidence for differences in the physicochemical properties of the estrogen receptor when liganded with antiestrogens versus estrogens.

EFFECTS OF ANTIESTROGENS ON PROLIFERATION OF BREAST CANCER CELLS IN VITRO

Studies with antiestrogens in human breast cancer cells in culture indicate that antiestrogens preferentially inhibit the proliferation of estrogen receptor–containing breast cancer cells. Hence, if one examines the effects of antiestrogens on the proliferation of three human breast cancer cell lines that differ in their estrogen receptor content, it is seen that their sensitivity to growth suppression by antiestrogens such as tamoxifen correlates well with their estrogen receptor content (Fig. 1). MCF-7 cells, which contain high levels of estrogen receptor, have their growth inhibited markedly by antiestrogens; T47D cells, which contain low levels of estrogen receptor, have their growth inhibited weakly by antiestrogens; and MDA-MB-231 cells, which contain no detectable estrogen receptors, have their growth unaffected by micromolar concentrations of antiestrogens. These findings are mirrored by the results with human breast cancer patients indicating that estrogen receptor–containing breast cancers are most sensitive to antiestrogen treatment (4).

In our studies with breast cancer cells in culture, we were struck by the curious observation that antiestrogens not only suppressed estradiol-stimulated cell proliferation, but that they also appeared to suppress the growth of estrogen receptor–positive "control" MCF-7 cells, even in the apparent absence of estrogens (15,19), suggesting that cells in the

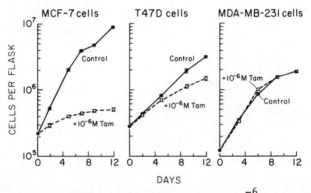

Fig. 1. Effect of tamoxifen (Tam; 10^{-6}M) on the growth of three different human breast cancer cell lines, MCF-7 cells, T47D cells, and MDA-MB-231 cells. Cells were grown in tissue culture media containing phenol red but with 5% charcoal dextran-treated calf serum in the continuous presence of tamoxifen, and media with fresh tamoxifen were renewed every other day. On the days indicated, triplicate flasks of cells were counted. Values are the means of the triplicate determinations. Bars represent SE. (From Miller and Katzenellenbogen, reference 20.)

210

control media might be inadvertently exposed to an estrogenic stimulus. Since we have gone to great lengths to eliminate sources of estrogens from the sera used in the cell cultures by charcoal treatment, frequently coupled with sulfatase treatment of serum, since some cells can hydrolyze estrogen sulfates to active estrogens, we considered that components of the cell culture media might themselves have hormonal activity.

In examining the potential source of estrogenic activity in the culture media, we noted that phenol red, the commonly used pH indicator in tissue culture media, bears some structural resemblance to certain non-steroidal estrogens. Since we have found that a variety of compounds with low affinity for the estrogen receptor can act as significant estrogens when present at high concentrations in a continuous fashion, as is the case in tissue culture in which there is no "clearance" of compounds, we sought to evaluate the estrogenic activity of phenol red. Indeed, we have found that phenol red preparations are estrogenic and that at the concentrations found in tissue culture media (15–45 μM), they cause significant stimulation of cell proliferation and specific protein synthesis in estrogen responsive cells (i.e., MCF-7 cells, but not in estrogen receptor-negative MDA-MB-2231 cells; 22). In addition, the antiestrogen suppression of cell proliferation under "control" conditions can be accounted for by the suppression of the phenol red stimulated activity.

Effects of Short-Term and Long-Term Estrogen (Phenol Red) Withdrawal on MCF-7 Cell Proliferation and Growth Responsiveness to Estrogen and Antiestrogen

Since we found that phenol red is a weak estrogen, we undertook to compare the proliferation and estrogen and antiestrogen responsiveness of MCF-7 breast cancer cells grown in the short-term and long-term absence of estrogens. Hence, cells were grown in medium without phenol red and with charcoal dextran-treated serum to eliminate all known sources of estrogens for brief and for extended periods of time.

As seen in Figure 2, control cells grown in the presence of phenol red (Fig. 2, left) proliferate at a rapid rate that is only slightly increased by estradiol. Hydroxytamoxifen decreased proliferation of these cells and hydroxytamoxifen inhibited the cell proliferation stimulated by 10^{-9}M estradiol, reducing the cell number to below that of the control.

MCF-7 cells exhibit a reduced growth rate when they are transferred to tissue culture medium that lacks phenol red. As seen in Figure 2 (middle bars), addition of estradiol (10^{-9}M) to cells grown in the absence of phenol red for several days (short-term phenol red-free cells) resulted in a marked increase in their proliferation rate, up to that seen in cells maintained in the presence of phenol red. Addition of the antiestrogen transhydroxytamoxifen (10^{-7}M) to these short-term phenol red-free cells had no effect on their proliferation rate, but antiestrogen did suppress the stimulatory effect of concomitant estradiol.

When MCF-7 cells were grown in the absence of phenol red for a period of 1 month prior to assay, their growth rate remained reduced, and their hormonal responsiveness to estradiol and transhydroxytamoxifen was similar to that seen in Figure 2, with short-term (approximately 1 week) phenol red withdrawn cells. The behavior of these short-term estrogen withdrawn cells is in contrast to that of cells maintained for much longer periods— 5 to 6 months—in the apparently complete absence of estrogens (no phenol red and with charcoal dextran-treated calf serum). These long-term estrogen-withdrawn cells (Fig. 2, right bars) have an increased rate of proliferation, and the addition of estradiol causes no further increase in

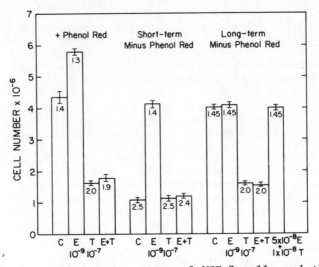

Fig. 2. Proliferation rates of MCF-7 cells and the effect of estradiol (E) and transhydroxytamoxifen (T) on the proliferation of MCF-7 cells grown in the continuous presence of phenol red (left-most bars); or grown in the short-term (1 week) or long-term (6 months) absence of phenol red. Cells grown in medium containing phenol red and cells grown for 1 week or for 6 months in phenol red-free medium were seeded into T-25 flasks, and at 2 days after cell seeding, triplicate flasks of cells were counted and each medium was then supplemented with 10^{-9} M E, 10^{-7} M T, E + T, control ethanol vehicle (0.1%, C), or with 5 x 10^{-8} M E + 1 x 10^{-8} M T. Media and hormones were changed every other day and on day 7, triplicate flasks of cells were counted. Values represent the mean ± SEM of the values for each group and are representative of 3 separate experiments. The numbers inside each bar indicate the cell doubling time in days. (From Katzenellenbogen et al., reference 23.)

this maximal rate of proliferation, but antiestrogen decreases proliferation (Fig. 2, right). The reduction of proliferation by transhydroxytamoxifen (10^{-8} M, which gave suppression equal to that seen with 10^{-7} M transhydroxytamoxifen) was reversed by estradiol (5 x 10^{-8} M, or 10^{-8} M).

Partial Agonistic Effect of Certain Antiestrogens

Additional studies were done to evaluate the effects of varying concentrations of antiestrogen on the proliferation of these MCF-7 cells (Fig. 3). In short-term estrogen withdrawn cells which are growing slowly (panel A), the antiestrogen transhydroxytamoxifen showed mixed partial agonist/antagonist activity. At low concentrations (10^{-10} and 10^{-9} M), transhydroxytamoxifen stimulated proliferation, although to a lesser extent than that evoked by 10^{-10} or 10^{-8} M estradiol (i.e., partial agonist), but transhydroxytamoxifen showed no stimulation at higher concentration (10^{-7} M), where it fully inhibited estradiol-stimulated proliferation (i.e., complete antagonist). We have also observed a similar, weak partial stimulation of proliferation with some other antiestrogens (23).

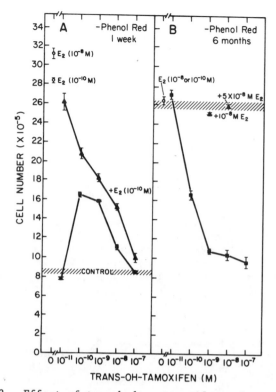

Fig. 3. Effect of transhydroxytamoxifen and estradiol on the proliferation of MCF-7 cells grown in the absence of phenol red for a short (1 week) or long (6 months) period of time. Cells were seeded into T-25 flasks and, at 2 days after cell seeding, triplicate flasks of cells were counted and media were then supplemented with either the indicated concentration of hydroxytamoxifen alone (■) or the indicated concentration of hydroxytamoxifen and estradiol (▲) or control ethanol vehicle (0.1%, hatched line). Media and hormones were changed every other day and on day 6, triplicate flasks of cells were counted. Values represent the mean ± SEM of values for each group and are from 3 separate experiments. (From Katzenellenbogen et al., reference 23.)

In contrast (Fig. 3, panel B), cells maintained for 6 months in the absence of estrogens showed a more rapid rate of cell proliferation (as noted by the higher control cell number, hatched line) and estradiol was unable to increase further the rate of proliferation, and antiestrogen showed only a dose-dependent suppression of proliferation which was reversible by estradiol (+ 10^{-8} or + 5 x 10^{-8} M E_2 points).

Estrogen Receptor and Progesterone Receptor Levels in Cells Grown in the Short-Term and Long-Term Absence of Estrogens

While cells grown in the short-term absence of estrogens have estrogen receptor levels similar to those of control cells (Table 1), cells grown in the long-term absence of estrogens have 3-times higher estrogen receptor levels (Table 1).

Table 1. Estrogen receptor concentrations in control MCF-7 cells and in MCF-7 cells grown in the short-term (5 days) or long-term (>6 months) absence of estrogens.

Cells	Estrogen Receptor (fmol per 1 x 10^6 cells)*
Control	59.3 ± 6.6 (n = 4)
Short-term Minus phenol red	65.5 ± 11.3 (n = 4)
Long-term Minus phenol red	204 ± 28.2 (n = 4)

*Estrogen receptor levels in MCF-7 cells were determined on late logarithmic phase cells by a whole cell receptor assay. Values represent the mean ± SEM from 4 separate experiments. (From Katzenellenbogen et al., 1987, reference 23.)

As expected, progesterone receptor levels were very low in cells grown in the absence of phenol red for either a short time (5 days, short-term minus phenol red) or a long time (greater than 5 to 6 months, long-term minus phenol red). As seen in Figure 4, the control level of progesterone receptor in the short-term and long-term phenol red-free cells was significantly lower than that of cells grown with phenol red. In addition, the fold stimulation of progesterone receptor by estradiol was much greater in both the short-term and long-term phenol red-free cells than in control cells (grown in charcoal dextran-treated calf serum plus phenol red). Hence, both the long-term and short-term phenol red-free cells have low progesterone receptor levels that are markedly stimulated by estrogen, but they differ in their growth rate, with the long-term phenol red-free cells showing a rapid proliferation rate.

Effects of Estradiol and Antiestrogen on the Synthesis of Secreted Proteins by MCF-7 Cells

When incorporation of [^{35}S]-methionine and [^{35}S]-cysteine into newly synthesized secreted protein was measured in MCF-7 cells grown in regular media (24), estradiol was found to increase the production of 3 secreted proteins over those of control cells. In addition to previously identified MW 160,000, and MW 52,000 proteins (16,17), estradiol increased production of an MW 32,000 protein. It is interesting to note that the MW 32,000 protein was observed to be increased by estradiol only when the secreted proteins were labeled both with [^{35}S]-methionine and [^{35}S]-cysteine, or with [^{35}S]-cysteine alone. When labeled only with [^{35}S]-methionine, only weak incorporation into the MW 32,000 protein was seen, suggesting that the MW 32,000 protein is probably rich in cysteine but low in methionine content. Trans-OH-tamoxifen (10 nM) stimulated the production of an MW 37,000 secreted protein over that of control cells, and it did so in a time-dependent fashion (see below).

Figure 5 shows that there is a rapid increase in the level of MW 37,000 radiolabeled protein after trans-OH-tamoxifen treatment of MCF-7 cells. A 6- to 12-h treatment with trans-OH-tamoxifen results in a half-maximal response and after 1 day, the level of the MW 37,000 protein has plateaued, changing little over the 24- to 96-h period. In contrast to the marked effect of this antiestrogen, estradiol alone at a high

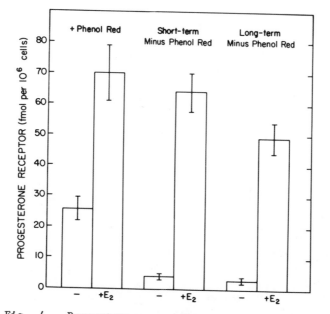

Fig. 4. Progesterone receptor concentrations in control and estradiol-treated MCF-7 cells grown in the continuous presence of phenol red, or in the short-term (1 week) or long-term (6 months) absence of phenol red. Progesterone receptor levels in these different MCF-7 cells were determined after 5 days of growth in the absence (−) or presence (+) of 1 nM estradiol. All media contained 5% charcoal dextran-treated calf serum, and fresh medium and hormone were added daily during the 5-day period. The cells were then harvested and assayed for progesterone receptor utilizing 10 nM [³H]R5020 in the absence and presence of a one hundredfold excess of radioinert R5020. Values indicate the mean ± SEM of data obtained from 3 separate experiments. (From Katzenellenbogen et al., reference 23.)

concentration (10^{-7}M) did not alter the synthesis of this MW 37,000 protein, yet estradiol very effectively blocked the stimulation of the MW 37,000 protein by trans-OH-tamoxifen. The production of this protein was stimulated by a variety of antiestrogens (but not by estrogens such as cis-tamoxifen; 24). These findings suggest that antiestrogen stimulation of the MW 37,000 secreted protein in MCF-7 cells is most likely mediated through the estrogen receptor system.

When cells are grown in estrogen-free conditions, i.e., in charcoal dextran-treated serum in medium lacking the estrogen phenol red, for several days, the basal level of synthesis of the MW 32,000, 160,000 and 52,000 proteins is extremely low so that estradiol-stimulation results in a tenfold increase in the production of the MW 32,000 protein with increases observable by 6 h, with maximal stimulation at 2 days. Interestingly, the basal level of synthesis of the MW 37,000 protein is high in the absence of estrogen and is then stimulated only minimally by the addition of antiestrogen, suggesting that this protein is clearly produced as an estrogen-antagonistic protein. Amino acid incorporation conducted in the presence of tunicamycin and endoglycosidase H indicate both of

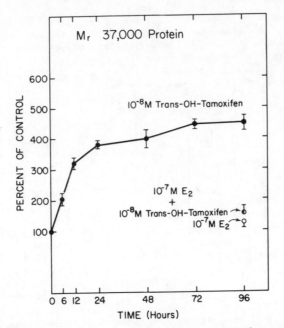

Fig. 5. Time course of MW 37,000 secreted protein following 10 nM trans-OH-tamoxifen treatment. Cells in medium containing phenol red and 5% charcoal dextran-treated calf serum were incubated for varying times with 10^{-8}M trans-OH-tamoxifen + 10^{-7}M estradiol (o), 10^{-7}M estradiol (●), or 10^{-8}M trans-OH-tamoxifen + 10^{-7}M estradiol (ⓞ). Proteins were labeled with $[^{35}S]$-cysteine and $[^{35}S]$-methionine, separated on SDS gels, and fluorograms were analyzed by densitometry. Each point represents the mean of 3 different experiments, bars, S.E. The level of MW 37,000 protein synthesis in the control cells was 1.3 ± 0.2% (n=3) of total $[^{35}S]$-methionine and $[^{35}S]$-cysteine incorporation into secreted proteins. (From Sheen and Katzenellenbogen, reference 24.)

these proteins are glycoproteins (24). These proteins should serve as useful markers for antiestrogen and estrogen action and may be involved in antiestrogen and estrogen modulation of cell proliferation and/or cell function. Hence, efforts are underway to purify and learn more about these proteins.

CONCLUSIONS: ESTROGEN-GROWTH FACTOR INTERRELATIONSHIPS

Our studies indicate that MCF-7 cells respond almost immediately to the lack of estrogens with a decreased proliferation rate. In these short-term withdrawn cells, estradiol stimulated cell proliferation markedly while the antiestrogen transhydroxytamoxifen showed mixed partial agonist/antagonist activity. It weakly stimulated proliferation at low concentrations, but had no effect on proliferation at high concentrations. In addition, transhydroxytamoxifen showed a dose-dependent antagonism of estradiol-stimulated cell proliferation. The reduced rate of proliferation in the absence of estrogens is maintained by MCF-7 cells for at least 1 month, but by 5-6 months of growth in a phenol red-free environment, the "basal" proliferation rate of the cells has increased, returning to that of control cells maintained in continuous phenol-red. While estradiol was not able to further stimulate the proliferation of these long-term withdrawn cells, antiestrogen was still inhibitory to cell proliferation and estradiol was able to reverse the hydroxytamoxifen inhibition.

These studies document that the proliferation rate of MCF-7 cells is modulated markedly by the conditions under which the cells are grown, and that MCF-7 cells increase their basal growth rate in the long-term absence of estrogens. It is possible that this may represent selection of a subpopulation of MCF-7 cells during long-term culture in the total absence of estrogenic stimulation. This possibility is being investigated presently. The increased proliferation rate of cells grown in the long-term absence of estrogen does not appear to be due to the acquisition of supersensitivity to possible low levels of estrogen, since the basal progesterone receptor content of the long term-withdrawn cells is very low. Indeed, these cells remain highly sensitive to estrogen since their progesterone receptor content is increased markedly by estradiol. In fact, their cellular estrogen receptor levels are increased approximately threefold, although the mechanism of this increase is not known. Welshons and Jordan have observed a similar increase in estrogen receptor levels in MCF-7 cells grown in the absence of phenol red (25).

It has been well documented that MCF-7 cells have receptors for many hormones and growth factors and have their growth influenced by many of these agents (26). Recent studies have also shown that MCF-7 cells produce a variety of growth factors (TGF-α/EGF, TGF-β, IGF-1 and probably others) and that the production of some of these growth factors and growth inhibitors is modulated by estrogen and antiestrogen (26,27). Hence, it is possible that in the long-term absence of estrogen, there is either an altered production and/or secretion of growth factors or a change in sensitivity to growth factors present in the serum or secreted by the MCF-7 cells in culture.

It is of note that antiestrogens show both agonistic and antagonistic effects on proliferation of MCF-7 cells grown in the short-term absence of estrogen, while antiestrogens display only a growth antagonistic action in MCF-7 cells grown in the long-term absence of estrogen. Cells grown in the short-term absence of estrogen are growing slowly and, under these conditions, we are able to observe an interesting, usually biphasic stimulatory effect of antiestrogens on cell proliferation. Antiestrogen is most stimulatory at low to moderate concentrations, while little or no stimulation is observed at higher concentrations.

Several previous studies have also noted an agonistic effect of tamoxifen when estrogen receptor-positive human breast cancer cells were growing slowly (28-30), and these researchers also observed more stimulation at low as opposed to higher tamoxifen concentrations. Indeed, from these findings, Reddel and Sutherland (28) made the intriguing proposal that low blood levels of tamoxifen might account for the "flare" observed occasionally during the start of antiestrogen therapy, and that achieving high concentrations of tamoxifen after continued dosing might well result then in the regression usually observed thereafter. Hence, in cells growing slowly in phenol red-free media, we are able to observe both the weak agonist and the antagonist activities of antiestrogen on growth that have been well known in other species and tissues, such as the rat uterus (1), and in MCF-7 cells grown in nude mice (31). Interestingly, however, when MCF-7 cells are growing rapidly as in the long-term absence of estrogen, proliferation is not increased further by estradiol, and hydroxytamoxifen then shows only a dose-dependent reduction of proliferation.

Hence, our studies reveal that MCF-7 cells increase their proliferation rate and grow rapidly in the long-term absence of estrogen while showing high levels of estrogen receptors, sensitivity to antiestrogen as measured by suppression of growth, and sensitivity to estrogen as measured by stimulation of cellular progesterone receptor levels. That antiestrogen is able to suppress this growth suggests that antiestrogens may suppress growth here by decreasing constitutive growth factor production or increasing growth inhibitors, a hypothesis that has been validated for control MCF-7 cells (27), and which needs to be examined in these long-term estrogen-free cells. Indeed, in addition to increasing TGF-β production, antiestrogens have been shown to increase the production of other proteins, such as the MW 37,000 protein, which might also function as possible growth inhibitors (24,32). Our observation that antiestrogens are able to suppress the growth of rapidly proliferating MCF-7 cells, i.e., long-term estrogen withdrawn MCF-7 cells growing in the absence of estrogen, is consistent with recent findings of Vignon et al. (33) who show that antiestrogens can suppress the stimulation of cell proliferation due to estradiol as well as other mitogens (growth factors such as EGF or insulin), and that in both cases the action of the antiestrogen is mediated via estrogen receptor sites.

ACKNOWLEDGMENTS

We are grateful for support of this research by NIH grants CA 18119 and HD 21524 (to B. S. K.). C. E. Snider was assisted by postdoctoral traineeship 5T32 HD 07028. Y. Berthois was supported in part by INSERM, France.

REFERENCES

1. Katzenellenbogen BS, Bhakoo HS, Ferguson ER, et al. Estrogen and antiestrogen action in reproductive tissues and tumors. Recent Prog Horm Res 1979; 35:259-300.
2. Katzenellenbogen BS, Miller MA, Mullick A, Sheen YY. Antiestrogen action in breast cancer cells: modulation of proliferation and protein synthesis, and interaction with estrogen receptors and additional antiestrogen binding sites. Breast Cancer Res Treat 1985; 5:231-43.
3. Aitken SC, Lippman ME. Effect of estrogens and antiestrogens on growth regulatory enzymes in human breast cancer cells in tissue culture. Cancer Res 1985; 45:1611-20.
4. McGuire WL. Steroid receptor sites in cancer therapy. Adv Intern Med 1979; 24:127-40.
5. Sheridan PJ, Buchanan JM, Anselomo VC, Martin PM. Equilibrium. The intracellular distribution of steroid receptors. Nature 1979; 282:579-84.
6. Welshons WV, Lieberman ME, Gorski J. Nuclear localization of unoccupied oestrogen receptors. Nature 1984; 307:747-9.
7. King WJ, Greene GL. Monoclonal antibodies localize oestrogen receptor in nuclei of target cells. Nature 1984; 307:745-7.
8. Katzenellenbogen BS. Dynamics of steroid hormone receptor action. Annu Rev Physiol 1980; 42:17-35.
9. Gorski J, Gannon F. Current models of steroid hormone action: a critique. Annu Rev Physiol 1976; 38:425-50.
10. Yamamoto KR. Steroid receptor regulated transcription of specific genes and gene networks. Annu Rev Genet 1985; 19:209-52.
11. Katzenellenbogen BS, Miller MA, Mullick A, Sheen YY. Antiestrogen action in breast cancer cells: modulation of proliferation and protein synthesis, and interaction with estrogen receptors and

additional antiestrogen binding sites. Breast Cancer Res Treat 1985; 5:231-43.

12. Coezy E, Borgna JL, Rochefort H. Tamoxifen and metabolites in MCF-7 cells: correlation between binding to estrogen receptor and inhibition of cell growth. Cancer Res 1982; 42:317-24.

13. Soule MD, Vazquez J, Long A, Albert S, Brennan M. A human cell line from a pleural effusion derived from a breast carcinoma. J Natl Cancer Inst 1973; 51:1409-13.

14. Lippman ME, Bolan G, Huff K. The effects of estrogen and antiestrogen on hormone-responsive human breast cancer in long-term tissue culture. Cancer Res 1976; 36:4595-601.

15. Katzenellenbogen BS, Norman MJ, Eckert RL, Peltz SW, Mangel WF. Bioactivities, estrogen receptor interactions, and plasminogen activator-inducing activities of tamoxifen and hydroxytamoxifen isomers in MCF-7 human breast cancer cells. Cancer Res 1984; 44: 112-9.

16. Westley B, May EB, Brown AM, et al. Effects of antiestrogens on the estrogen regulated pS2 RNA and 52 and 160 kilodalton proteins in MCF-7 cells and two tamoxifen resistant sublines. J Biol Chem 1984; 259:10030-5.

17. Westley B, Rochefort H. A secreted glycoprotein induced by estrogen in human breast cancer cell lines. Cell 1980; 20:353-9.

18. Edwards DP, Adams DJ, McGuire WL. Estradiol stimulates synthesis of a major intracellular protein in the human breast cancer cell line MCF-7. Breast Cancer Res Treat 1981; 1:209-15.

19. Miller MA, Sheen YY, Mullick A, Katzenellenbogen BS. Antiestrogen binding to estrogen receptors and additional antiestrogen binding sites in human breast cancer cells. In: Jordan VC, ed. Estrogen/antiestrogen action and breast cancer therapy. University of Wisconsin Press, 1986:127-48.

20. Miller MA, Katzenellenbogen BS. Characterization and quantitation of antiestrogen binding sites in estrogen receptor-positive and -negative human breast cancer cell lines. Cancer Res 1983; 43:3094-100.

21. Sheen YY, Simpson DM, Katzenellenbogen BS. An evaluation of the role of antiestrogen binding sites in mediating the growth modulatory effects of antiestrogens: studies using t-butylphenoxyethyl diethylamine, a compound lacking affinity for estrogen receptor. Endocrinology 1985; 117:561-4.

22. Berthois Y, Katzenellenbogen JA, Katzenellenbogen BS. Phenol red in tissue culture media is a weak estrogen: implications concerning the study of estrogen-responsive cells in culture. Proc Natl Acad Sci USA 1986; 83:2496-500.

23. Katzenellenbogen BS, Kendra KL, Norman MJ, Berthois Y. Proliferation, hormonal responsiveness, and estrogen receptor content of MCF-7 human breast cancer cells grown in the short-term and long-term absence of estrogens. Cancer Res 1987; 47:4355-60.

24. Sheen YY, Katzenellenbogen BS. Antiestrogen stimulation of the production of a 37,000 molecular weight secreted protein and estrogen stimulation of the production of a 32,000 molecular weight secreted protein in MCF-7 human breast cancer cells. Endocrinology 1987; 120:1140-51.

25. Welshons WV, Jordon VC. Adaptation of estrogen-dependent MCF-7 cells to low estrogen (phenol red-free) culture. Eur J Cancer Clin Oncol 1987 (in press).

26. Dickson RB, Lippman ME. Estrogenic regulation of growth and polypeptide growth factor secretion in human breast carcinoma. Endocr Rev 1987; 8:29-42.

27. Knabbe C, Lippman ME, Wakefield LM, et al. Evidence that transforming growth factor-β is a hormonally regulated negative growth factor in human breast cancer cells. Cell 1987; 48:417-28.

28. Reddel RR, Sutherland RL. Tamoxifen stimulation of human breast

cancer cell proliferation in vitro: a possible model for tamoxifen tumor flare. Eur J Cancer Clin Oncol 1984; 20:1419-24.

29. Sonnenschein C, Papendorp JT, Soto AM. Estrogenic effect of tamoxifen and its derivatives on the proliferation of MCF-7 human breast tumor cells. Life Sci 1985; 37:387-94.

30. Darbre PD, Curtis S, King RJB. Effect of estradiol and tamoxifen on human breast cancer cells in serum-free culture. Cancer Res 1984; 44:2790-3.

31. Osborne CK, Hobbs K, Clark GM. Effect of estrogens and antiestrogens on growth of human breast cancer cells in athymic nude mice. Cancer Res 1985; 45:584-90.

32. Bronzert DA, Silverman S, Lippman ME. Estrogen inhibition of a M_r 39,000 glycoprotein secreted by human breast cancer cells. Cancer Res 1987: 47:1234-8.

33. Vignon F, Bouton MM, Rochefort H. Antiestrogens inhibit the mitogenic effect of growth factors on breast cancer cells in the total absence of estrogens. Biochem Biophys Res Commun 1987; 146:1502-8.

16

AN ESTROGEN INDUCED PROTEASE IN BREAST CANCER:

FROM BASIC RESEARCH TO CLINICAL APPLICATIONS

Henri Rochefort, Patrick Augereau, Pierre Briozzo,
Francoise Capony, Vincent Cavailles, Marcel Garcia,
Muriel Morisset, Gilles Freiss, and Francoise Vignon

Unite d'Endocrinologie Cellulaire et Moleculaire (U 148)
INSERM and Universite de Montpellier, Faculte de Medecine
60, rue de Navacelles, 34090 Montpellier, France

In the cascade of events following the interaction of estrogens with their nuclear receptors in breast cancer cells, some of them are involved in the hormonal stimulation of cell growth. Their identification may improve both our understanding of the mechanism by which tumor growth is controlled and the monitoring and treatment of breast cancer.

Several breast cancer cell lines can be used to define these events, some of which require estrogens to grow (MCF7, T47D, ZR75-1) and others grow without estrogens (MDA-MB231, BT20, etc.) and have no estrogen receptors (ER). The proteins and peptides induced by estrogens before growth stimulation, and secreted into the culture medium, are particularly interesting since some of them may act as mediators of estrogen action to stimulate the growth and/or the invasion of breast cancer cells by an autocrine and/or paracrine mechanism (for review, see 1-4). We here summarize the studies from our laboratories which have concentrated on one of these proteins, named 52K based on its molecular weight in denaturing polyacrylamide gel electrophoresis, leading to its identification and showing its possible function in mammary carcinogenesis. Lastly, we review the clinical potential of this protein, which can be detected and assayed in the mammary tissue and tumors of patients.

BIOLOGY OF THE 52K PROTEIN IN MCF7 CELLS

First Description and Purification

The 52K protein was first detected by labeling protein of MCF7 cells with [^{35}S]methionine and analyzing the secreted protein by SDS-polyacrylamide gel electrophoresis (5,6). While estradiol increased the total amount of secreted proteins two- to threefold, some of the proteins (mainly a 160K and a 52K species) were more specifically increased by estradiol at concentrations as low as 1 to 10 picomoles. The 52K protein is secreted in small amounts into the culture medium by estrogen-treated MCF7 cells (5 ng/10^6 cells/hour) and by other ER-positive breast cancer cells under estrogen control (T47D, ZR75-1). It is constitutively produced without estrogen in ER-negative cell lines (MDA-MB231, BT20) (7). In ER-positive cells, the protein is specifically regulated by hormones

(estrogens and high doses of androgens) that can bind to and activate the
estrogen receptor, but not by glucocorticoids, progestins, or androgens at
low concentrations (6). The effects of the antiestrogens tamoxifen and
hydroxytamoxifen suggested that this protein was in some way related to
the mitogenic activity of estrogens. In wild-type MCF7 cells, antiestrogens totally inhibited the synthesis of the protein, whereas they
partially stimulated the synthesis of the progesterone receptor. By
contrast, in the antiestrogen-resistant variants of MCF7 cells (R27 and
RTx6) cloned for their ability to grow in 1 μM tamoxifen, the antiestrogens became able, like estrogens, to increase the production of the 52K
protein, but remained unable, as in wild-type MCF7 cells, to stimulate the
production of the estrogen-regulated 160K secreted proteins and pS2 mRNA
(8). In these cell lines, the 52K protein was therefore a better candidate for being a mitogen than the pS2 or 160K proteins. A possible
mechanism for the antiestrogen resistance was acquisition by the cells of
a growth advantage, due to the tamoxifen-induced increase in the production of autocrine growth factors such as the 52K protein.

Using concanavalin-A sepharose chromatography, we partially purified
the 52K protein from 22 liters of conditioned medium from MCF7 cell
cultures. From this fraction, we obtained several mouse monoclonal
antibodies to the 52K protein (9). Finally, using an immunoaffinity
column, we purified the 52K protein to apparent homogeneity (1,000-fold
purification) both in its secreted and cellular forms (10). The purification of 52K protein made it possible to determine its structure, identity,
and biological activities.

The MCF7-52K protein is an inactive pro-cathepsin-D (11,12) which can
be autoactivated when secreted, or processed successively into a one chain
(48K) and two chains (34K+14K) mature enzyme. The processed forms of
cathepsin-D in normal fibroblasts (13) and in MCF7 breast cancer cells are
very similar if not identical.

Structure and Identification as a Cathepsin-D

Study of the co- and posttranslational modifications of the 52K
protein helped us to define its structure and enzymatic activity. After
exposure of cultured MCF7 cells to ^{32}P, the 52K protein was intensely
labeled. However, most of this label could be removed by endoglycos-
idase-H treatment, which deleted the two N-glycosylated chains of the
protein. Mannose-6-P signals were then identified on the chains (11).
Pulse-chase experiments and Western blot showed that the 52K protein is
the precursor of a lysosomal enzyme that accumulates in lysosomes as a
stable 34K protein (Fig. 1) (12). About 40% of the cellular 52K precursor
is secreted while about 60% is successively processed into a 48K and a
34K+14K protein. Part of the secreted 52K protein can be taken up and
processed by MCF7 cells, but its binding is specifically inhibited by
mannose-6-P and not by other sugars.

The presence of mannose-6-P signals indicated that the protein is
normally routed to lysosomes where it exerts its usual function (13,14).
In testing several enzymatic activities corresponding to lysosomal hy-
drolases of similar molecular weight, we found that both the purified
secreted 52K protein and the corresponding cellular proteins (52K,48K,
34K+14K) displayed strong proteolytic activity at acidic pH, which was
mostly inhibited by pepstatin. Comparison with the previously described
ubiquitous cathepsin-D revealed close similarities (11). Antibodies to
the 52K protein interact with liver cathepsin-D, while anti-cathepsin-D
immunoprecipitates the 52K protein. The pH and inhibitor sensitivities of
the two proteases are very similar, as are their molecular weights. In

addition, the first 15 amino acids determined by microsequencing the N-terminal of the molecules are identical (P. Ferrara, unpublished).

Cloning, Sequencing and Comparison with Normal Pro-Cathepsin-D

Cloning and sequencing of cDNA were needed to determine indirectly the complete sequencing of the 52K-cathepsin-D and compare it with that of normal human cathepsin-D (15). Using both monoclonal antibodies to the secreted 52K protein of MCF7 cells and a synthetic oligonucleotide obtained from partial sequencing of the protein, we screened a gtll cDNA library of MCF7 cells. Four clones (p1-p6-p8 and p9] were isolated and sequenced. They covered the whole coding sequence of 52K-mRNA. By comparing this sequence with that of the pro-cathepsin-D of normal human kidney (16), we found only 5 nucleotide changes giving only one amino acid substitution in the pro-fragment. At present, it is not known whether this change explains the slower processing and increased secretion of the pro-cathepsin-D observed in MCF7 cells, or whether it is due to a trivial polymorphism. The differences with the previously characterized cathepsin-D of normal tissue at present appear to be mostly quantitative and linked to its hormonal regulation. The concentration of this enzyme is very high in some breast cancers and melanomas (see clinical studies), and its precursor is secreted in greater amounts by breast cancer cells (30 to 40%) than by normal mammary epithelial cells or fibroblasts in culture (2 to 10%) (Capony et al., in preparation). Moreover, to our knowledge, a specific regulation of cathepsin-D by estrogens has never been observed in normal cells. In the rat uterus, the regulation is mostly triggered by progesterone (17) while progestins have no effect on the gene in breast cancer cells (6).

Mechanism of Regulation by Estrogens

The 52K protein was first defined according to the inducibility of the secreted form by estrogens. We then showed that the intracellular protein was also increased and that there was no specific regulation of glycosylation or phosphorylation (12). The 52K-λp9 cDNA probe could then be used to quantify the 52K-mRNA by hybridization after Northern blotting. The accumulation of 2.2 kb pre-pro-cathepsin-D mRNA was shown to be increased approximately tenfold by estradiol treatment of MCF7 cells. This increase was rapid for 3 h and optimal at 72 h (Fig. 2a); it was specific for estrogen receptor ligands since other classes of steroids were in-

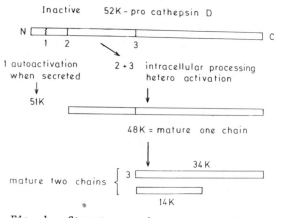

Fig. 1. Structure and processing of the 52K-cathepsin D.

active (18). The concentration of estradiol required to induce this mRNA corresponded to its affinity for the estrogen receptor (Fig. 2b).

The 52K-mRNA was not increased by the antiestrogen tamoxifen. Cyclo-heximide did not inhibit the induction and run-on transcription assay indicating that the stimulation was direct (18). As in the case of other steroid-induced responses, the regulation of cathepsin-D by estradiol was transcriptional. However, we also found that estradiol decreased by approximately twofold the processing of intracellular 52K-pro-cathepsin-D by an unknown posttranslational mechanism (12). The 52K-cathepsin-D gene is now being cloned to study the mechanism of its regulation and define the estrogen-responsive elements in both normal and cancerous cells. In situ hybridization of the 52K-λp9 cDNA probe has localized the 52K-cathepsin-D gene on the extremity of the short arm of chromosome 11 (band p.15) (20).

Biological Activities

The 52K-cathepsin-D secreted by MCF7 cells displays in vitro both a mitogenic activity on MCF7 cells (21) and a proteolytic activity on proteoglycans (22) and basement membrane (23) when activated at an acidic pH. These two activities suggest that it may have major function(s) in mammary carcinogenesis, stimulating tumor growth and/or invasion via its proteolytic activity (Fig. 2).

Mitogenic activity. The concept of estrogen-induced growth factors secreted by hormone-responsive cancer cells was first proposed in 1980 at the First International Congress on Hormones and Cancer (24) (Fig. 3).

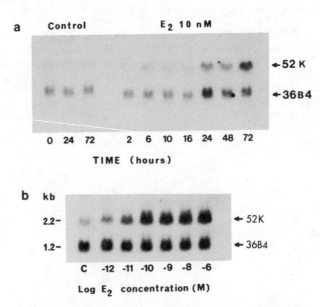

Fig. 2. Effect of estradiol on the accumulation of the 52K-cath-D mRNA (18). Hybridization with the ^{32}P labeled 52K-p9 cDNA clone. The 36B4 cDNA probe corresponds to an mRNA which is not regulated by estrogens (19). It allows a correction for the amount of RNA analyzed. (a) Time-course experiment. (b) Dose-response.

The first experimental evidence for a mitogenic effect of conditioned media prepared from estrogen-stimulated MCF7 cells was provided by Vignon et al. in 1983 (25). Since then, several groups have confirmed this mitogenic activity of estrogen-induced factors (26-27). There is, however, no consensus on the identity of the molecules responsible for this activity. Lippman, Dixon, and colleagues have found several growth factor-like activities to be stimulated by estrogens in these media (26). Some of them also appear to be active in vivo on the growth of MCF7 cells transplanted into nude mice (28). Taking a different approach, we purified the secreted 52K-protein and found that this fraction stimulated the growth of estrogen-deprived MCF7 cells (21). This stimulation was dose-dependent and occurred at concentrations (1 to 10 nM) similar to those found in the culture medium. However, time-course experiments indicated that both estradiol and 52K protein required the same lag (18 h) before stimulating [³H]thymidine incorporation. The in vitro mitogenic activity of purified 52K protein was in agreement with an estrogen-regulated autocrine mechanism. However, the mechanism of this mitogenic activity of 52K-cathepsin-D is unknown. It does not appear to be a classical growth factor since it contains its own enzymatic activity, whereas growth factors are peptides which indirectly stimulate the activity of another protein (enzyme or transporter) through their interaction with a membrane receptor. We have eliminated large contaminations of the purified 52K protein by growth factors and residual estrogens (21). Contamination by a very weak proportion ($\cong 10^{-3}$) of a potent growth factor, acting in the picogram range, remains a possibility, though unlikely. There are, however, examples of proteases acting as mitogens, such as trypsin or thrombin (29). Like other proteases, cathepsin-D may act indirectly via its enzymatic activity by releasing growth factors from precursors or from extracellular matrix and/or by activating growth factor receptors. For instance, proteolytic cleavages are needed to detach the TGFα precursor from membrane (30) and cathepsin-D may be involved in the activation of TGFβ (31). However, it is not certain that the mitogenic activity of the 52K-cathepsin-D observed at physiological pH (7.5) is due to its proteolytic activity, which is only observed in vitro at pH ≤5.5. It is thus possible that the protease directly stimulates a membrane receptor, since

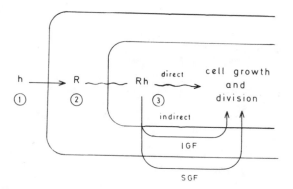

Fig. 3. Control of cell proliferation by a steroid hormone. A steroid hormone (h) such as estradiol acting via its specific receptor (R) stimulates cell growth and division in a breast cancer cell either directly or indirectly by inducing intracellular (IGF) or secreted (SGF) endogenous growth factor(s). Studies with conditioned media have supported the third pathway via SGF. Reproduced from Hormone and Cancer (1980) by permission (24).

homologies between growth factors and certain domains of proteases have been described (32). Further work is required to discriminate between these mechanisms.

  Proteolytic activity. Cathepsins normally function in lysosomes at very low pH, where they degrade endogenous proteins. Since a pro-cathepsin-D enzyme is secreted in large amounts at the periphery of cancer cells, we proposed that the enzyme may acquire abnormal functions, such as facilitating cancer cell migration and invasion by digesting basement membrane, extracellular matrix, and connective tissue. We therefore tested the ability of the purified 52K-pro-cathepsin-D and of conditioned media to digest in vitro [³H]proline-labeled extracellular matrix prepared from bovine corneal endothelial cells (23). The 52K cathepsin-D is secreted as an inactive proenzyme, but at acidic pH it can be auto-activated by the removal of a small part of the N-terminal pro-fragment. Both the purified 52K-cathepsin-D and media conditioned by estrogen-stimulated MCF7 cells were found to digest proteoglycans (22) and bovine endothelial extracellular matrix (23) at pH 4 to 5 but not at pH 7. Moreover, the degradation of extracellular matrix by secreted proteases was mostly due to cathepsin-D since it was totally inhibited by pepstatin. When MCF7 cells were cultured at pH 7.4 on this matrix, part of the degradation was also due to cathepsin-D (M. Morisset, Ph.D. thesis). However, other proteases inhibited by leupeptin and trasylol also appear to play a role in this degradation. Most cancer cells tested at present appear to secrete a pepstatin-inhibited protease (i.e., aspartyl protease) which appears to be one of the most abundant protease secreted by the epithelial cancers (23).

  Although the involvement of cathepsin-D in breast cancer metastasis has not yet been directly demonstrated, clinical studies performed in collaboration with several cancer centers, have strongly supported this hypothesis.

CLINICAL POTENTIAL OF 52K-CATHEPSIN-D AS A PROGNOSTIC TISSUE MARKER

Tissue Distribution of Immunoperoxidase Staining

  Using monoclonal antibodies to the mature 34K enzyme (9), we have examined frozen sections of several human tissues (33) with the peroxidase-antiperoxidase technique of Sternberger. Most of the staining was granular in the cytoplasm of epithelial cells and corresponded to lysosomes. No staining was observed in fibroblasts. Among the normal tissues studied, the protein appeared to be mostly concentrated in sweat glands and liver, but not in normal uterus or normal resting mammary glands collected during reduction mammoplasties. By contrast, immunostaining was observed in 43% of 127 biopsies of benign mastopathies. Gynecomastias, fibroadenomas, fibrous lesions, and lobular structures (adenosis, sclerosing adenosis, atypical lobular hyperplasia) were usually negative. The two groups of mastopathies that were highly stained were cysts over 3 mm in diameter and ductal hyperplasia.

  When the different histological types of mastopathy were pooled into proliferative (high-risk) and nonproliferative (low-risk) lesions, according to criteria defined by Dupont and Page (34), we found a significant correlation between proliferation and 52K protein staining. The use of 52K protein staining in predicting high-risk (proliferative) mastopathies may therefore be useful and complementary to histopathology, since 91.5% of the 52K-protein-negative lesions were nonproliferative and 60.5% of the 52K-protein-positive (noncystic) lesions were proliferative.

We also studied 52K-immunostaining of breast cancer tissue in an attempt to correlate its positivity with steroid-receptor content and other prognostic markers. The study included 232 primary breast carcinomas collected from April to September 1985, in three French cancer centers (Institut Gustave Roussy, Villejuif; Centre A. Lecassagne, Nice; Centre Paul Lamarque, Montpellier). The 52K protein was evaluated in frozen sections by immunohistochemistry, and the concentrations of estrogen receptors and progesterone receptors were assayed in cytosol by the classical dextran-coated charcoal method (7). The 52K protein was detected in 64% of the 232 tumor biopsies. No statistical correlation, either positive or negative, was observed between the estrogen or progesterone receptor concentration and the amount of 52K-positive cells.

The absence of correlation between these two types of markers was also shown directly using fine-needle aspirates of breast carcinomas to perform double immunohistochemical staining of the nuclear ER and cytoplasmic 52K protein in the same sample (35). There were tumor cells with detectable 52K protein and without ER staining, and others with ER and without detectable 52K protein. Among the other cancers examined, some melanomas were found to be positive, while benign nevi were generally negative (33) suggesting that this marker may be useful in detecting melanoma. Since histochemical parameters are difficult to quantify, we completed the study by immunoenzymatic assay of the 52K-cathepsin-D.

Immunoassay in Soluble Extracts

Using two combinations of antibodies that recognize two domains of the pro-enzyme, both the precursor (52K) and its cellular products (48K + 34K) can be assayed in the culture medium or in soluble extracts such as breast cancer cytosol. The validity and characteristics of the immunoassay are described separately (38,37). The production and secretion of the 52K protein were compared in several ER-positive and ER-negative cell lines. All ER-positive cell lines tested at confluency produced the 52K protein in the presence of estradiol, but its secretion varied markedly according to the cell line and the subspecies. For instance, the secretion of 52K protein by two MCF7 subspecies was quite different, but its regulation by estrogens was found in all ER-positive cell lines (7).

Interestingly, 52K-cathepsin-D was also produced and secreted by the two ER-negative breast cancer cell lines (BT20, MDA-MB231). The secretion and intracellular concentration of 52K protein in ER-negative cell lines were even higher than in some ER-positive cell lines, but were not regulated by estrogens.

Breast cancer cytosol is routinely used to determine estrogen and progesterone receptor levels. Several laboratories and cancer centers have collected banks of frozen cytosol which allow retrospective clinical studies with new markers. We therefore adapted the immunoassay of 52K-cathepsin-D for use with the breast cancer cytosol routinely used for receptor assays. We recently assayed in this cytosol the level of total cathepsin-D-like protein (using antibodies to the mature 34K enzyme) (36) and that of the 52K precursor alone (using one antibody to the pro-fragment) (37). In each case, a solid-phase double-determinant immunoenzymatic assay was used. Three studies have recently been completed. The first is a prospective study on 183 cytosols of pre- and postmenopausal primary breast cancers (38) collected in Montpellier between February 1985 and June 1986. The concentration of total cathepsin-D-like enzyme varied markedly according to the patient, from 3 to 167 pmoles cytosol protein, as did the proportion of the 52K precursor (0 to 38%). The absence of correlation with estrogen receptor concentration was confirmed (r=0.15). The significantly higher proportion of invaded axillary lymph nodes when the primary tumors contained ≥42 pmoles/mg protein suggested that the assay of total enzyme in cytosol may be valuable as a prognostic marker for predicting the degree of invasiveness of breast cancers. However, these tumors represented only 18% of the total population, and no correlation between 52K protein concentration and lymph node invasion was observed in the total population. Moreover, there was no correlation with Scarff and Bloom grading, tumor size, and age of patients. The other two studies were retrospective and performed in collaboration with the Finsen Institute of Copenhagen (S. Thorpe and C. Rose) on patients of the Danish Breast Cancer Cooperative Group. We assayed total 52K-cath-D in breast cancer cytosol collected at surgery 6 to 10 years earlier and kept at -70°C (S. Thorpe et al., submitted for publication) without knowledge of their clinical evolution or other prognostic parameters. In 154 postmenopausal patients, a significant correlation (P=0.039) was found between tumors with high (>24 pmole/mg protein) 52K-cath-D concentrations and short recurrence-free survival. In this study, the 52K protein parameter was found to be independent of other prognostic parameters in a final Cox multiparametric analysis. The receptor concentration and status, and the degree of lymph node invasiveness were not correlated with the 52K-cath-D concentration (39). In 237 premenopausal patients, preliminary analysis indicates similar results. There is a significant (P=0.046) correlation with relapse-free survival. In this case, however, the 52K-cath-D status is directly correlated with the estrogen receptor status (P=0.0125). The concentration of the cath-D precursor alone compared to that of total 52K protein is less correlated with the relapse-free survival of patients but more correlated with estrogen and progesterone receptor concentrations.

These first clinical studies indicate that 52K-cathepsin-D may be an important additional prognostic marker useful in monitoring breast cancer patients at the time of surgery. However, these results will have to be confirmed and extended in further studies and compared with those of other new prognostic markers. Since 52K-cath-D is independent of other parameters, it may particularly be useful in lymph-node-negative patients, where high 52K-cath-D concentrations may orientate towards an adjuvant therapy not otherwise used. Moreover, these clinical data are consistent with biological studies on cell lines suggesting a role of 52K-cath-D in the process of tumor invasion and metastasis. It now must be determined whether the mitogenic activity, the proteolytic activity, or both activities of this pro-cathepsin-D are actually responsible for the poorer prognosis of tumors expressing the highest level of the enzyme.

CONCLUSIONS

Estrogens participate in mammary carcinogenesis by stimulating the growth of cancer cells; they may also be involved in tumor invasion. Some distal metastases such as bone metastasis are particularly estrogen-responsive. The mechanism of cell metastasis is unknown and involves several steps, i.e., the digestion of basement membrane, the migration of tumor cells, and the homing and multiplication of metastasized cells (40). The first steps most likely involve proteases. The most frequent proteases thought to play a role are collagenases, plasminogen activator and cathepsin-B (41-43). Some of these proteases may act at the plasma membrane level, possibly by interacting with an anchorage membrane receptor as in the case of plasminogen activator (32). Other proteases may act directly at distant sites after secretion. Cathepsins are normally active in lysosomes at an acidic pH. Since the secreted precursor is enzymatically inactive, it must be secreted in an acidic micro-environment to be able to digest basement membrane. Cathepsin-B has previously been shown to be regulated by estrogen in uterus (44) and to be secreted in excess by metastatic melanoma cells (41). In breast cancer, at least two proteases, tissue plasminogen activator (45) and pro-cathepsin-D, are induced by estrogens and secreted by breast cancer cells. Future studies will aim at determining the respective roles of these proteases (and others) in cooperation with several growth factors (Fig. 4).

Increased cathepsin activity has previously been implicated in the process of tumor regression after castration in animal models (47). It is therefore an apparent paradox that in human breast cancer cells, cathepsin-D appears to be involved in stimulating tumor growth and invasion. The estrogen regulation of cath-D synthesis and processing in breast cancer cells in culture provides an interesting model for studying the mechanism regulating gene expression by estrogens in human cells, and the mechanism by which estrogens stimulate the initial steps of carcinogenesis in estrogen target tissues. It remains to be determined whether pro-cath-D can be activated extracellularly or intracellularly, whether it is able to favor metastatic process in vivo and whether specific inhibition of its activity could be a new therapeutic approach to breast cancer. Two major clinical applications are, in fact, anticipated by these studies. In the short term, the assay of 52K-cath-D in primary breast cancer appears to be of prognostic value for indicating a more appropriate adjuvant therapy. In the longer term, discovery of the way in which this protease stimulates cell growth and eventually digests basement membrane, may lead to specific ways of inhibiting these activities. This could then be applied to new therapeutic approaches to cancers that secrete large amounts of this protease.

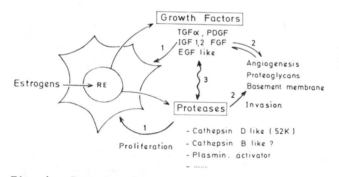

Fig. 4. Putative functions of estrogen-regulated secreted proteins, and peptides secreted by breast cancer cells. Estrogens, via their nuclear receptors (ER), induce several proteins and factors which are secreted by breast cancer cells. One category (growth factors) may act as autocrine factors stimulating the growth of the same cells. Other proteins, such as proteases, may act as mitogens either directly or via their enzymatic activity and may also facilitate tumor cell invasion. Proteases and growth factors may act cooperatively and it is essential to determine the relationship between the two types of protein: induction of proteases by growth factors, activation of growth factor precursors or receptors by proteases, interaction on similar membrane receptors via homologous sequences, etc. Reproduced with permission (46).

ACKNOWLEDGMENTS

We would like to thank members of our laboratory who have contributed to several parts of this work and E. Barrie for her skillful preparation of the manuscript. We are grateful to SANOFI Laboratory (B. Pau, F. Paolucci) for monoclonal antibodies, P. Chambon (Strasbourg) and F. Rougeon (Pasteur, Paris) for 52K-cDNA cloning, P. Ferrara, P. Louisot, A. Barrett, for protein structure studies, G. Mattei for chromosome mapping and to several scientists (Drs. M. Lippman, M. Rich, I. Keydar, and the Mason Research Institute) for their gifts of mammary cell lines. Clinical studies have been performed with the help of several clinical centers in Copenhagen (Finsen Institute, Dr. S. Thorpe), Montpellier (Professors H. Pujol, J. L. Lamarque, F. Laffargue), Villejuif (Drs. G. Contesso, Delarue) and Nice (Drs. Duplay, Namer).

This work was supported by the "Institut National de la Sante et de la Recherche Medicale," the Faculty of Medicine of Montpellier, the "Association pour la Recherche sur le Cancer," the "Federation Nationale des Centres de Lutte contre le Cancer" and a grant INSERM-SANOFI n° 81039.3.

REFERENCES

1. Adams DJ, Edwards DP, McGuire WL. Estrogen regulation of specific proteins as a mode of hormone action in human breast cancer; vol 11. In: Biomembranes, 1983:389.
2. Rochefort H, Chalbos D, Capony F, et al. Effect of estrogen in breast cancer cells in culture: released proteins and control of cell proliferation. In: Gurpide E, Calandra R, Levy C, Soto RJ, eds. Hormones and cancer; vol 142. New York: Alan R. Liss, Inc., 1984:37.
3. Vignon F, Rochefort H. The regulation by estradiol of proteins released by breast cancer cells. In: Hollander VP, ed. Hormone responsive tumors. New York: Academic Press, 1985:135.
4. Lippman ME, Dickson RB, Bates S, et al. Autocrine and paracrine growth regulation of human breast cancer. Breast Cancer Res Treat 1986; 1:59.
5. Westley B, Rochefort H. Estradiol induced proteins in the MCF7 human breast cancer cell line. Biochem Biophys Res Commun 1979; 90:410.
6. Westley B, Rochefort H. A secreted glycoprotein induced by estrogen in human breast cancer cell lines. Cell 1980; 20:352.
7. Garcia M, Contesso G, Duplay H, et al. Immunohistochemical distribution of the 52K protein in mammary tumors: a marker associated to cell proliferation rather than to hormone responsiveness. J Steroid Biochem 1987; 26 (in press).
8. Westley B, May FEB, Brown AMC, et al. Effects of antiestrogens on the estrogen regulated pS2 RNA, 52-kDa and 180-kDa protein in MCF7 cells and two tamoxifen resistant sublines. J Biol Chem 1984; 259:10030.
9. Garcia M, Capony F, Derocq D, Simon D, Pau B, Rochefort H. Monoclonal antibodies to the estrogen-regulated Mr 52,000 glycoprotein: characterization and immunodetection in MCF7 cells. Cancer Res 1985; 45:709.
10. Capony F, Garcia M, Capdevielle J, Rougeot C, Ferrara P, Rochefort H. Purification and characterization of the secreted and cellular 52-kDa proteins regulated by estrogens in human breast cancer cells. Eur J Biochem 1986; 161:505.
11. Capony F, Morisset M, Barrett AJ, et al. Phosphorylation, glycosylation and proteolytic activity of the 52K estrogen-induced protein secreted by MCF7 cells. J Cell Biol 1987; 104:253.

12. Morisset M, Capony F, Rochefort H. Processing and estrogen regulation of the 52-kDa protein inside MCF7 breast cancer cells. Endocrinology 1986; 119:2773.

13. Von Figura K, Hasilik A. Lysosomal enzymes and their receptors. Annu Rev Biochem 1985; 55:167.

14. Barrett AJ. Purification of isoenzymes from human and chicken liver. Biochem J 1970; 117:601.

15. Augereau P, Garcia M, Cavailles V, Chalbos D, Capony F, Rochefort H. cDNA cloning and regulation of the messenger RNA for the estrogen-regulated 52K protease in human breast cancer. Proceedings of the Endocrine Society Meeting, The Endocrine Society, Bethesda, 1987 (in press).

16. Faust PL, Kornfeld S, Chirgwin JM. Cloning and sequence analysis of cDNA for human cathepsin D. Proc Natl Acad Sci USA 1985; 82:4910.

17. Moulton BC, Koenig BB. Progestin increases cathepsin D in uterine luminal epithelial cells. Am J Physiol 1983; 244:E442-6.

18. Cavailles V, Augereau P, Garcia M, Rochefort H. Estrogens induce the mRNA coding for a pro-cathepsin-D secreted by breast cancer cells. Submitted for publication.

19. Chambon P, Dierich A, Gaub MP, et al. Promoter elements of genes coding for proteins and modulation of transcription by estrogens and progesterone. In: Greep O, ed. Recent Progress in Hormone Research. New York: Academic Press, 1984; 40:1.

20. Augereau P, Garcia M, Mattei MG, et al. Cloning and sequencing of the 52K cathepsin D cDNA of MCF7 breast cancer cells and mapping on chromosome 11. Mol Endocrinol 1987 (in press).

21. Vignon F, Capony F, Chambon M, Freiss G, Garcia M, Rochefort H. Autocrine growth stimulation of the MCF7 breast cancer cells by the estrogen-regulated 52K protein. Endocrinology 1986; 118:1537.

22. Morisset M, Capony F, Rochefort H. The 52-kDa estrogen-induced protein secreted by MCF7 cells is a lysosomal acidic protease. Biochem Biophys Res Commun 1986; 138:102.

23. Briozzo P, Morisset M, Capony F, Rougeot C, Rochefort H. Cathepsin D is the major acidic protease secreted by cultured breast cancer cells and able to degrade extracellular matrix in vitro. Submitted for publication.

24. Rochefort H, Coezy E, Joly E, Westley B, Vignon F. Hormonal control of breast cancer in cell culture. In: Iacobelli S, et al., eds. Hormones and cancer. New York: Raven Press, 1980:21.

25. Vignon F, Derocq D, Chambon N, Rochefort H. Endocrinologie. Les proteines oestrogeno-induites secretees par les cellules mammaires cancereuses humaines MCF7 stimulent leur proliferation. C R Acad Sci [III] (Paris) 1983; 296:151.

26. Lippman ME, Dickson RB, Bates S, et al. Breast Cancer Res Treat 1986; 1:59-70.

27. Manni A, Wright C, Feil P, et al. Autocrine stimulation by estradiol-regulated growth factors of rat hormone-responsive mammary cancer: interaction with the polyamine pathway. Cancer Res 1986; 46:1594-9.

28. Dickson RB, McManaway ME, Lippman ME. Estrogen-induced factors of breast cancer cells partially replace estrogen to promote tumor growth. Science 1986; 232:1540.

29. Low DA, Wiley HS, Cunningham DD. In: Feramisco J, Ozanne B, Stiles B, eds. Cancer cells 3. Growth factors and transformation. Cold Spring Harbor, New York: Cold Spring Harbor Laboratory, 1985:401-8.

30. Derynck R, Roberts AB, Winkler ME, Chen EY, Goeddel DV. Human transforming growth factor-β: precursor structure and expression in E. Coli. Cell 1984; 38:287.

31. Lawrence DA, Pircher R, Jullien P. Conversion of a high molecular weight latent β-TGF from chicken embryo fibroblasts into a low molecular weight active β-TGF under acidic conditions. Biochem Biophys Res Commun 1985; 133:1026.

32. Appella E, Robinson EA, Ullrich SJ, et al. The receptor-binding sequence of urokinase. A biological function for the growth-factor module of proteases. J Biol Chem 1987; 262:4437.

33. Garcia M, Salazar-Retana G, Pages A, et al. Distribution of the Mr 52,000 estrogen-regulated protein in benign breast diseases and other tissues by immunohistochemistry. Cancer Res 1986; 46:3734.

34. Dupont WD, Page DL. Risk factors for breast cancer in women with proliferative breast disease. N Engl J Med 1985; 312:146.

35. Cavailles V, Garcia M, Salazar G, et al. Immunodetection of estrogen receptor and 52K protein in fine needle aspirates of breast cancer. J Natl Cancer Inst 1987; 79:245.

36. Rogier H, Freiss G, Paolucci F, Garcia M, Pau B. An immunoenzymometric assay for determining 52K protein in the cytosol of breast cancer tissues. Submitted for publication.

37. Freiss G, Rochefort H, Maudelonde T, Cavalie G, Khalaf S, Vignon F. Characterization and properties of two monoclonal antibodies to the pro-fragment of the 52K estrogen-regulated protease. Proceedings of the Endocrine Society, The Endocrine Society, Bethesda, 1987 (in press).

38. Maudelonde T, Khalaf S, Garcia M, et al. Immunoenzymatic assay of 52K cathepsin D in 182 breast cancer cytosols. Low correlation with other prognostic parameters. Cancer Res 1987 (in press).

39. Thorpe S, et al. The 52K-cathepsin-D, a novel independent prognostic factor in breast cancer. Submitted for publication.

40. Liotta LA, Tryggvason K, Garbisa S, Hart I, Foltz CM, Shafie S. Metastatic potential correlates with enzymatic degradation of basement membrane collagen. Nature 1980; 284:67.

41. Goldfarb RH. Proteolytic enzymes in tumor invasion and degradation of host extracellular matrices. In: Honn KV, Powers WE, Sloane BF, eds. Mechanisms of cancer metastasis. Boston: Martinus Nijhoff Publishing, 1986:341.

42. Ossowski L, Reich E. Antibodies to plasminogen activator inhibit human tumor metastasis. Cell 1983; 35:611.

43. Poole AR. Tumor lysosomal enzymes and invasive growth. In: Dingle JT, Fell HB, eds. Lysosomes in biology and pathology. New York: American Elsevier Publishing Company, 1979:304.

44. Pietras RJ, Szego CM. Estrogen-induced membrane alterations and growth associated with proteinase activity in endometrial cells. J Cell Biol 1979; 81:649.

45. Butler WB, Kirkland WL, Jorgensen TL. Induction of plasminogen activator by estrogen in a human breast cancer cell line (MCF7). Biochem Biophys Res Commun 1979; 90:1328-34.

46. Rochefort H, Capony F, Garcia M, et al. Estrogen-induced lysosomal proteases secreted by breast cancer cells: a role in carcinogenesis? J Cell Biochem 1987; 35-7.

47. Cho-Chung YS, Gullino PM. Mammary tumor regression. V. Role of acid ribonuclease and cathepsin. J Biol Chem 1973; 248:4743.

17

NUCLEAR ACCEPTOR SITES: INTERACTION WITH ESTROGEN- VERSUS ANTIESTROGEN-RECEPTOR COMPLEXES

Thomas S. Ruh, Mary F. Ruh, and Raj K. Singh

Department of Physiology
St. Louis University School of Medicine
St. Louis, MO 63104

INTRODUCTION

Although it is generally accepted that an interaction between steroid hormone receptors and nuclear acceptor sites is necessary for steroid induction of gene expression, the components of specific nuclear acceptor sites are still being investigated. There have been numerous models for steroid receptor interaction with target cell nuclear components, such as binding to nuclear membranes, RNA, nuclear matrix, DNA sequences and acceptor protein-DNA complexes. None of these models are mutually exclusive of one another.

Enhanced binding of steroid hormone receptor complexes to selected DNA sequences, termed hormone response elements, in or immediately upstream from steroid regulated genes has been reported (1-4). Sequence insertion and deletion experiments have suggested an important role for several of these regions of DNA in in vivo steroid action on gene transcription (5-7). However, these hormone response elements do not demonstrate the high affinity and specificity expected of hormone receptor-acceptor sites. In fact, glucocorticoid response elements bind progesterone receptors as well as glucocorticoid receptors (3,8). In tissues possessing several different hormone receptors, the mechanisms whereby a given steroid hormone only elicits the response specific to that hormone must still be elucidated. In addition, recent reports also indicate that receptors bound by agonist or antagonist bind in vitro to the same DNA sequences with the same order of preference, yet in vivo provide very different biological responses (9).

Advances in understanding the structure of steroid hormone receptors have indicated that all steroid hormone receptors can be divided into at least four regions (10): steroid binding domain, hinge region, DNA binding domain, and immunological region (N-terminus). Steroid hormone receptors with overlapping steroid binding activity show greater homology in the steroid binding domain than with those steroid receptors with little overlap in steroid binding. The hinge region may be responsible for exposing the DNA binding region, a process that occurs with ligand binding and termed transformation or activation (11,12). The DNA binding domain shows a great deal of homology (> 90%) for several receptors within a group, i.e., glucocorticoid, mineralocorticoid and progesterone receptors versus estrogen and vitamin D receptors (10). Whereas the DNA binding domain itself is insufficient to induce significant gene expression in transfection experiments using modified receptor forms, the immunological region, which shows little homology (< 15%) among receptors, is essential for induction of gene expression (8,10). Could part of this region of the receptor interact with specific chromosomal proteins, allowing the DNA binding region to come in contact with hormone response elements, which then results in gene transcription? In other words, is protein-protein interaction the key to high affinity binding of receptors to acceptor sites and does such binding allow for target tissue and hormone receptor specificity? It could well be that certain nonhistone chromosomal proteins are needed to confer receptor binding specificity to such systems.

Our laboratory has chosen to study nonhistone chromosomal acceptor proteins as candidate components of acceptor sites for steroid receptors (Fig. 1). The term "acceptor site" as used in this review will signify nonhistone protein-DNA complexes which confer high affinity binding in the interaction with steroid receptor complexes. In our approach to the study of the mechanisms of action of steroid hormones, we have used receptor binding to acceptor protein-DNA sites termed nucleoacidic protein (NAP). NAP is defined as either that partially deproteinized chromatin fraction with enhanced acceptor activity (native NAP) or certain chromosomal nonhistone proteins reconstituted to DNA forming an acceptor protein-DNA complex with enhanced acceptor activity (reconstituted NAP) (13,14).

It is still not known whether acceptor sites (nonhistone protein-DNA sequences) are near structural genes or regulatory genes. Those regions immediately upstream from structural genes may not represent the acceptor sites for steroid receptors (15). It is quite possible that the receptor could bind an acceptor site near a regulatory gene and induce a response in that regulatory gene a long distance from the structural gene that characterizes the biological response to the hormone (Fig. 1). With DNA looping where a regulatory gene may be in close proximity to a structural gene, such a postulate is easy to envision. Alternately, a product of a regulatory gene (RNA or protein) could regulate a structural gene at some distance. Of course, the steroid receptor may also bind to acceptor sites neighboring related structural genes. The availability of acceptor sites for binding by steroid receptor may itself be regulated by removal of "masking proteins," nonhistone proteins which render a gene unavailable for induction (15,16). Therefore, multiple acceptor sites could become available as the biological response proceeds.

We have found that acceptor sites for the estrogen receptor can distinguish estrogen receptors bound by estrogens versus antiestrogens (16-20). Since antiestrogens can stimulate certain cellular responses but can also inhibit estrogen action (mixed agonists/antagonists), the study of the interaction of estrogen- versus antiestrogen-receptor complexes with chromatin acceptor sites may help us to better understand both estrogen and antiestrogen action. Also, antiestrogens may be useful probes for helping to elucidate the general mechanisms whereby steroid hormones alter gene expression.

CHROMATIN ACCEPTOR SITE CHARACTERISTICS

Our initial studies, designed to study estrogen receptor acceptor sites in chromatin, utilized selectively deproteinized chromatin fractions obtained with chaotropic agents. This approach served two functions: (i) removing specific proteins which mask acceptor sites; and (ii) extraction or removal of the acceptor protein components of these same sites. The technique (21) for immobilizing chromatin on an insoluble matrix in order

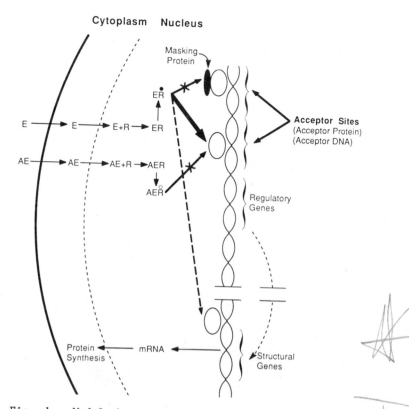

Cytoplasm   Nucleus

Masking Protein

ER

Acceptor Sites
(Acceptor Protein)
(Acceptor DNA)

E ⟶ E ⟶ E+R ⟶ ER

AE ⟶ AE ⟶ AE+R ⟶ AER

AER

Regulatory Genes

Protein Synthesis ⟵ mRNA ⟵

Structural Genes

Fig. 1. Model depicting the potential mechanism of action of estrogens versus antiestrogens. Antiestrogens (AE) compete with estrogens (E) for binding to the estrogen receptor (R), resulting in an altered receptor conformation. The AER is unable to bind certain nuclear acceptor sites necessary for maximal cell stimulation. The estrogen receptor may bind directly to acceptor sites in association with structural genes or the receptor may bind acceptor sites that induce an intermediate signal (regulatory gene) which in turn induces the structural gene.

to unmask acceptor sites was utilized (Fig. 2). Chromatin was prepared and linked to cellulose and the chromatin-cellulose resin was partially deproteinized using increased concentrations of the chaotropic agent guanidine hydrochloride (Gdn·HCl). Essentially all of the histones and 80% nonhistone proteins were extracted by 2 M Gdn·HCl and 3-8 M Gdn·HCl extracted approximately 1% nonhistone proteins with each increase in molarity (Fig. 3). The washed chromatin resins were assayed for high affinity binding (acceptor activity) by interaction with partially purified radiolabeled steroid hormone receptor complexes.

Experiments utilizing partially deproteinized chromatin fractions from a variety of systems have demonstrated the specific interaction of steroid receptors with acceptor sites. We have found that acceptor sites can distinguish structural/conformational changes induced in the estrogen receptor by estrogens versus antiestrogens (Fig. 4). For the rabbit uterine system (A) the binding of [^{3}H]estradiol-receptor complexes ([^{3}H]ER) displayed 3 high affinity binding sites which were unmasked with 1 M, 4 M and 6 M Gdn·HCl (17). Because of the high affinity of [^{3}H]H1285

235

Methods

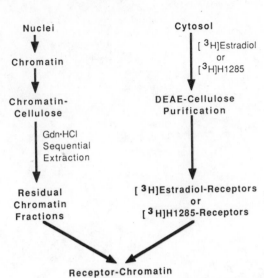

Fig. 2. Procedure for the chromatin–cellulose binding assay for nuclear acceptor sites. The preparations of partially deproteinized chromatin-cellulose and partially purified estrogen receptors are outlined.

(22) for the calf and rabbit uterine as well as MCF-7 cell estrogen receptors, we were able to partially purify [^{3}H]H1285–receptor complexes ([^{3}H]HR) and use these as probes for the actions of antiestrogens at the chromatin level in order to better understand the differing biological responses of estrogens and antiestrogens. Acceptor site activity for

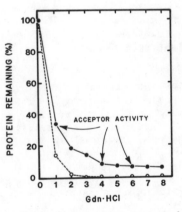

Fig. 3. Extraction of histone and nonhistone proteins from rabbit uterine chromatin-cellulose by Gdn·HCl. Chromatin-cellulose was extracted with 0-8 M Gdn·HCl and washed extensively to remove the Gdn·HCl. The pellet was assayed for histone (o---o) and nonhistone (•——•) proteins. Arrows denote residual fractions which contain acceptor site activity. Reprinted from reference 17.

antiestrogen-receptor complexes in rabbit uterus was markedly decreased at sites unmasked by 4 M and 6 M Gdn·HCl. Results similar to those obtained with the rabbit uterus were found with MCF-7 cells (B). Partially deproteinized chromatin from antiestrogen-sensitive cells revealed maximal binding activity unmasked by 1 M and 6 M Gdn·HCl for [³H]ER (18). In contrast, antiestrogen-receptor complexes bound maximally to the 1 M site and to a new 4 M site, with negligible binding to the 6 M site. Of special interest was the finding that antiestrogen-receptor complexes could not detect a 4 M site in chromatin prepared from antiestrogen-resistant MCF-7 cells.

Using the chromatin-cellulose assay, we were also able to determine that steroid receptors bind in a saturable manner to select residual chromatin fractions, allowing direct calculation of Kd's and sites per

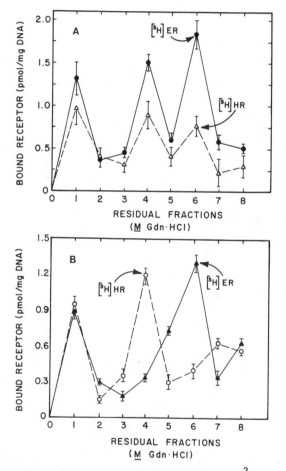

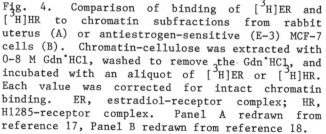

Fig. 4. Comparison of binding of [³H]ER and [³H]HR to chromatin subfractions from rabbit uterus (A) or antiestrogen-sensitive (E-3) MCF-7 cells (B). Chromatin-cellulose was extracted with 0-8 M Gdn·HCl, washed to remove the Gdn·HCl, and incubated with an aliquot of [³H]ER or [³H]HR. Each value was corrected for intact chromatin binding. ER, estradiol-receptor complex; HR, H1285-receptor complex. Panel A redrawn from reference 17, Panel B redrawn from reference 18.

cell. Using the same procedures, receptor binding to intact double-stranded DNA is linear and not saturable. High affinity of receptor for acceptor sites in several systems has been reported by our laboratory, i.e., calf (23) and rabbit uterus (17), MCF-7 cells (18), mouse B lymphocytes (24), shark testis (25), mouse mammary glands (26,27). Several chromatins appear to possess multiple high affinity and low capacity binding sites for steroid receptors. The Kd's for most systems are in the 0.1 nM range. The number of sites per cell is in agreement with the number of binding sites for steroid hormones in target tissue nuclei. High affinity binding of steroid receptors for nuclear acceptor sites has also been reported by others (see 14,15 for review).

Specificity and saturability of nuclear acceptors has also been studied in a variety of steroid hormone responsive systems by our laboratory. A summary of the various criteria applied to nuclear acceptor sites is given in Table 1. Just as competition for binding by nonradiolabeled ligand for radiolabeled ligand is a criterium for steroid receptors, so also should competition by nonradiolabeled receptor complexes for binding to chromatin by radiolabeled receptor complexes be a criterium for defining nuclear acceptor sites. For example, binding of [^{3}H]ER or [^{3}H]HR in the presence of unlabeled ligand-receptor complexes was determined for those fractions of deproteinized chromatin demonstrating the greatest acceptor activity (18,28). A twofold excess of radioinert ER or HR was able to compete with and displace the appropriate radiolabeled receptor complex with a respective decrease of approximately 70% which compares well to a theoretical maximum of 67% for a twofold excess radioinert receptor. These results indicate not only that the receptor binding to chromatin acceptor sites is competable but also that these sites can be quite specific for a particular ligand-receptor complex, i.e., ER or HR.

We have also demonstrated the necessity for intact, activated and functional receptor complexes. Chromatin binding of salt-activated but not molybdate-stabilized nonactivated receptors has been shown (17,24). Free radioligand or heat-denatured receptors will not bind (17,23,24). Chromatin acceptor sites are receptor-specific, i.e., glucocorticoid receptors will not bind estrogen receptor acceptor sites and vice versa (21,27). There is a positive relationship between the specific interaction of steroid receptors with chromatin acceptor sites and hormone sensitivity of the target tissue (21). In addition, chromatin acceptor sites demonstrate target tissue vs. nontarget tissue specificity (17,25, 26). In some systems acceptor site specificity is distinct between species and tissues (25,26).

Thus, several parameters of the specific interaction of receptor with acceptor sites have been determined using the chromatin-cellulose binding assay. In addition, the different binding characteristics of antiestrogen-receptor complexes (compared with estrogen-receptor complexes) to chromatin acceptor sites suggests mechanisms whereby antiestrogens induce both agonistic and antagonistic responses in many tissues.

CHARACTERIZATION OF ACCEPTOR PROTEINS

The chromatin-cellulose assay described previously suggests that certain salt concentrations remove masking proteins, which allows for increased acceptor activity, and the next subsequent higher salt concentrations remove these exposed acceptor site proteins. Support for these results requires characterization of the removed acceptor proteins. To do this, the chromosomal proteins (CP) conferring acceptor activity must be extracted using the next higher concentrations of a chaotropic agent, the proteins must be fractionated, and these proteins must be assayed for

Table 1. Specificity of nuclear acceptor sites.

Acceptor sites:
  display high affinity for receptors
  are saturable (competition)
  display steroid receptor specificity
  require intact, activated receptors
  require functional receptors
  distinguish receptors bound by agonist vs. antagonist
  display target tissue vs. nontarget tissue specificity
  display species and target tissue preference

acceptor activity by reconstituting onto DNA. The latter step allows these highly hydrophobic proteins to be soluble in low salt buffers and therefore allows for receptor binding assays. Using methods originally described by Spelsberg's laboratory (13,14), results from our laboratory (Fig. 5) have demonstrated that the interpretation of the chromatin-cellulose studies is supported by reconstitution studies. For example, 2M, 5M and 7M Gdn·HCl removed the proteins involved in conferring acceptor activity to the acceptor sites unmasked by 1M, 4M and 6M Gdn·HCl, respectively.

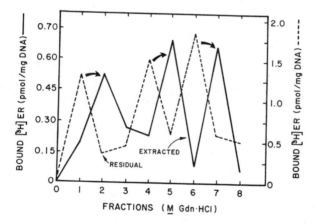

Fig. 5. Comparison of the binding of [³H]ER to native and reconstituted chromatin acceptor sites in rabbit uterus. [³H]ER were partially purified by DEAE-cellulose chromatography. In one series of experiments, chromatin-cellulose was extracted stepwise with 0-8 M Gdn·HCl, washed to remove the Gdn·HCl and incubated with [³H]ER. After washing, radioactivity was extracted with absolute ethanol and counted (--). Each of these values was corrected for intact chromatin binding. For reconstitution studies, histones were removed by 3 M NaCl and uterine chromatin non-histone proteins were fractionated from chromatin-hydroxylapatite by step-elution using Gdn·HCl (1-8 M). Samples of the extracted proteins were reconstituted to rabbit spleen DNA by reverse gradient dialysis. The receptor complexes were then incubated with each reconstituted nucleoacidic protein (NAP) or rabbit DNA. Acceptor activity for [³H]ER was then assayed using the streptomycin filter assay (13). Binding to DNA was subtracted from these values.

Chromatin from rabbit uterus or MCF-7 cells was bound to hydroxy-lapatite, and the histones were removed with 3 M NaCl and the nonhistone chromosomal proteins (CP) were removed with a series of step-elutions by 1-8 M Gdn·HCl and termed CP1 through CP8 on the basis of molarities of the salt (Fig. 6). Samples of nonhistone protein fractions were then reconstituted to rabbit DNA to form nucleoacidic protein (NAP) fractions. The reconstituted NAP fractions were assayed for their ability to bind [^{3}H]ER and [^{3}H]HR using the streptomycin assay (13).

Antiestrogen-sensitive MCF-7 Cells

We investigated the characteristics of MCF-7 chromatin proteins from antiestrogen-sensitive cells. Results revealed enhanced [^{3}H]ER binding to protein-DNA complexes reconstituted with CP2 and CP7 (Fig. 7). However, [^{3}H]HR bound not only to the reconstituted CP2 site but in addition bound to a new CP5 site, whereas binding to the CP7 site was nearly absent as compared to [^{3}H]ER. These results support our previous findings of unmasked acceptor sites in residual chromatin subfractions. The reconstituted CP5 and CP7 sites were saturable (Fig. 8) for their respective receptor complexes with Kd's of 0.17 and 0.35 nM, respectively, the concentration of acceptor sites was approximately 4000 sites/cell. In addition, a twofold excess of unlabeled ER, but not HR, competed with [^{3}H]ER for the CP7 site whereas a twofold excess unlabeled HR, but not ER, competed with [^{3}H]HR for the CP5 site (Fig. 9). Specific binding is estimated to be about 50% of total binding.

Rabbit Uterus

Chromosomal protein fractions CP2, CP5 and CP7 when reconstituted to rabbit DNA showed increased binding for [^{3}H]ER (Fig. 10), whereas [^{3}H]HR did not bind significantly to the acceptor sites formed with CP7. Satura-

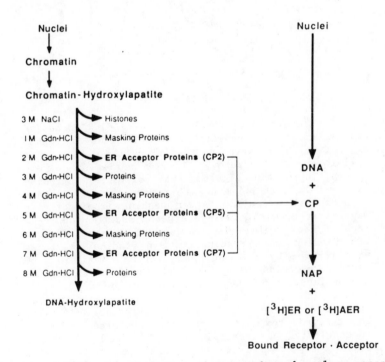

Fig. 6. Outline for the assay of reconstituted nuclear acceptor sites. NAP = nucleoacidic proteins, CP = chromosomal proteins.

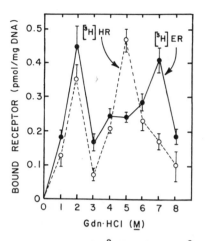

Fig. 7. Binding of [3H]ER and [3H]HR to
reconstituted chromatin acceptor sites in
MCF-7 antiestrogen-sensitive cells. Samples
of the Gdn·HCl extracted proteins were reconstituted to human DNA by reverse gradient
dialysis. The receptor complexes were then
incubated with each reconstituted nucleoacidic
protein (NAP). Binding was then assayed using
the streptomycin filter assay. Binding to DNA
was subtracted from these values. ER, estradiol-receptor complex; HR, H1285-receptor
complex. Reprinted from reference 29.

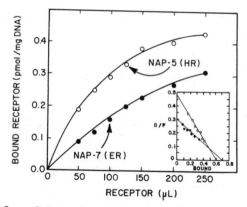

Fig. 8. Saturation kinetics for binding of
[3H]ER and [3H]HR to NAP from chromatin protein
fractions CP7 and CP5, respectively. MCF-7 nonhistone proteins fractionated from chromatin
between 4M and 5M Gdn·HCl and between 6M and 7M
Gdn·HCl were reconstituted to DNA by reverse
gradient dialysis. Increasing concentrations of
[3H]ER or [3H]HR were incubated with reconstituted NAP from CP7 or CP5 and binding assayed.
Bound is expressed as pmol/mg DNA. Scatchard
analysis of binding experiments. ER, estradiol-
receptor complex; HR, H1285-receptor complex.
Redrawn from reference 20.

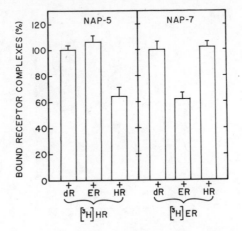

Fig. 9. Competitive binding of MCF-7 cell estrogen-receptor complexes to reconstituted NAP from CP5 and CP7. Partially purified [^{3}H]ER or [^{3}H]HR were used to determine binding to NAP from CP7 and CP5, respectively, in the absence of (100%) or in the presence of twofold excess unlabeled ER or HR. Protein content was kept constant with heat-denatured receptor preparations (dR). ER, estradiol-receptor complex; HR, H1285-receptor complex. Reprinted from reference 20.

tion analysis of the reconstituted CP7 acceptor sites with [^{3}H]ER yielded a Kd of approximately 10^{-9} M whereas [^{3}H]ER binding to rabbit DNA was nonsaturable (Fig. 11A). Saturability and specificity of [^{3}H]ER for the CP7-DNA complex was confirmed by competition studies. CP7 reconstituted to rabbit DNA was incubated with [^{3}H]ER in the absence or presence of twofold excess nonradiolabeled ER or HR (Fig. 12). Unlabeled ER but not HR competed with [^{3}H]ER for binding to this acceptor site. Both [^{3}H]ER and [^{3}H]HR bound the acceptor sites formed with CP5 (Fig. 11B) and CP2 (Fig. 11C) with Kd's in the 10^{-9} M range. Again, binding of either complex to DNA was nonsaturable. The number of binding sites for these reconstitution studies ranged from 8,000-10,000 sites/cell.

To further characterize the protein components of these acceptor sites, CP fractions were subjected to molecular sieve chromatography using CL-Sepharose 6B (Fig. 13). Two protein subfractions of the CP7 (approximate MW 50,000 and MW 12,000) were isolated which, when reconstituted to rabbit DNA, yielded high affinity sites for [^{3}H]ER (Fig. 13A). No protein subfractions from CP7 yielded high affinity sites for [^{3}H]HR. In addition, the nonhistone proteins in CP5 contained two species of acceptor proteins (Fig. 13B). When reconstituted to DNA, one protein (approximate MW 30,000) bounds only [^{3}H]HR while another protein (approximate MW 12,000) binds only [^{3}H]ER. Furthermore, CP2 contained two subsets of acceptor proteins (approximate MW 45,000 and MW 9,000) which seemed to bind [^{3}H]HR and [^{3}H]ER equally well (Fig. 13C).

DISCUSSION

We have reviewed the data from our laboratory which demonstrate the characteristics of the specific interaction of steroid hormone receptors with acceptor sites and we have summarized our findings that estrogen- and

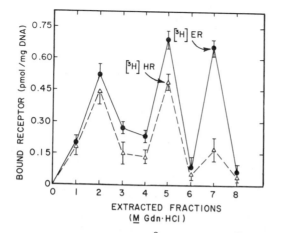

Fig. 10. Binding of [³H]ER and [³H]HR to
reconstituted rabbit uterine chromatin acceptor
sites. Samples of extracted proteins were
reconstituted to rabbit DNA by reverse gradient
dialysis. The receptor complexes were then
incubated with each reconstituted NAP or rabbit
DNA and acceptor activity measured. Samples of
extracted spleen (nontarget tissue) chromosomal
proteins were also reconstituted to DNA; however, no acceptor activity was detected. ER,
estradiol-receptor complex; HR, H1285-receptor
complex. Reprinted from reference 16.

antiestrogen-receptor complexes differ in their chromatin binding characteristics. These results were obtained using two different approaches,
i.e., binding of receptor to partially deproteinized residual chromatin
fractions and to reconstituted nucleoacidic protein fractions. In summary, estrogen receptors interact in a saturable manner with intact or
partially deproteinized chromatin subfractions as well as reconstituted
NAP. Specific chromosomal proteins appear to be associated with acceptor
site activity, since removal of these proteins by salt (or pronase)
decreases receptor binding to residual fractions, and only specific
protein fractions when reconstituted to DNA enhance acceptor activity.
That chromatin acceptor sites can distinguish structural/conformational
changes induced in the estrogen receptor by estrogens versus antiestrogens
supports our previous findings (30) which suggested that estrogen receptor
bound by estrogen undergoes activation to a different degree when compared
with estrogen receptor bound by antiestrogen. Antiestrogen binding may
affect the monomer-dimer equilibrium of the receptors (31-34) as well as
conformational changes in the receptors which may ultimately be responsible for the altered chromatin binding. This, then, may result in the
antagonistic actions of antiestrogen.

It is possible that acceptor activity which is similar for both
estrogens and antiestrogens may involve the agonistic biological responses
obtained with both classes of compounds, whereas acceptor sites which only
interact with estrogen-bound receptor may be responsible for the complete
or maximal responses obtained with estradiol. Antiestrogens, when bound
to the estrogen receptor, would fail to interact with this set of acceptor
sites and, thus, would not yield maximal effects. Since antiestrogens
compete with estrogens for the estrogen receptors, there would not be
sufficient ER to interact with the estrogen specific acceptor sites to
elicit maximal growth and cellular responses. In addition, our results

lend support to the idea that antiestrogens have effects of their own on cells in addition to acting as estrogen antagonists and, in some cases, agonists.

Our current chromatin binding data demonstrate that antiestrogen-receptor complexes bind uterine or MCF-7 chromatin in a way that is

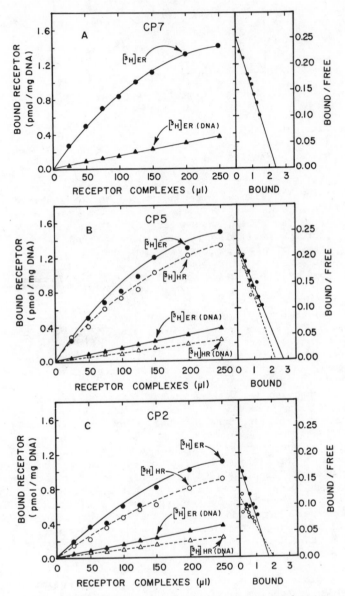

Fig. 11. Saturation kinetics for binding of receptor complexes to nucleo-acidic proteins (NAP) from chromatin fractions. Rabbit uterine nonhistone proteins fractionated from chromatin between 6 M and 7 M (A) 4 M and 5 M (B) and 1 and 2 M (C) Gdn·HCl were reconstituted to rabbit spleen DNA by reverse gradient dialysis. Increasing concentrations of [³H]ER or [³H]HR were incubated with either DNA or reconstituted NAP and binding assayed. Data were also analyzed by Scatchard plots. ER, estradiol-receptor complex; HR, H1285-receptor complex. Panel A reprinted from reference 16.

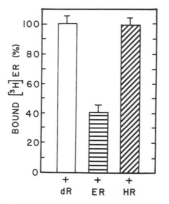

Fig. 12. Specificity of binding of [³H]ER complexes to rabbit uterine NAP from CP7. Partially purified [³H]ER were used to determine binding to NAP from CP7 in the absence of (100%) or in the presence of twofold excess unlabeled ER or HR. Protein content was kept constant with heat-denatured receptor preparations (dR). Reprinted from reference 16.

similar to estrogen-receptor complexes, such as the 1 M site (CP2), but also in ways that are different, such as less binding to a 6 M site (CP7) and specific binding to a protein component of the 4 M site (CP5). That antiestrogen-receptor binding to a distinct site may have a role in inhibition of proliferation is supported by our finding that MCF-7 clone RR, which is resistant to growth inhibition by antiestrogens but is still sensitive to estrogens, appears to lack that portion of the chromatin binding (4 M site or CP5) which is unique for antiestrogen-receptor complexes (18). It could be that antiestrogens increase the production of some inhibitor such as a tumor growth inhibiting factor (35) which is triggered by the binding of conformationally altered receptor complexes to the appropriate acceptor sites for that function.

It is clear that the binding of receptors to specific nonhistone protein-DNA complexes is physiologically significant and may be involved in allowing the appropriate developmental and time specific regulations by steroids. However, it is not known whether one, ten or even a hundred acceptor sites are needed for steroid receptors to control a single gene (14). Moreover, it is still not known whether acceptor sites are near structural genes, regulatory genes, or both (Fig. 1). The availability of acceptor sites for binding by steroid receptor may itself be regulated by removal of "masking proteins," nonhistone proteins which render an acceptor site unavailable for receptor binding. Therefore, multiple acceptor sites could become available as the biological response proceeds. Although we use in our studies a chaotropic agent, Gdn·HCl, as an in vitro tool to expose certain chromatin acceptor sites, it is quite possible that in vivo some acceptor sites are made available (unmasked) at different times during the several hours of a response to steroids by subtle but specific alterations in nonhistone masking proteins. These alterations may be enzymatic, may include changes in the degree of phosphorylation or acetylation, may be the result of peptide cleavage or subunit loss, or may be the result of other conformational changes in nonhistone proteins induced by steroid receptor binding to a few initially open sites. These processes may alter the supercoiled structure of chromatin causing a disruption of condensed chromatin and unfolding into a configuration that permits access of RNA polymerase II molecules, allowing initiation of transcription. Thus, both the masking and unmasking of acceptor sites in vivo would be envisioned as physiological events. Increased availability of unmasked acceptor sites for ER have been measured in intact chromatin

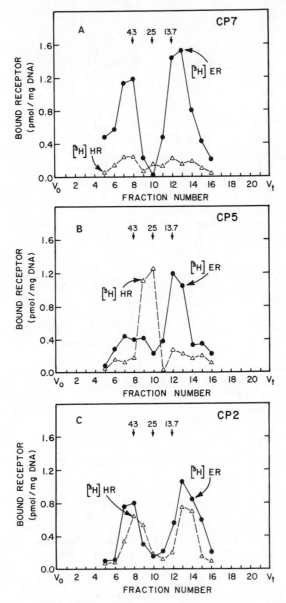

Fig. 13. Molecular sizing of rabbit uterine CP7 (A), CP5 (B) and CP2 (C) proteins and analysis of acceptor activity for [³H]ER or [³H]HR. The CP protein fractions were suspended in 7.5 M Gdn·HCl and applied to a 0.9 x 30 cm column of CL-Sepharose 6B. A sample of the eluted fractions was then reconstituted to rabbit DNA and assayed for acceptor activity. Molecular weight markers were ovalbumin, chymotrypsinogen, and ribonuclease A (43, 25, and 13.7 kDa, respectively). ER, estradiol-receptor complex; HR, H1285-receptor complex. Panel A reprinted from reference 16.

when comparing immature to mature rabbit uterine chromatin. Also, un-masked progesterone receptor acceptor sites in chick oviduct intact chromatin increase fourfold after estrogen injection (36). Recently, results obtained in the hamster uterus suggest that progesterone treatment decreases available estrogen receptor-acceptor sites (37,38).

It has been clearly demonstrated that estrogen receptors must be bound within nuclei with high affinity for prolonged periods in order to achieve maximal DNA synthesis and cell proliferation (39). Such studies have suggested a "sequential" or "ratchet" model of hormone action (40). Data from such studies as well as results from our own laboratory have led us to speculate that in vivo some nuclear acceptor proteins would be sequentially unmasked and masked with time after exposure to hormone bound receptor, i.e., availability of acceptor sites for binding by receptor is variable. The ability of antiestrogens to elicit some agonist responses, inhibit some estrogen-induced responses and to have unique actions can be explained by this model (Fig. 14). Both estrogen- and antiestrogen-receptor complexes could elicit early responses by binding unmasked acceptor sites in intact chromatin. However, only estrogens would allow complete stimulation upon continued exposure to estrogen by binding of receptor to newly unmasked acceptor sites. In addition, antiestrogens could initiate inhibitory responses of their own by interacting with different sites.

The receptor/acceptor interactions described in our studies fulfill many of the criteria of a physiologically significant binding system.

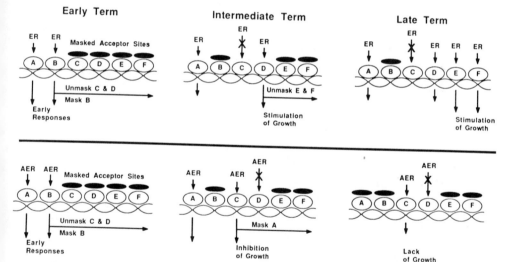

Fig. 14. Model suggesting the effects of unmasking and masking of nuclear acceptor sites in vivo. Acceptor proteins A-F would be sequentially unmasked and masked with time after exposure of target tissue to estrogen or antiestrogen. Receptor complexes initially bind to available unmasked sites which initiate early responses. With time some of these sites may become masked while others become unmasked to initiate other sets of responses. Antiestrogen-receptor complexes would be unable to bind certain acceptor sites (i.e., D), thus preventing completion of agonist responses, resulting in "anti-estrogenicity." It is also possible that antiestrogens initiate inhibitory responses of their own by interacting with different sites (i.e., C).

What is unknown is the exact nature of the protein and DNA components of the acceptor site. Does the estrogen receptor bind to a nonhistone protein-DNA complex, to a nonhistone protein alone or to a DNA sequence alone? Nonetheless, from previous and current evidence, it is clear that certain nonhistone proteins are implicated in the specificity of acceptor sites for steroid receptors. Ultimately the acceptor site components will have to be isolated and highly purified to determine the role these sites may have in steroid hormone action.

Also of interest are the studies suggesting that specific acceptor sites are localized in the nuclear matrix (41,42) where DNA replication and transcription sites are located. Since nuclear proteins are believed to be critical factors involved in regulating the structure and function of DNA, the nuclear matrix which is predominantly nonhistone proteins plus approximately 1% DNA is an attractive model. Although the chemical nature of the nuclear matrix acceptor sites is not yet known, it is possible that the nonhistone protein-DNA acceptor sites discussed above are an integral part of the nuclear matrix.

In summary, what is beginning to emerge is a picture of steroid receptor action in which the effect of a ligand on a cell depends on at least three factors: the ligand (agonist or antagonist), the nature of the receptor (ligand specificity, chromatin affinity and other properties when a ligand is bound), and the state of the available chromatin acceptor sites (unmasked or masked, present or absent). Changes in any one of these can affect the range of responses of a cell to steroid hormone or related ligand.

REFERENCES

1. Payvar F, Wrange O, Carlstedt-Duke J, Okret S, Gustafsson J-A, Yamamoto KR. Purified glucocorticoid receptors bind selectively in vitro to a cloned DNA fragment where transcription is regulated by glucocorticoids in vivo. Proc Natl Acad Sci USA 1981; 78:6628-32.
2. Compton JG, Schrader WT, O'Malley BW. DNA sequence preference of the progesterone receptor. Proc Natl Acad Sci USA 1983; 80:16-20.
3. Mulvihill ER, LePennec J-P, Chambon P. Chicken oviduct progesterone receptor: location of specific regions of high affinity binding in cloned DNA fragments of hormone-responsive genes. Cell 1982; 24: 621-32.
4. von der Ahe D, Janich S, Scheidereit C, Renkawitz R, Schutz G, Beato M. Glucocorticoid and progesterone receptors bind to the same sites in two hormonally regulated promoters. Nature 1985; 313:706-9.
5. Chandler V, Maler B, Yamamoto K. DNA sequences bound specifically by glucocorticoid receptor in vitro render a heterologous promoter hormone responsive in vivo. Cell 1983; 33:489-99.
6. Lee F, Mulligan R, Berg P, Ringold G. Glucocorticoids regulate expression of dehydrofolate reductase cDNA in mouse mammary tumour virus chimaeric plasmids. Nature 1981; 294:228-32.
7. Payvar F, Firestone GL, Ross SR, et al. Multiple specific binding sites for purified glucocorticoid receptors on mammary tumor virus DNA. J Cell Biochem 1982; 19:241-7.
8. Beato M. DNA regulatory elements for steroid hormone receptors. Biochem Actions Horm 1987; 14:1-26.
9. Miller PA, Ostrowski MC, Hagar GL, Simons SS Jr. Covalent and noncovalent receptors-glucocorticoid complexes preferentially bind to the same regions of the long terminal repeat of murine mammary tumor virus proviral DNA. Biochemistry 1984; 23:6883-9.
10. Arriza JL, Weinberger C, Cerelli G, et al. Closing of human mineralocorticoid receptor complementary DNA: structural and functional

kinship with the glucocorticoid receptor. Science 1987; 237:268-75.

11. Giguere V, Hollenberg SM, Rosenfeld MG, Evans RM. Functional domains of the human glucocorticoid receptor. Cell 1986; 46:645-52.

12. Green S, Chambon P. Oestradiol induction of a glucocorticoid-responsive gene by a chimaeric receptor. Nature 1987; 325:75-8.

13. Spelsberg T. Chemical characterization of nuclear acceptors for the avian progesterone receptor. Biochem Actions Horm 1982; 9:141-204.

14. Spelsberg TC, Littlefield BA, Seelke R, et al. Role of specific chromosomal proteins and DNA sequences in the nuclear binding sites for steroid receptors. Recent Prog Horm Res 1983; 39:463-517.

15. Spelsberg TC, Horton M, Fink K, et al. A new model for steroid regulation of gene transcription using chromatin acceptor sites and regulatory genes and their products. In: Moudgil VK, ed. Molecular mechanisms of steroid hormone action: recent advances II. Berlin: Walter de Gruyter, 1987:59-63.

16. Spelsberg TC, Ruh T, Ruh M, et al. Nuclear acceptor sites for steroid hormone receptors: comparisons of steroids and antisteroids. In: Pasqualini J, ed. Antisteroids. New York: Raven Press, 1987 (in press).

17. Singh RK, Ruh MF, Ruh TS. Binding of [^{3}H]estradiol- and [^{3}H]H1285-receptor complexes to rabbit uterine chromatin. Biochim Biophys Acta 1984; 800:33-40.

18. Singh RK, Ruh MF, Butler WB, Ruh TS. Acceptor sites on chromatin for receptor bound by estrogen versus antiestrogen in antiestrogen-sensitive and -resistant MCF-7 cells. Endocrinology 1986; 118:1087-95.

19. Ruh TS, Keene JL, Ross P Jr. Estrogen receptor binding parameters of the high affinity antiestrogen ^{3}H-H1285. In: Agarwal MK, ed. Hormone antagonists. Berlin: Walter de Gruyter and Co., 1982:163-77.

20. Ruh TS, Ruh MF, Singh RK. Antiestrogen action in MCF-7 cells. In: Agarwal MK, ed. Receptor mediated hormone antagonisms. New York: Walter de Gruyter and Co., 1987 (in press).

21. Webster RA, Pikler GM, Spelsberg TC. Nuclear binding of progesterone to hen oviduct: role of acidic chromatin proteins in high affinity binding. Biochem J 1976; 156:409-19.

22. Ruh TS, Ruh MF. The agonistic and antagonistic properties of the high affinity antiestrogen-H1285. Pharmacol Ther 1983; 21:246-74.

23. Ruh TS, Ross P Jr, Wood DM, Keene JL. The binding of [^{3}H]estradiol-receptor complexes to calf uterine chromatin. Biochem J 1981; 200:133-42.

24. Ruh MF, Singh RK, Bellone CJ, Ruh TS. Binding of [^{3}H]triamcinolone acetonide-receptor complexes to chromatin from the B-cell leukemia line, BCL$_1$. Biochim Biophys Acta 1985; 844:24-33.

25. Ruh MF, Singh RK, Mak P, Callard GV. Tissue and species specificity of unmasked nuclear acceptor sites for the estrogen receptor of Squalus testis. Endocrinology 1986; 118:811-8.

26. Shyamala G, Singh RK, Ruh MF, Ruh TS. Relationship between mammary estrogen receptor and estrogenic sensitivity. II. Binding of cytoplasmic receptor to chromatin. Endocrinology 1986; 119:819-26.

27. Ruh MF, Singh RK, Ruh TS, Shyamala G. Binding of glucocorticoid receptors to mammary chromatin acceptor sites. J Steroid Biochem 1987 (in press).

28. Ruh TS, Ruh MF, Singh RK, Butler WB. Nuclear acceptor sites for the mammalian estrogen receptor: effects of antiestrogens. In: Spelsberg TC, Kumar R, eds. Steroid and sterol hormone action. Boston: Martinus Nijhoff Publishing, 1987; 131-48.

29. Ruh MF, Ruh TS. Specificity of chromatin acceptor sites for steroid hormone receptors. In: Sheridan PJ, Blum K, Trachtenberg MC, eds. Steroid receptors and disease: cancer, autoimmune, bone and circulatory disorders. New York: Marcel Dekker, Inc., 1987 (in press).

30. Singh RK, Ruh MF, Ruh TS. Activation of [^{3}H]estradiol- and [^{3}H]-H1285-receptor complexes: effect of molybdate-stabilized estrogen receptors. J Steroid Biochem 1984; 21:205-8.

31. Katzenellenbogen BS, Miller MA, Mullick A, Sheen YY. Antiestrogen action in breast cancer cells: modulation of proliferation and protein synthesis, and interaction with estrogen receptors and additional antiestrogen binding sites. Breast Cancer Res and Treatment 1985; 4:231-43.

32. Keene JL, Ruh MF, Ruh TS. Interaction of the antiestrogen [^{3}H]H1285 with the two forms of the molybdate-stabilized calf uterine estrogen receptor. J Steroid Biochem 1984; 21:625-31.

33. Jasper TW, Ruh MF, Ruh TS. Estrogen and antiestrogen binding to rat uterine and pituitary estrogen receptor: evidence for at least two forms of the estrogen receptor. J Steroid Biochem 1985; 23:537-45.

34. Sheen YY, Ruh TS, Mangel WF, Katzenellenbogen BS. Antiestrogenic potency and binding characteristics of the triphenylethylene H1285 in MCF-7 human breast cancer cells. Cancer Res 1985; 45:4192-9.

35. Knabbe C, Lippman ME, Wakefield LM, et al. Evidence that transforming growth factor-B is a hormonally regulated negative growth factor in human breast cancer cells. Cell 1987; 48:417-28.

36. Martin-Dani G, Spelsberg T. Proteins which mask the nuclear binding sites of the avian oviduct progesterone receptor. Biochemistry 1985; 24:6988-97.

37. Cobb A, Leavitt WW. Chromatin binding sites for the estrogen receptor: mechanism of progesterone down regulation. J Cell Biol 1986; 103:44A.

38. Cobb AD, Leavitt WW. Novel mechanisms for regulation of mammalian estrogen and progesterone receptors. In: Spelsberg TC, Kumar R, eds. Steroid and sterol hormone action. Boston: Martinus Nijhoff Publishing, 1987:61-78.

39. Clark JH, Anderson JN, Peck EJ Jr. Nuclear receptor-estrogen complexes of rat uteri: concentration-time-response parameters. In: O'Malley BW, Means AR, eds. Receptors for reproductive hormones; vol 36. Advances in experimental medicine and biology. New York: Plenum Press; 1973: 15-59.

40. Stack G, Gorski J. Relationship of estrogen receptors and protein synthesis to the mitogenic effect of estrogens. Endocrinology 1985; 117:2024-32.

41. Barrack ER. The nuclear matrix of the prostate contains acceptor sites for androgen receptors. Endocrinology 1983; 113:430-2.

42. Barrack ER, Coffey DS. The specific binding of estrogens and androgens to the nuclear matrix of sex hormone responsive tissues. J Biol Chem 255:7265-75.

18

ANTISTEROID HORMONES, RECEPTOR STRUCTURE AND

HEAT-SHOCK PROTEIN MW 90,000 (HSP 90)

Etienne-Emile Baulieu

INSERM U 33 and Faculte de Medecine Paris-Sud Lab Hormones
94275 Bicetre Cedex, France

SUMMARY

Antisteroid hormones compete for hormone binding at the receptor level and prevent the hormonal response. A new parameter is proposed for explaining both antiglucocorticosteroid and antiprogesterone activities of RU 486, a synthetic derivative of high affinity for receptors. It is based on the antagonist ability to stabilize the hetero-oligomeric 8S-form of the glucocorticosteroid (in the chick oviduct) and progesterone (in the rabbit uterus) receptors. These 8-S complexes involve the interaction of the ~94,000 and ~120,000 Da receptor with the heat-shock protein of MW ~90,000 (hsp 90). It is proposed that hsp 90 caps the DNA binding site of the receptor, preventing it from interaction with the DNA of hormone regulatory elements (HRE) and thus from modifying transcription of regulated genes. In contrast, hormone agonists induce the dissociation of the hetero-oligomeric form of receptors, thus unmasking their functional DNA binding domain. Whether other differences between agonist- and antagonist-receptor complexes are involved in the expression of hormone and antihormone effects also is discussed in this paper.

INTRODUCTION

Selective and safe suppression of the effects of a given steroid hormone can be medically useful. Antiprogesterone (to interrupt the luteal phase and early pregnancy), antiglucocorticosteroid (to decrease deleterious consequences of corticosteroids produced in excess by some tumors), antiestrogens (active in "receptor +" breast cancers), antialdosterone (frequently used in cases of high blood pressure) and antiandrogens (for treating hypersexualism and prostate cancers) have been successfully prescribed in human beings. These antihormones are not designed to decrease steroid production or availability to target cells. They are not addressed to postreceptor event which would not be specific enough, most cellular activities being under multisignal controls. Indeed, antihormones are, by definition, acting at the receptor level, and presently only steroid analogues, binding to the same site of the receptor as the corresponding endogenous steroids, have been synthesized. Their prevailing binding pattern, even though not definitively demonstrated, seems of competitive nature vs. agonists.

It is conceivable that, in the future, other drugs may interact specifically with a "postbinding region" of the receptor. They would not compete for hormone binding, but oppose a crucial step following ligand–receptor interaction and probably be chemically very different from steroids. Search for them will be only possible when we know more about the tridimensional structure of receptors and their interactions with DNA and other components. These potential "antireceptor" molecules should not be confused with antihormones discussed in this presentation which, however, have postbinding effect(s) on receptor structure and thus function (Fig. 1).

A number of studies of antisteroid hormones medically used (Table 1) are already available. In contrast to previous hypothesis, low affinity for the corresponding receptor is not predictive of an antagonist property. Low affinity antagonist may be very useful if their metabolism is slow (e.g., tamoxifen). However and conversely, a high affinity antagonist may be not medically convenient because of too high clearance rate (e.g., 4-hydroxytamoxifen). The effect of an antihormone is often more complex than a simple attenuation of hormone activity. Most (maybe all) antihormonal compounds display mixed agonist/antagonist activities, probably due to the homologous structural features shared with the corresponding agonists in order to fit the receptor binding site (Fig. 2); further in this paper, we offer an hypothesis to explain some available data. Other results remain puzzling, as for instance the estrogenic activity of tamoxifen in the chick oviduct system acquired in specific target organs in presence of other hormones (1), and the nonantiestrogenic properties of triphenylethylene derivatives (2).

STEROID RECEPTOR: HETERO–OLIGOMERIC 8S–STRUCTURE INCLUDING
HEAT–SHOCK PROTEIN MW 90,000 (HSP 90) RELEASED DURING
HORMONE–INDUCED TRANSFORMATION

In the absence of steroid hormone, all or a very large fraction of any steroid receptor is found in the cytosol, i.e., supernatant fraction of target tissue homogenates made in low ionic strength buffer (3,4). All receptors thus obtained sediment as an 8-10S hormone-binding entity (designated as 8S-R), of apparent MW ~300kDa (5) and not binding to DNA. If the homogenate has been obtained with high ionic strength buffer (usually >0.25 M KC1), or if secondarily the 8S-R is exposed to such a salt-containing medium, the hormone-binding peak sediments with an ~4S sedimentation coefficient (4S-R), which corresponds to the estrogen (E)-, progesterone (P)-, glucocorticosteroid (G)- or mineralocorticosteroid receptors whose cDNAs have been recently sequenced or to the androgen

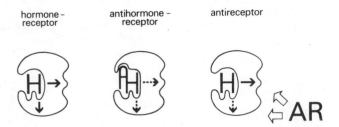

Fig. 1. The figure represents steroid hormone (H), antisteroid hormone (AH) and antireceptor (AR) actions at the receptor level. H has induced the release of hsp 90, AH competes with the steroid binding site of the receptor and when bound, it stabilizes the hetero-oligomer hsp 90-receptor. AR opposes the function of the hormone-receptor complexes.

Table 1. Main antisteroid hormones.

Antihormones	Binding affinity*	Biological affinity**	Clinical usefulness
antiandrogens			
flutamid and anandron	±	+	good
cyproterone acetate	+	+	good
antiestrogens			
tamoxifen	+	++	excellent
4-hydroxytamoxifen	+++	+++	not used
antimineralocorticosteroids			
spironolactones	+	nt	good
antiglucocorticosteroid			
RU 486	++++	+++	excellent
antiprogesterone			
RU 486	+++	+++	excellent

*Three crosses refer to approximative affinity of the correspond-
ing natural hormone. ± means very weak affinity.
**In cultured cells. Three crosses refer to very high antihor-
monal activity. nt: nontested.

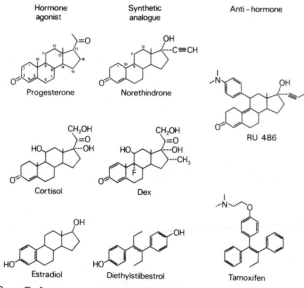

Hormone agonist   Synthetic analogue   Anti-hormone

Progesterone   Norethindrone

Cortisol   Dex   RU 486

Estradiol   Diethylstilbestrol   Tamoxifen

Fig. 2. Endogenous steroid hormones, synthetic analogues
and antagonists. Note the structure of tamoxifen with an
extracycle as compared to active estrogens. We suggested
looking for a similar chemical addition to the progestogen
overall steroidal structure, based on the probable homologies between steroid receptor binding sites. The antiglucocorticosteroid activity of RU 486 is not clinically a
concern when the compound is used for fertility control,
since there is compensatory increase of cortisol by
derepression of the hypothalamus-pituitary adrenal axis
(50,51).

receptor. The purification by hormone affinity chromatography of the chick oviduct 8S-PR, stabilized by molybdate ions, has allowed to obtain a monoclonal antibody (6) which recognizes a protein moiety not binding steroid (7). This protein was characterized as hsp 90 by biochemical and cloning techniques (8,9), in accord with results obtained by D. Toft, W. Pratt and their collaborators (10,11). A number of arguments indicate that all 8S-Rs include the same hsp 90 molecule. Sequence data of the chick hsp 90 cDNA (N. Binart et al., in preparation) and of the corresponding protein in E. coli, yeast, Drosophila, mouse and human indicate not only overall evolutionary conservation, but also (not in E. coli) a remarkable charged sequence(s) of aminoacids able to form an α-helix with alignment of negative residues (M. G. Catelli, N. Binart, J. Garnier and E. E. Baulieu, unpublished results). It was therefore postulated that this segment can interact with the DNA binding domain of steroid receptors, that is the region having highest degree of homology in the proteins belonging to the erb-A-related superfamily (12,13). This homology is >50% between different steroid hormone receptors and >90% between receptors for the same steroid hormone in different species. The postulated finger structure, as in TFIIIA and other DNA-binding metalloproteins (14), probably contains a divalent metal (likely Zn^{2+}). Using 1,10-phenanthroline and EDTA, two metal chelators, it was observed that the 5S-ER (dimer of the 65 kDa-ER which binds to DNA and likely is its active form [15]), is irreversibly prevented from binding DNA-cellulose after metal removal (16). In receptor reassociation experiments (17), treatment by phenanthroline precluded the ~40% recombination to 8-9S-ER of 5S-ER with hsp 90 (16). Further (unpublished) experiments of G. Redeuilh and M. Sabbah have improved the reassociation conditions (obtaining ~100%), and yet the phenanthroline inhibition effect is observed. Therefore, we propose that there is a stabilizing effect of Zn^{2+} on the receptor structure, permitting binding to both DNA and hsp 90.

Hsp 90 is constitutively present in most if not all cells, whatever target or not for steroid hormones. Contrary to other heat-shock proteins, there is a sizable constitutive concentration, in absence of heat-shock or stress, in the 0.1-2% range of cytosoluble proteins. Hsp 90 is essentially a cytoplasmic protein, and, upon purification, obtained as a dimer (18, and unpublished data of P. Aranyi, M. G. Catelli, C. Radanyi, G. Redeuilh and M. Renoir), not dissociated by KCl and which does not bind hormone or DNA. A small fraction of hsp 90 appears to be located in the nucleus (unpublished immunocytochemical data of J. M. Gasc at both the light and electron microscopy levels), which may account for the nuclear localization of steroid hormone receptors in their nontransformed 8S-form in absence of hormone (19-25).

8S-Rs are notoriously unstable, but, with the use of stabilizing molybdate ions (26), we were able to purify 8S-PR (27) and 8S-ER (28). That molybdate ions do not create an artefactual binding of receptor to hsp 90 is indicated by experiments where 8S-PR was found, by immunological criteria, to contain hsp 90, even in a medium made 0.15 M KCl, thus approaching the physiological ionic strength (19), and also by cross-linking experiments performed in nonmolybdate containing cytosol (29). 8S-Rs are present in absence of ligand in target cell cytosol (17). Cross-linking was obtained with bisimidates, which create lysine-lysine bonds and are rapidly hydrolyzed, preventing the formation of fortuitous protein-protein interactions. The most effective was dimethyl pimelimidate, of effective 0.73 nm reagent length. Even in presence of 0.4 M KCl and absence of molybdate ions, conditions under which the transformation 8S → 4S should occur, the cross-linked 8S-PR of chick oviduct remained intact, by criteria of size and hsp 90 content. No 8S-PR was stabilized by cross-linking if cytosol was made in 0.3 M KCl. When the 8S-PR was purified in absence of cross-linking and secondarily exposed to dimethyl pimelimidate and studied by HPLC, a ~200 kDa structure was obtained, containing the receptor and presumably a single molecule of hsp 90 (detected immunologically). These cross-linking experiments suggest that receptor-hsp 90 interaction is very specific, and in no case another protein was detected within the cross-linked material. The possibility that other (minor) components participate in the nontransformed receptor, that is, interact with the R-hsp complex in the cell, remains open, including for a still undefined 60 kDa protein (30).

Intracellular occurrence of 8S-PR, before cell homogenization which may create artefacts, has not been directly demonstrated. The 8S-form is still observed when technical precautions to obtain rapidly cytosol are taken (31,32). The increased resistance of the receptor against a number of physicochemical denaturation factors (29) adds a circumstantial argument, and indeed protection of the unliganded receptor in target cells may be of biological significance. The 8S → 4S transformation induced in warming up the receptor is dependent on hormone binding, contrary to the dissociation of 8S-complexes provoked by salt (33-35). It has been observed, in cultured cells, that the transformation of 10S-GR to 4S-GR is hormone-dependent, while upon steroid withdrawal, there is reversal to the large form (36). This result is in favor of a reversible equilibrium, in accord with our cell-free experiments (see above). The absence of hormone favors the non-DNA binding form, and thus this form of the receptor presumably is prevented to be active by binding hsp 90. Constitutively active mutants (37) should, according to this concept, be correlated with a lack of hsp 90 interaction with their DNA binding site. Recent transfection experiments, performed with the c-DNA of this GR C-terminal truncated forms, led to only observe 4S forms of the receptors, that is devoid of hsp 90 interaction (38). These results suggest that the mechanism by which the C-terminal, steroid-binding domain of receptors represses their function involves hsp 90. With reference to the present discussion, they also favor the possibility that the inhibitory interaction of receptor with hsp 90 is operative in vivo.

It is therefore proposed that hsp 90 is a "cap" for the steroid receptors, interacting with their DNA-binding site (Fig. 1). R-hsp complexes would form in the cytoplasm during/just after receptor biosynthesis, therefore precluding interaction of the receptor with the DNA until the incoming hormone intervenes. This could explain the finding of 8S-receptors in the cytosol, the non-DNA binding receptor leaking out easily from the cell nuclei. In addition to the lack of direct proof for such a concept, presently available data still leave unresolved the mode of interaction of the 8S-R constituents. The 65 kDa ER is in a dimeric structure, with which two hsp 90 molecules complete the 8S-ER (28). The receptor dimerization interface resides in the C-terminal region of the receptor molecules, since the "trypsin 4-S" molecule (39,17), which can be obtained after enzymatic treatment of both the 5S-ER or 8-9S-ER, is formed of two ~30 kDa identical peptides, binding estrogen and not DNA (G. Redeuilh and M. Sabbah, unpublished experiments). Transfection studies with mutated cDNAs from P. Chambon laboratory, have indicated that the DNA-binding putative domain is involved in the formation of 8S-ER (B. Chambraud et al., unpublished experiments). Differently from 8S-ER, 8S-PR both in the chick (27) and the rabbit (40), and rat 8S-GR (41) likely contain one molecule of hormone-DNA binding receptor and two of hsp 90. Transfection experiments (38) have indicated that, besides the involvement of putative DNA-binding domain, there is an obligatory participation of the C-terminal portion of the molecule receptor to obtain a 8S-GR form. The nt^- GR mutant (~40,000 kDa), which binds strongly to a DNA upon hormone binding, is practically devoid of the N-terminal domain and forms a 8S-structure (42). Conversely, the calcitriol and thyroid receptors which have a very small N-terminal domain but shares ~40-50% homology in the putative DNA-binding site with other steroid hormone receptors, have not yet been found associated to hsp 90. Uneven stability of the different 8S-receptors has been recorded (GR is more stable than PR and ER, and chick PR is more stable than rabbit PR) and it cannot be excluded that better technology will demonstrate interaction of all erb-A related molecules with hsp 90.

It is proposed that, upon hormone binding, the hormone-binding unit of the receptor is physiologically trans(con)formed. This change of structure is responsible for hsp release, and the putative DNA binding site may then interact with either nonspecific DNA and/or specific hormone regulatory elements (HRE) of DNA (Fig. 3). It is not known if hormone binding, besides being responsible for the release of hsp 90, does or does not lead to a change of the structure and then of the properties of the DNA-binding site of the receptor. For instance, the latter could acquire higher affinity for nonspecific and/or HRE DNA. It is now known that the receptor, separated from hsp 90, has affinity for both nonspecific and HRE DNA, including in absence of hormone (48, and see later) or when binding an antihormone. The triple binding equilibrium of the receptor with hsp 90, available nonspecific DNA and HRE DNA is likely to be important to hormone action. Kinetic differences in the transformation of 8S-R to 4S-R, when bound to agonist or antagonist respectively, may have to be considered when envisaging quantitatively the effect of a given hormone/ antihormone. They may differ in different target cells and furthermore, one has to consider different components of the hormonal response (e.g., mRNA and protein half lives). Whether or not the receptor, after triggering the response, is recycled back to 8S-R form with the participation or not of an energy-dependent step, is unknown. Changes of phosphorylation of the receptor and/or hsp 90 may also be involved. Indeed, we do not know to which macromolecular structure the hormone-free receptor is loosely bound in the nucleus (and possibly in the cytoplasm for GR), and if activated hormone-receptor complexes (4S-R) only bind to HRE-DNA. Besides precluding DNA binding of the receptor, hsp 90 may play a role in protecting the receptor against denaturation and in positioning the 8S-R in the cell (hsp 90 binds to actin). When binding to specific HRE, the hormone-receptor complex perturbates the chromatin structure, and studies with the MMTV-papilloma virus system (43) suggest opening of a nucleosome and intervention of (at least) a transcription factor (TF).

A ROLE FOR HSP 90 IN THE ANTIGLUCOCORTICOSTEROID AND ANTIPROGESTERONE EFFECTS OF RU 486

RU 486 (a 19-norsteroid, see Fig. 2, [reviews in 44]) binds with high affinity to the chick GR, and antagonizes ovalbumin and conalbumin synthesis induced by glucocorticosteroids in oviduct glandular cells (references in 45). The system is convenient to study glucocorticosteroid effect since RU 486 does not bind to chick PR. In contrast, it binds with high affinity to the rabbit PR and antagonizes progesterone induced uteroglobin synthesis. Recent studies (45) have indicated that RU 486, contrary to the strong agonist triamcinolone acetonide (TA), stabilizes the 8S form of GR, as assessed by studies in oviduct explants and in cell free extracts using gradient sedimentation, HPLC and appropriate binding and immunological techniques. However, in vitro TA- and RU 486-4S-GR show comparable DNA-binding activity. These results agree with recent findings indicating that agonist-bound, antagonist-bound and ligand-free GR and PR bind to HREs in mouse mammary tumor virus long terminal repeat (MMTV-LTR) DNA and uteroglobin gene promoter, respectively. They explain also the DNA-binding data showing that RU 486-GR complexes are less transformed than TA-GR and behave in some aspects like agonist-nt⁻ GR complexes (46). Even if alternative explanation may be presented (47), our data may

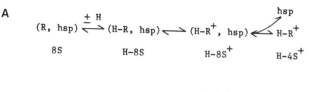

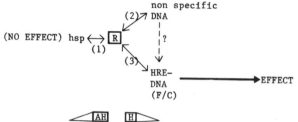

Fig. 3. (A) Series of reactions leading from hetero-
oligomeric 8S receptor (inactive) to active hormone
receptor complexes. The stoichiometry of R and hsp in
the 8S-R is not indicated (see text). The $+$ indicates
that there is some activation of the receptor within
the 8S complex (see text). Released H-R$^+$ is able to
interact with DNA and possibly chromatin proteins.
(B) Triple putative interaction of receptor R (4S)
with hsp 90, nonspecific DNA, and DNA of hormone-
regulatory element HRE. In addition, we have indicated, by F and C, factors and chromatin features which
are implicated in the hormonal response, besides HRE--
DNA binding. At the bottom, AH and H suggest that, in
the presence of antihormone AH, the system is driven
to the left (no effect), while the binding of hormone
H drives it to the right (effect).

reconcile the apparent contradiction between the in vitro comparable
DNA-binding activity of agonist- and antagonist-4S-R complexes and the in
vivo mandatory presence of hormone for receptor-DNA interaction to occur,
while no HRE occupancy is detected in its absence or in presence of an
antagonist (48). However, it is difficult to assess that the antisteroid
activity of RU 486 is only related to the stabilization of the inactive
8S-receptors. Indeed, even attributable to experimental conditions
generating artefacts, in both the chick oviduct and the rabbit uterus PR
systems, some dissociation of 8S-receptor and thus release of DNA-binding
RU 486-receptor complexes have been observed. If this occurs in the cell,
the next problem is to decide whether they are active or nonactive complexes. It is not yet excluded that their binding to DNA, similar to that
of agonist-receptor complex binding to HRE, may actually differ in a way
undetected by available methodology. Another possibility is that the RU
486-receptor complexes are not active due to lack of appropriate receptor
transconformation, thus precluding required transcription factor(s) to
bind to DNA (Fig. 4). However, in vitro ovalbumin and conalbumin gene
transcription is enhanced when adding purified preparation of GR complexes
with either TA or RU 486 in chick oviduct nuclear preparation, and therefore RU 486-transformed receptor complexes may be active (F. Cadepond, G.
Schweizer-Groyer, et al., unpublished experiments). The lack of agonist
activity in vivo would thus rely entirely on hsp 90-receptor interaction.
Hsp 90 may then be considered as a protein acting as a transcription
regulator, which itself does not bind to DNA but precludes the DNA-binding
receptor to do so. The steroid receptor systems will involve several
proteins, as it is the case for other regulatory protein systems. For

example, the cAMP-dependent protein kinases are also composed of two proteins, but here the ligand binding unit and the effector moiety, are different molecules and upon cAMP binding to the cAMP-binding unit, the catalytic part is released in active form. Carboxamide-antiglucocortico-steroids stabilize the 8S-form of rat liver GR, as does also RU 486 (32). Other antiglucocorticosteroids have not been studied in detail. However, available results with dexamethasone-mesylate are not in favor of the mechanism involving stabilization of the 8S-GR form (H. Richard-Foy, personal communication). With various antiestrogens, a decreased trans-formation of the receptor related to antihormone binding has been reported in several cases. However, in the context of the pure antiestrogenic effect of tamoxifen in the chick, we found ~80% as much nuclear estrogen receptor after tamoxifen as compared to after estradiol. Data have indi-cated that estradiol- and tamoxifen (hydroxytamoxifen)-receptor complexes differ by several physicochemical criteria (partition coefficient, inter-action with monoclonal antibody, size and rate of ligand association, and lack of the decrease of hydroxytamoxifen dissociation from the 8S-R under conditions slowing down that of estradiol [references in 49]).

MULTISTEP MECHANISM FOR ANTIHORMONE ACTION AT THE RECEPTOR LEVEL

Based on available evidence, we can suggest a few molecular targets for antihormone action. Limited knowledge of the tertiary structure and posttranslational modifications of receptor and hsp 90, as well as the many unknown features of multiple HREs, chromatin structure, transcription factors, etc., make this list incomplete.

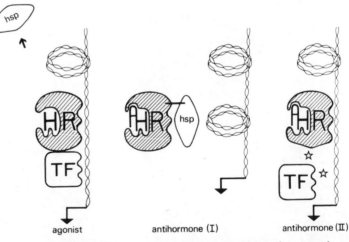

Fig. 4. Schematic representation of hormone (agonist) and antihormone (antagonist) mechanisms of action. It is pos-tulated that active H-R (4S) complex releases a nucleosome and allows a transcription factor(s) (TF) to intervene. Note hsp which has been detached from the receptor after hormone binding. Two mechanisms for antihormone action are represented. I suggests that hsp 90 binding to the receptor is reinforced by AH binding. There is no inter-action with chromatin element. II represents an alter-native class of mechanisms. AH-R interact with DNA; data, however, suggest that the same chromatin modification as with H-R do not occur. In any case, we have arbitrarily represented the lack (☆) of efficient interaction of the transcription factor with the receptor and DNA (see text).

(1) Antihormones can stabilize the 8S-hetero-oligomer, preventing the release of the active receptor. This does not insure that 100% of the nonactive form of the receptor will remain as such, and one has to integrate this effect within the context of receptor turnover and response kinetics. (2) If stabilization of the 8S-receptor is incomplete or absent, there is release of antihormone-receptor complexes with high affinity for nonspecific and specific DNA. High affinity for nonspecific DNA may decrease availability of the receptor for binding to HRE and/or antihormone receptor complexes may have qualitatively abnormal binding to HRE as compared to hormone-receptor complex binding. (3) If antihormone-receptor complexes bind to HRE identically to agonist-receptor complexes, they may be unable to promote the necessary change of chromatin and/or interaction with transcription factor(s) implicated in the transcriptional response.

This analysis is thus characterized by a cascade of potential consequences of antihormone binding to the receptor, each of them being possibly operational in antihormone activity. They are probably not the same for all antihormones and receptors. Naturally if the stabilization of the hetero-oligomer were efficient at 100%, the other putative mechanisms would not play any role. However, stabilization is only limited. If the fraction of released antihormone-receptor complexes binds well to DNA and has agonist activity, the model predicts the mixed agonist/antagonist activity of the ligand, depending on the equilibrium 8S/4S reached after antisteroid binding. Theoretically, a compound which induces several of the above-cited mechanisms could be more efficient than another able to provoke only one of them. Some of these possibilities are experimentally testable, offering a novel molecular approach to test steroid hormone antagonists.

In summary, the main point here discussed is a new concept involving the stabilization by antihormone of the nonactive hetero-oligomeric 8S-form of steroid receptors, where the DNA-binding site is capped by the heat-shock protein hsp 90. Hsp 90 has then the potential of a transcription modulator which itself does not bind to DNA but acts by preventing a DNA-binding protein interacting with hormone regulatory elements of the DNA. Several of this and other mechanisms proposed for antihormone action are already testable experimentally.

REFERENCES

1. Binart N, Mester J, Baulieu EE, Catelli MG. Combined effects of progesterone and tamoxifen in the chick oviduct. Endocrinology 1982; 111:7-16.
2. Sutherland RL, Wattz CKW, Ruenitz PC. Definition of two distinct mechanisms of action of antiestrogens on human breast cancer cell proliferation using hydroxytriphenylethylenes with high affinity for the estrogen receptor. Biochem Biophys Res Commun 1986; 140:523-9.
3. Toft D, Shyamala G, Gorski J. A receptor molecule for estrogens: studies using a cell free system. Proc Natl Acad Sci USA 1967; 57:1740-3.
4. Baulieu EE, Alberga A, Jung I, et al. Metabolism and protein binding of sex steroids in target organs: an approach to the mechanism of hormone action. Recent Prog Horm Res 1971; 27:351-419.
5. Sherman MR, Moran MC, Tuazon FB, Stevens YW. Structure, dissociation, and proteolysis of mammalian steroid receptors. J Biol Chem 1983; 258:10366-77.
6. Radanyi C, Joab I, Renoir JM, et al. Monoclonal antibody to chicken oviduct progesterone receptor. Proc Natl Acad Sci USA 1983; 80: 2854-8.

7. Joab I, Radanyi C, Renoir JM, et al. Immunological evidence for a common non hormone-binding component in "non-transformed" chick oviduct receptors of four steroid hormones. Nature 1984; 308:850-3.

8. Catelli MG, Binart N, Jung-Testas I, et al. The common 90-kd protein component of non-transformed "8S" steroid receptors is a heat-shock protein. EMBO J 1985; 4:3131-5.

9. Catelli MG, Binart N, Feramisco JR, Helfman D. Cloning of the chick hsp 90 cDNA in expression vector. Nucleic Acids Res 1985; 13:6035-47.

10. Schuh S, Yonemoto W, Brugge J, et al. A 90,000-dalton binding protein common to both steroid receptors and the rous sarcoma virus transforming protein, pp60^{v-src}. J Biol Chem 1985; 260:14292-6.

11. Housley PR, Sanchez E, Westphal HM, et al. The molybdate-stabilized L-cell glucocorticoid receptor isolated by affinity chromatography or with a monoclonal antibody is associated with a 90-92-kDa non-steroid-binding phosphoprotein. J Biol Chem 1985; 260:13810-7.

12. Weinberger C, Hollenberg SM, Rosenfeld MG, Evans RM. Domain structure of human glucocorticoid receptor and its relationship to the v-erb-A oncogene product. Nature 1985; 318:670-2.

13. Krust A, Green S, Argos P, et al. The chicken oestrogen receptor sequence: homology with v-erbA and the human oestrogen and glucocorticoid receptors. EMBO J 1986; 5:891-7.

14. Miller J, McLachlan AD, Klug A. Repetitive zinc-binding domains in the protein transcription factor IIIA from Xenopus oocytes. EMBO J 1985; 4:1609-14.

15. Notides AC, Nielsen S. The molecular mechanism of the in vitro 4S to 5S transformation of the uterine estrogen receptor. J Biol Chem 1974; 249:1866-73.

16. Sabbah M, Redeuilh G, Secco C, Baulieu EE. DNA and hsp 90 binding activity of estrogen receptor is dependent on receptor bound metal. J Biol Chem 1987; 262:8631-5.

17. Rochefort H, Baulieu EE. Effect of KCl, CaCl$_2$, temperature and oestradiol on the uterine cytosol receptor of oestradiol. Biochimie 1971; 53:893-907.

18. Welsch W, Feramisco JR. Purification of the major mammalian heat-shock proteins. J Biol Chem 1982; 257:14949-59.

19. Baulieu EE, Binart N, Buchou T, et al. Biochemical and immunological studies of the chick oviduct cytosol progesterone receptor. In: Eriksson H, Gustafsson JA, eds. Steroid hormone receptors: structure and function. Nobel Symposium n°57. Amsterdam: Elsevier, 1983:45-72.

20. Gasc JM, Ennis BW, Baulieu EE, Stumpf WE. Recepteur de la progesterone dans l'oviducte de poulet: double revelation par immunohistochimie avec des anticorps antirecepteur et par autoradiographie a l'aide d'un progestagene tritie. C R Acad Sci [III] (Paris) 1983; 297:477-82.

21. Gasc JM, Renoir JM, Radanyi C, et al. Progesterone receptor in the chick oviduct: an immunohistochemical study with antibodies to distinct receptor components. J Cell Biol 1984; 99:1193-201.

22. King WJ, Greene GL. Monoclonal antibodies localize oestrogen receptor in the nuclei of target cells. Nature 1984; 307:745-7.

23. Welshons WV, Krummer BM, Gorski J. Nuclear localization of unoccupied receptors for glucocorticoids, estrogens, and progesterone in GH$_3$ cells. Endocrinology 1985; 117:2140-7.

24. Isola J, Ylikomi T, Tuohimaa P. Immunoelectron microscopic localization of chick progesterone receptor [Abstract]. J Cell Biochem 1987; (suppl 11A):108.

25. Perrot-Applanat M, Logeat F, Groyer-Picard MT, Milgrom E. Immunocytochemical study of mammalian progesterone receptor using monoclonal antibodies. Endocrinology 1985; 116:1473-84.

26. Leach KL, Dahmer MK, Hammond ND, et al. Molybdate inhibition of

glucocorticoid receptor in activation and transformation. J Biol Chem 1979; 254:11884-90.

27. Renoir JM, Buchou T, Mester J, et al. Oligomeric structure of the molybdate-stabilized, non-transformed "8S" progesterone receptor from chicken oviduct cytosol. Biochemistry 1984; 23:6016-23.

28. Redeuilh G, Moncharmont B, Secco C, Baulieu EE. Subunit composition of the molybdate-stabilized "8-9S" non-transformed estradiol receptor purified from calf uterus. J Biol Chem 1987; 262:6969-75.

29. Aranyi P, Radanyi C, Renoir M, et al. Covalent stabilization of the non-transformed chick oviduct cytosol progesterone receptor by chemical cross-linking. Biochemistry 1987 (in press).

30. Tai PK, Maeda Y, Nakao K, et al. A 59-kilodalton protein associated with progestin, estrogen, androgen, and glucocorticoid receptors. Biochemistry 1986; 25:5269-75.

31. Mendel DB, Bodwell JE, Gametchu B, et al. Molybdate-stabilized nonactivated glucocorticoid-receptor complexes contain a 90-kDa non-steroid-binding phosphoprotein that is lost on activation. J Biol Chem 1986; 261:3758-63.

32. Sablonniere B, Danze PM, Formstecher P, et al. Physical characterization of the activated and non-activated forms of the glucocorticoid-receptor complex bound to the steroid antagonist [^{3}H]RU 486. J Steroid Biochem 1986; 25:605-14.

33. Yang CR, Mester J, Wolfson A, et al. Activation of the chick oviduct progesterone receptor by heparin in the presence or absence of hormone. Biochem J 1982; 208:399-406.

34. Moudgil K, Eessalu TE, Buchou T, et al. Transformation of chick oviduct progesterone receptor in vitro: effects of hormone, salt, heat, and adenosine triphosphate. Endocrinology 1985; 116:1267-74.

35. Tienrungroj W, Meshinchi S, Sanchez ER, et al. The role of sulfhydryl groups in permitting transformation and DNA binding of the glucocorticoid receptor. J Biol Chem 1987; 262:6992-7000.

36. Raaka BM, Samuels HH. The glucocorticoid receptor in GH1 cells: evidence from dense amino acid labeling and whole cell studies for an equilibrium model explaining the influence of hormone on the intracellular distribution of receptor. J Biol Chem 1983; 258:417-25.

37. Hollenberg SM, Giguere V, Segui P, Evans RM. Co-localization of DNA-binding and transcriptional activation functions in the human glucocorticoid receptor. Cell 1987; 49:39-46.

38. Pratt WB, Jolly DJ, Pratt DV, et al. A region in the steroid binding domain determines formation of the non-DNA-binding, 9S glucocorticoid receptor complex. J Biol Chem 1988 (in press).

39. Erdos T. Properties of a uterine oestradiol receptor. Biochem Biophys Res Commun 1968; 32:338-43.

40. Renoir JM, Buchou T, Baulieu EE. Involvement of a non-hormone binding 90kDa protein in the non-transformed 8S form of the rabbit uterus progesterone receptor. Biochemistry 1986; 25:6405-13.

41. Denis M, Wikstrom AC, Gustafsson JA. The molybdate-stabilized nonactivated glucocorticoid receptor contains a dimer of M_r 90,000 non-hormone-binding protein. J Biol Chem 1987; 262:11803-6.

42. Gehring U, Arndt H. Heteromeric nature of glucocorticoid receptors. FEBS Lett 1985; 179:138-42.

43. Cordingley MG, Riegel AT, Hager GL. Steroid-dependent interaction of transcription factors with the inducible promoter of mouse mammary tumor virus in vivo. Cell 1987; 48:267-70.

44. Baulieu EE, Segal SJ, eds. The antiprogestin steroid RU 486 and human fertility control. New York: Plenum Press, 1985.

45. Groyer A, Schweizer-Groyer G, Cadepond F, et al. Antiglucocorticosteroid effects suggest why steroid hormone is required for receptors to bind DNA in vivo but not in vitro. Nature 1987; 328:624-6.

46. Bourgeois S, Pfahl M, Baulieu EE. DNA binding properties of glucocorticosteroid receptors bound to the steroid antagonist RU 486. EMBO J 1984; 3:751-5.

47. Green S, Chambon P. A superfamily of potentially oncogenic hormone receptors. Nature 1986; 324:615-7.

48. Becker PB, Gloss B, Schmid W, et al. In vivo protein-DNA interactions in a glucocorticoid response element require the presence of the hormone. Nature 1986; 324:686-8.

49. Baulieu EE. Steroid hormone antagonists at the receptor level. A role for the heat-shock protein MW 90,000 (hsp 90). J Cell Biochem 1987; 24 (in press).

50. Gaillard RC, Riondel A, Muller MF, et al. RU 486: a steroid with antiglucocorticosteroid activity that only disinhibits the human pituitary-adrenal system at a specific time of day. Proc Natl Acad Sci USA 1984; 81:3879-82.

51. Bertagna X, Bertagna C, Luton JP, et al. The new steroid analog RU 486 inhibits glucocorticoid action in man. J Clin Endocrinol Metab 1984; 59:25-8.

VI. PHARMACOLOGICAL AND CLINICAL CORRELATIONS

19

NEURAL ESTROGEN AND PROGESTIN RECEPTORS AND THE NEUROCHEMISTRY OF REPRODUCTIVE BEHAVIOR AND SEXUAL DIFFERENTIATION

Bruce S. McEwen

Laboratory of Neuroendocrinology
Rockefeller University,
1230 York Avenue, New York, NY 10021

INTRODUCTION

Gonadal steroids are secreted in response to signals emanating from the brain, and the signals in the brain are the integrated output of incoming information from internal and external stimuli. Among the external stimuli are the light-dark cycle and season of the year, as well as the presence and behavior of other animals who may represent competitors or potential sexual partners. The internal stimuli are comprised of interoceptive neural input, circulating hormones and the psychological state of the animal related to such states as sexual arousal and anxiety or depression.

The actions of the secreted gonadal hormones on target tissues of the reproductive tract and brain help to coordinate and synchronize behavioral and endocrine events leading to successful reproduction, of which territorial, mate-finding and copulatory behaviors are the most interesting and complex. Although behavior is often regarded as too complex for quantitative analysis and study of underlying mechanism, it has nevertheless been possible by judicious selection of the behavior to gain considerable insight into cellular and neurochemical mechanisms by which steroids regulate behavior. The behavior which we have studied is lordosis behavior of the female rat, the copulatory response to the mounting attempts of the male, which is induced in female rats by estradiol (E) followed by progesterone (P). This paper presents a progress report of our understanding of the role of E and P in the control of lordosis.

NEURAL LOCALIZATION OF THE CONTROL OF LORDOSIS

The lordosis response of the female rat is activated by circulating E and P during the evening of proestrus which occurs every 4 or 5 days in the estrous cycle [1]. This can be mimicked in ovariectomized rats by sequential administration of microgram quantities of E for 24 h, followed by 0.5 mg of P acting over several hours. Studies of E and P action in the brain with respect to lordosis began 25 years ago with the measurement of neural sites of uptake and retention of 3H steroids [1,2]. Neural sites of uptake and retention of 3H E and 3H progestins turned out to be neurons containing receptor-like macromolecules which are attached to cell nuclei (2). Mapping of these receptors in brain occurred in parallel with functional studies in which E and P implants were used to probe sites of hormonal control over dependent behaviors like lordosis. These studies revealed that the basal hypothalamus and, more particularly, neurons in the ventrolateral portion of the ventromedial nuclei (VMN) are the key to E and P induction of lordosis (2). Additional studies with RNA and protein synthesis inhibitors led to the demonstration that genomic activity was undoubtedly required for E and P to bring about the lordosis response of the female to mating attempts by the male (2-4).

EVIDENCE OF GENOMIC ACTIVITY AND MORPHOLOGICAL ALTERATIONS IN VMN NEURONS

Thus, induction of lordosis by E plus P involves hormonal activation of the genome of a group of neurons in the VMN. We have found that genomic activation by E in VMN is very rapid, with increases in nucleolar and nuclear size and chromatin structure evident within 2 h of initial E exposure (5). Altered patterns of labeling of newly synthesized proteins are also seen within this time frame (6). Also within 6 h or less of E exposure, increased levels of ribosomal RNA are seen in VMN, and there are also increases in labeling of total RNA by 3H uridine (7,8). The rapid genomic response of VMN neurons to E is consistent with the fact that 6 h of E exposure is sufficient to induce lordosis 24 h later and with the fact that RNA and protein synthesis inhibitors and anti-estrogens, given 6 h or more after E exposure begins, do not block lordosis induction (2,9).

Although the initial genomic events are rapid in response to E, the actual ability to show lordosis response does not occur for 18-24 h (1,2). Intervening cellular events are presumed to account for this lag, including axonal transport of newly synthesized proteins to presynaptic terminals of VMN neurons in the midbrain central gray, which is the head of a reflex arc governing lordosis (1-3,6).

SYNAPTIC AND NEUROCHEMICAL RESPONSES TO E

By 48 h after E, and possibly sooner, the VMN shows an increase in density of synaptic terminals (10). There are also changes in densities of various neurotransmitter receptor types and alterations in the level of the mRNA for at least one putative neuromodulator. E induces increased densities of oxytocin receptors in VMN (11), as well as muscarinic cholinergic receptors labeled by the antagonist, 3H QNB (12,13). E induces decreased densities of high affinity GABAa receptors labeled by 3H muscimol (14), as well as decreased densities of CCK receptors (15). E also induces increased levels of proenkephalin mRNA in VMN (16). Thus, the microcosm of the VMN demonstrates a heterogeneity of response to E treatment which implies that a number of putative neurotransmitters play a role in the control of lordosis. The functional significance of changes in receptor density is not clear although it appears likely that both acetylcholine and oxytocin may facilitate lordosis responding, whereas GABA and CCK may inhibit it (6). The direction of change in receptor densities is consistent with this possibility although more data is required before any firm conclusion is reached. The significance of the proenkephalin mRNA is also not clear although a related peptide, leumorphin, facilitates lordosis when infused into VMN (16).

SIGNIFICANCE OF THE PROGESTIN RECEPTOR AND ITS INDUCTION BY E

Physiological levels of E priming do not induce lordosis without sequential secretion or administration of P (18). In the absence of E

266

priming, P does not induce lordosis. Clearly, from the discussion above, there are many neurochemical events, as well as synaptic features, which are primed by E so that the P can be effective. One of the priming effects of E is to induce P receptors in the VMN and in other E-sensitive brain regions (19). The induction of P receptors shows many of the temporal requirements as far as E priming as the induction of the lordosis response itself, and it is dependent on protein synthesis (3,19).

P administration to an E-primed female rat induces lordosis responding within as little as 1 h, and this induction, though rapid, is blocked by inhibiting protein synthesis. P induction of lordosis also shows a rapid termination, particularly when protein synthesis is blocked after initiation (19). This is most likely explained by P-induced proteins having a short half-life. Another aspect of P action is the delayed induction of sequential inhibition, the inability of the female rat while still E primed to respond to a second P treatment 24 h after a previous P exposure. Sequential inhibition may be due to the delayed induction of proteins by P since protein synthesis inhibitors block the sequential inhibition phase (20).

SEX DIFFERENCES IN LORDOSIS AND IN PROGESTIN RECEPTOR INDUCTION BY E IN VMN

Male rats which are castrated as adults and given E priming fail to show substantial lordosis, and they are particularly refractory to the effects of P (19). Male rat brains contain E receptors with the same levels and distributions as in the female brain, and P receptor induction by E is more or less the same in male and female brains (21). However, there is an exception, and this exception may be important for the sex difference in lordosis induction. Specifically, the VMN shows a substantially higher induction of progestin receptors in the female compared to the male (22,23). Thus, the refractoriness of male rats to P may be due, in part, to the inadequate supply of P receptors induced by E.

Sex differences in lordosis responding can be altered developmentally by manipulating testosterone (T) levels or by interfering with the conversion of T to E (23). Thus, T suppresses developmentally (i.e., defeminizes) the ability to show lordosis and does so by conversion to E in the brain. Blockade of the T to E conversion (aromatization) blocks defeminization, and administration of T or E to newborn female rats causes defeminization (23). In parallel, blockade of aromatization in newborn males results in female-like inducibility of P receptors by E in genetic males at the same time as blocking defeminization of lordosis (24). And administration to newborn females results in male-like induction of P receptors by E in genetic females at the same time as inducing defeminization or lordosis (24).

SEX DIFFERENCES IN NEUROCHEMICAL RESPONSES TO E PRIMING

Sex differences in P receptor induction by E in VMN raise the possibility that other responses to E may differ between males and females. Thus far, only some of the E effects cited above have been investigated in this regard. Specifically, E induction of putative muscarinic receptors labeled by 3H QNB is deficient in VMN and hypothalamus of adult castrated male rats (12,13), but the induction of oxytocin receptors by E in VMN does not appear to differ between males and females (Coirini, Johnson and McEwen, unpublished). Thus, only some of the effects of E in the VMN may be influenced by the early actions of T which lead to sex differences in lordosis responding.

FUTURE DIRECTIONS IN THE STUDY OF THE VMN AND ITS RESPONSE TO E AND P AND ROLE IN LORDOSIS

It has become evident in the course of our studies that the VMN of the female and male rat is a structure worthy of intensive further investigation in relation to hormone action and sex differences. This nucleus shows a diversity of responses to E treatment which reflects its neurochemical complexity. Undoubtedly what we have found thus far is only the tip of the proverbial iceberg. We are especially interested in mapping the neuroanatomical distribution of effects of E on diverse neurotransmitter systems throughout the rostral-caudal extent of the nucleus, as well as ascertaining the heterogeneity of responses to E within the dorsal-ventral and medial-lateral extent of the nucleus. One of the pressing questions is whether the sex differences in response to E reflect the heterogeneity of neurochemical cell types or are differential responses of the same cell types. Preliminary data for P receptors induced by E in VMN suggests that there may be certain neurons within the VMN with very high levels of P receptors that are more prevalent in females than in males (Gerlach and McEwen, unpublished). Thus, the apparent lack of sex difference in oxytocin receptor induction by E may be due to a different distribution of these receptors among cell types within the VMN. This hypothesis requires careful and painstaking mapping and requires the application of quantitative anatomical methods with high resolution.

ACKNOWLEDGMENTS

Research support is acknowledged from NIH Grant NS07080.

REFERENCES

1. Pfaff DW. Estrogens and brain function. New York: Springer-Verlag, 1980.
2. McEwen BS, Davis P, Parsons B, Pfaff DW. The brain as a target for steroid hormone action. Annu Rev Neurosci 1979; 2:65-112.
3. McEwen BS, Pfaff DW. Hormone effects on hypothalamic neurons: analyzing gene expression and neuromodulator action. TINS 1985; 8:105-8.
4. Yahr P, Ulibarri C. Estrogen induction of sexual behavior in female rats and synthesis of polyadenylated messenger RNA in the ventromedial nucleus of the hypothalamus. Mol Brain Res 1986; 1:153-65.
5. Jones KJ, Pfaff DW, McEwen BS. Early estrogen-induced nuclear changes in rat hypothalamic ventromedial neurons: an ultrastructural and morphometric analysis. J Comp Neurol 1985; 239:255-66.
6. McEwen BS, Jones K, Pfaff DW. Hormonal control of sexual behavior in the female rat: molecular, cellular and neurochemical studies. Biol Reprod 1987; 36:37-45.
7. Jones KJ, McEwen BS, Pfaff DW. Regional specificity in estradiol effects on 3H uridine incorporation in rat brain. Mol Cell Endocrinol 1986; 45:57-63.
8. Jones K, Chikaraishi D, Harrington C, McEwen BS, Pfaff DW. In situ hybridization detection of estradiol-induced changes in ribosomal RNA levels in rat brain. Mol Brain Res 1986; 1:145-52.
9. Meisel R, Dohanich G, McEwen BS, Pfaff DW. Antagonism of sexual behavior in female rats by ventromedial hypothalamic implants of antiestrogen. Neuroendocrinology 1987; 45:201-7.
10. Carrer H, Aoki A. Ultrastructural changes in the hypothalamic ventromedial nucleus of ovariectomized rats after estrogen treatment. Brain Res 1982; 240:221-33.
11. De Kloet ER, Voorhuis DA, Boschma Y, Elands J. Estradiol modulates

density of putative "oxytocin receptors" in discrete rat brain regions. Neuroendocrinology 1986; 44:415-21.

12. Rainbow T, Snyder L, Berck D, McEwen BS. Correlation of muscarinic receptor induction in the ventromedial hypothalamic nucleus with the activation of feminine sexual behavior by estradiol. Neuroendocrinology 1984; 39:476-80.

13. Dohanich G, Witcher J, Weaver D, Clemens L. Alteration of muscarinic binding in specific brain areas following estrogen treatment. Brain Res 1982; 241:347-50.

14. O'Connor L, Nock B, McEwen BS. Regional specificity of GABA receptor regulation by estradiol. Neuroendocrinology 1987 (in press).

15. Akesson T, Mantyh PW, Mantyh CR, Matt D, Micevych P. Estrous cyclicity of ^{125}I-cholecystokinin octapeptide binding in the ventromedial hypothalamic nucleus. Neuroendocrinology 1987; 45:257-62.

16. Romano G, Harlan R, Shivers B, Howells R, Pfaff DW. Estrogen increases proenkephalin mRNA in the mediobasal hypothalamus of the rat [Abstract]. In: Abstr Soc Neurosci 1986; 12:188.17.

17. Sakuma Y, Akaishi T. Leumorphin, a novel opioid peptide, promotes lordosis in female rats. Brain Res 1987; 407:401-4.

18. Boling J, Blandau R. The estrogen-progesterone induction of mating responses in the spayed female rats. Endocrinology 1939; 25:359-64.

19. McEwen BS, Davis P, Gerlach JL, et al. Progestin receptors in the brain and pituitary gland. In: Bardin CW, Mauvais-Jarvis P, Milgrom E, eds. Progesterone and progestin. New York: Raven Press, 1983: 59-76.

20. Parsons B, Rainbow T, MacLusky N, McEwen BS. Progestin receptor levels in rat hypothalamic and limbic nuclei. J Neurosci 1982; 2:1446-52.

21. Rainbow T, Parsons B, McEwen BS. Sex differences in rat brain oestrogen and progestin receptors. Nature 1982; 300:648-9.

22. Brown T, Clark A, MacLusky N. Regional sex differences in progestin receptor induction in the rat hypothalamus: effects of various doses of estradiol benzoate. J Neurosci 1987; 7:2529-36.

23. McEwen BS, Biegon A, Davis P, et al. Steroid hormones: humoral signals which alter brain cell properties and functions. In: Recent progress in hormone research. New York: Academic Press, 1982:41-92.

24. Parsons B, Rainbow T, McEwen BS. Organizational effects of testosterone via aromatization on feminine reproductive behavior and neural progestin receptors in rat brain. Endocrinology 1984; 115:1412-7.

ESTROGEN ACTIONS ON ENDOMETRIAL ADENOCARCINOMA

Erlio Gurpide, Christian F. Holinka, Yuzuru Anzai,
Hiroki Hata,* Hiroyuki Kuramoto*, Sharon Kassan,
and Leszek Markiewicz

Departments of Obstetrics, Gynecology and Reproductive
Science, Mount Sinai School of Medicine, New York, NY,
and *Department of Obstetrics and Gynecology, Kitasato
University, Kanagawa-Ken, Japan

Information about the role of hormones in the development of endometrial adenocarcinoma has been collected from a variety of sources. Epide-
miologic studies have shown that the risk for endometrial cancer increases
under conditions of chronic stimulation with estrogens, unopposed by progesterone (1). These conditions arise in some endocrinopathies resulting
in anovulation (2) or during exogenous administration of estrogenic drugs,
mostly for climacteric syndrome (3-5). Treatment of endometrial cancer
with progestins (6,7) or, more recently, with antiestrogens (8), causes
remissions in a significant proportion of patients with metastatic tumors;
these results have been interpreted to indicate hormonal responsiveness in
at least some endometrial adenocarcinomas. In fact, there is a convincing
relation between presence of estrogen or progesterone receptors in metastatic tumors and responsiveness to hormone-related therapy, as shown in
Table 1, and unresponsiveness to chemotherapy (13). Similarly, patients
with primary endometrial adenocarcinoma tumors containing steroid receptors have a better prognosis for survival (Fig. 1). All of these correlations involving receptor levels suggest that estrogens and progestins
affect tumor growth and invasiveness by acting as hormones. However, the
effects of progestins used for therapy are obtained at such large drug
concentrations that their actions may have to be considered cytotoxic or
cytostatic rather than hormonal. Furthermore, the prognostic value of
hormone receptor levels may be more a reflection of the relation of these
levels to the degree of differentiation of the tumor, as shown in Table 2,
than to any hormonal involvement in its development. It may then be
reasonable to consider an alternative concept for the interpretation of
these findings, namely that the presence of steroid receptors characterizes a physiologic state of the cancer cell and is associated with, rather
than responsible for, responses to therapy.

A considerable amount of work has been devoted to a search for
similarities and differences in biochemical characteristics and responsiveness to hormones of normal endometrium and endometrial adenocarcinoma.
These studies have included incubations of endometrial fragments under
organotypic culture conditions as well as examination of epithelial cells
isolated from normal endometrium and endometrial cancer cell lines.
Results obtained with these systems are reviewed here.

Table 1. Relationship between response of recurrent or advanced endometrial adenocarcinoma to progestins.*

Series	Responders		Nonresponders	
	PR(+)	PR(−)	PR(+)	PR(−)
Ehrlich et al. (9)	7	1	1	15
McCarty et al. (10)	4	0	1	8
Martin et al. (11)	13	1	0	6
Benraad et al. (12)	6	2	0	5
Total	30(88%)	4(12%)	2(6%)	34(94%)

*Adapted from Ehrlich et al. (9).

Human endometrial and mammary tissues have in common their responsiveness to the ovarian hormones. This similarity may explain the sharing of epidemiologically identified risk factors for development of mammary or endometrial cancer (17) and the applicability of hormone-related therapeutic modalities to both neoplasias. In spite of obvious differences in the genes that are regulated by ovarian hormones in endometrial and mammary tissues, and of differences in responsiveness to other steroid and protein hormones, biochemical analogies or contrasts in the effects of steroids on these tumors have complementary value in the study of hormonal influences on cancer.

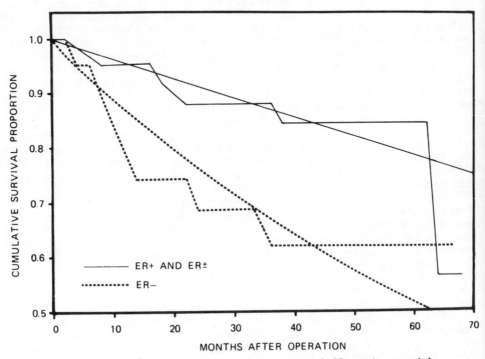

Fig. 1. Cumulative survival proportion of 87 patients with adenocarcinoma of the endometrium. From Martin et al. (14), with permission.

Table 2. Correlation of tumor differentiation with
cytosolic receptor content.[a]

	Primary tumor			Metastases and recurrences (%)	References
	Grade 1 (%)	Grade 2 (%)	Grade 3 (%)		
ER-	5(n=20)	29(n=17)	62(n=8)	64(n=1)	McCarty et al. (10)[b]
	18(n=22)	16(n=37)	22(n=9)		Ehrlich et al. (9)[c]
	7(n=70)	8(n=12)	32(n=22)	30(n=10)	Kauppila et al. (15)[d]
PR-	15(n=20)	29(n=17)	50(n=8)	73(n=11)	McCarty et al. (10)
	23(n-22)	43(n=37)	89(n=9)		Ehrlich et al. (9)
	9(n=70)	17(n=12)	41(n=22)	20(n=10)	Kauppila et al. (15)
ER+/PR+	85(n=20)	59(n=17)	13(n=8)	18(n=11)	McCarty et al. (10)
	68(n=22)	54(n=37)	11(n=9)		Ehrlich et al. (9)
	90(n=70)	75(n=12)	59(n=22)	60(n=10)	Kauppila et al. (15)

[a] From Gurpide et al. (16), with permission.
[b] Cutoff levels: 10 fmol/mg protein (dextran-coated charcoal method).
[c] Cutoff levels: 6 fmol/mg protein for ER, 50 fmol/mg protein for PR
(dextran-coated charcoal method).
[d] Cutoff levels: 3 fmol/mg protein for ER, 6 fmol/mg protein for PR
(dextran-coated charcoal method).

Many of these studies are carried out on human cell lines. Several
estrogen responsive mammary cancer cell lines, most prominently MCF-7,
have been used to identify markers associated with transformation, effects
of hormone on the production of autocrine growth factors expected to
affect cell proliferation, synthesis of specific proteins or changes in
enzymatic activities in response to the addition of hormones to the
medium. A critical review of these effects has been recently published
(18). In contrast to the abundance of estrogen responsive mammary cell
lines, relatively few, mostly unresponsive, endometrial cancer cell lines
are available. Results obtained in our laboratory with an estrogen
responsive endometrial cell line are also described here.

IN VITRO EFFECTS OF ESTROGENS ON ENDOMETRIAL TUMORS AND
ENDOMETRIAL CANCER CELLS

Cell Proliferation and Tumor Growth

Effects of estrogens on tumor growth in patients with endometrial
cancer are not verifiable experimentally. However, effects of estradiol
have been demonstrated on tumors developed in nude mice by implantation of
fragments of endometrial cancer tissue (19).

Effects of estradiol on MCF-7 cell proliferation were observed only
under conditions of growth restriction created by the addition of an
antiestrogen (20) and estrogenic effects on proliferation in serum-free
cultures could not be obtained (21). The requirement for serum to obtain
mitogenic responses to estrogens has provided support to the hypothesis
that actions of estradiol on cell proliferation involve neutralization of
growth inhibitory factors present in serum, as proposed by Soto and
Sonnenschein (22). However, it has recently been announced that elimina-
tion from the medium of phenol red, a pH indicator found to have estrogen-

ic activity, and removal of estrogens from serum by charcoal adsorption or by the use of serum-free media, allowed the demonstration of direct effects of estradiol on proliferation of these cells (18). A mechanism of estrogen action mediated by hormonal influences on the production of autocrine growth factors that stimulate or inhibit mitogenesis is supported by measurements of the levels of factors released to the medium by MCF-7 cells, as reviewed by Dickson and Lippman (18). That review also describes effects of estradiol-free conditioned media from cultures of MCF-7 cells treated with estradiol, on the growth of human breast tumors in nude mice and of breast cancer cells in soft agar. Such results provide further support for the model of hormonally regulated output of autocrine growth factors.

We have obtained clear effects of estradiol on Ishikawa cell proliferation, even in serum-free medium. The Ishikawa endometrial cancer cell line, established by Nishida et al. (23) from a specimen of well differentiated adenocarcinoma of a 39-year-old patient, has been shown to respond to estradiol by increasing DNA polymerase α (24) and alkaline phosphatase (25) activities, as well as progesterone receptor levels (26). When these cells were cultured in MEM containing 15% charcoal-treated fetal bovine serum, a plateau cell density was achieved in control cultures in about 10 days, whereas the number of cells in parallel cultures containing estradiol continued to increase, reaching densities 2-3 times greater in about 14-20 days (Fig. 2). Furthermore, addition of estradiol to control cultures at plateau densities resulted in resumption of growth (26,27). No effects on rates of cell proliferation during the exponential growth phase, when cells were dividing rapidly (doubling time approximately 27 h), could be detected in these experiments (27).

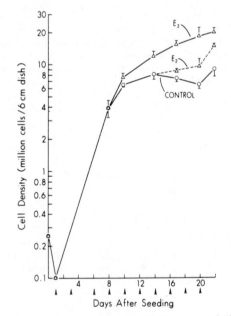

Fig. 2. Effects of estradiol on proliferation of Ishikawa cells grown in MEM-15% charcoal-treated FBS with (triangles) or without (circles) estradiol (10^{-8}M). Medium was changed at the times indicated by the arrows. Dotted line: estradiol added at day 14. Mean ± SD, n=3. From Holinka et al. (27), with permission.

We have recently found that Ishikawa cells can proliferate in serum-free medium (phenol red-free DMEM-Ham's F13, 1:1, with additional HEPES and glutamine), doubling their numbers approximately every 40 h during the logarithmic growth phase (Holinka CF, Hata H, Anzai Y, and Gurpide E, unpublished). Significant effects of estradiol on these serum-free cultures, as well as in cultures containing 1% or 15% charcoal-treated FBS, were evident from cell counting after about 6 days in culture (Fig. 3, Anzai Y, Holinka CF, Kuramoto H, Gurpide, E, unpublished). We have noted a dependence of colony formation efficiency on cell density, likely a reflection of autocrine factor production (27). Also consistent with autocrine regulation are our results on cell proliferation in the absence of serum and the stimulatory effects of estradiol added to cultures at plateau cell density (26,27).

Prostaglandin Production

As shown in Table 3, fragments of endometrial adenocarcinoma can respond to estradiol (10^{-8} M) by increasing $PGF_{2\alpha}$ output, and to progesterone (10^{-7} M) by decreasing the production of this prostaglandin under organ culture conditions (Markiewicz L and Gurpide E, unpublished). These results suggest another test for responsiveness of endometrial tumors to ovarian hormones. The basal output of $PGF_{2\alpha}$ in the specimens shown in Table 3 is much lower than those observed both in proliferative and secretory normal endometrium, which averaged 340+/-52 (n=17) and 120+/-18 (n=27) ng/mg prot x d, respectively (28-31). These results are in agreement with a previous report, based on another series of experiments, from which we concluded that the $PGE_2/PGF_{2\alpha}$ output ratio is lower in specimens of neoplastic endometrium than in normal tissue mainly due to a decrease in $PGF_{2\alpha}$ production (32).

Histologically normal secretory endometrium is very responsive to estrogens in vitro as evaluated by measuring $PGF_{2\alpha}$ output (28-30). Since one of the proposed approaches to reduce levels of circulating estrogens in postmenopausal cancer patients is to administer aromatase inhibitors (33) in order to prevent the conversion of androstenedione to estrogens, we have used the endometrial system to test for direct in vitro effects of adrenal C_{19} steroids (34). We found that dehydroepiandrosterone, its sulfate and its acetate, as well as 5-androstene-3β,17β-diol, can mimic the stimulatory effects of estradiol on $PGF_{2\alpha}$ output by interacting with the estrogen receptor, as indicated by the ability of the antiestrogen 4-hydroxytamoxifen to neutralize their actions (Table 4). It should, therefore, be considered that aromatase inhibitors may not suppress

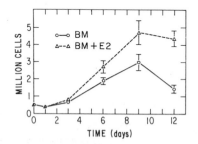

Fig. 3. Effects of estradiol on proliferation of Ishikawa cells grown in phenol red-free, serum-free basal medium (DMEM-Ham's F12, 1:1, with additional glutamine and HEPES), in the presence (triangles) or absence (circles) of estradiol (10^{-8} M). Anzai et al. (unpublished).

275

Table 3. $PGF_{2\alpha}$ production by fragments of endometrial
adenocarcinoma and responsiveness to estradiol (E_2)
and progesterone (P) added to the culture medium.

Specimen Number	Basal (ng/mg protxd)	$+E_2(10^{-8}M)$ (% of basal)	$+P(10^{-7}M)$ (% of basal)
Grade 1			
2	29	69	52
5	18	200	25
8	2.9	410	110
9	14		78
11	120	125	100
22	150	170	43
24	11	640	
28	21	170	57
29	71	140	48
35	150	280	65
36	95	750	61
38	37	510	84
Av±SE(n=12)	60±16		
Grade 2			
1	71	210	
13	14	140	
21	16	150	100
30	5.6	150	78
34	12	1000	54
Av±SE(n=5)	24±12		
Grade 3			
3	34	110	
4	0.86	300	140
20	6.4		59
AV±SE(n=3)	14±10		

estrogenic actions of dehydroepiandrosterone sulfate on endometrial tumors
since the steroid can exceed micromolar concentrations in plasma under
normal physiological conditions.

Lipocortin Production

Fragments of human endometrium in organotypic culture secrete lipocortins, closely related to 36-38K calpactins, that inhibit the action of
phospholipases and the release of arachidonic acid necessary for the
synthesis of $PGF_{2\alpha}$, other prostaglandins and leukotrienes (35,36).
Antiinflammatory effects of glucocorticoids have been considered to be
mediated by active lipocortins (37). Since dexamethasone (30) as well as
progestins (28,29) have been shown to inhibit in vitro production of $PGF_{2\alpha}$
by the endometrium, we looked for the presence of lipocortin in the media
of endometrial cultures and tested for the effects of these steroids at
$(10^{-8}-10^{-6}M)$ concentrations. Lipocortin radioimmunoassays were performed
in Dr. F. Hirata's laboratories. It was found that endometrium secretes
lipocortin and that the rates of output are increased by dexamethasone and
decreased by progesterone (30). If lipocortins are actually involved in
the regulation of the synthesis of arachidonic acid derivatives in endome-

Table 4. Estrogen-mediated in vitro effects of dehydroepiandrosterone and its sulfate on endometrial $PGF_{2\alpha}$ output.

Steroid added	$PGF_{2\alpha}$ output (% of control ± SE)	
	Uninhibited	+ Antiestrogen*
None	100 ± 19	140 ± 16
Estradiol (10^{-8}M)	340 ± 52	180 ± 15
DHEA (10^{-6}M)	200 ± 23	140 ± 20
DHEA-sulfate (10^{-6}M)	240 ± 43	110 ± 80

*4-hydroxytamoxifen (10^{-6}M)

trial tissue, these findings would indicate that glucocorticoids and progestins inhibit $PGF_{2\alpha}$ output by different mechanisms. However, the RIA employed does not distinguish between lipocortin and its phosphorylated (inactive) form.

SOURCES AND SINKS FOR ESTROGENS IN ENDOMETRIAL TISSUE

If it is accepted that estradiol at physiologic levels can stimulate the growth of endometrial tumors, it is most relevant to identify the sources of the intracellular hormone and the metabolic routes for its removal from endometrial cells. On the basis of arguments presented in previous publications, it seems clear that the activity of the hormone is determined by the levels of both the amount of receptor and by the intra-cellular concentration of unbound estradiol, which in turn is fully determined at the steady state by the rate of intracellular synthesis and metabolism of the hormone (38,39). Estradiol can be taken up as such or can be formed intracellularly from circulating precursors, mainly estrone, estrone sulfate and androstenedione. Estrone is converted to some extent to estradiol by action of 17β-hydroxy oxidoreductase (40), estrone sulfate is hydrolyzed to estrone by aryl sulfatase (41) in endometrial epithelial cells and androstenedione can be aromatized in stromal cells (42). Met-abolic processes involved in the removal of estradiol in endometrial cells include a sulfotransferase (43-45) leading to the formation of estrone and estradiol sulfates, and the 17β-hydroxysteroid oxidoreductase converting estradiol to estrone, a compound that is not estrogenic in target cells unless it is reduced to estradiol (38,46).

Experiments carried out with the Ishikawa endometrial cancer cells have shown that estradiol added to the culture medium at 10^{-8}M concentra-tions is rapidly and almost completely converted to estradiol-3- sulfate: after 24 h of incubation practically all of the initial estradiol in the medium is replaced by the sulfate (47). However, if estradiol is added at a 10^{-6}M concentration, it is metabolized much more slowly and mainly to estrone. These results can be explained by considering the relative Michaelis constants of the sulfotransferase (approximately nanomolar) and the oxidoreductase (approximately micromolar) (45,48). At very low concentrations of the substrate, most of it will be converted to sulfates if sulfatase activity is low, whereas at higher concentrations the 17β-dehydrogenase becomes relatively more important. Another observation made in these experiments was that a large proportion of the radioactivity in the cells at the end of the incubation period was in the form of fatty acid esters of estradiol, which have been described in Hochberg et al.

(49) and studied by Adams et al. in breast cancer cells (50). The role of these derivatives of the hormone is still undefined although it is postulated that they may function as reservoirs from which estradiol can be recovered.

ESTROGEN RECEPTOR IN ENDOMETRIAL CANCER CELLS

Estrogen receptors are currently expected to mediate all actions of the hormone by forming an activated complex that is able to bind to regulatory elements of specific genes, likely by interacting with specific acceptor proteins, to affect transcription (i.e., DNA-dependent RNA synthesis). Before fully embracing this concept in the discussion to follow, it may be appropriate to mention some experimental results which suggest the possibility that estrogen, in addition to affecting transcription, could act directly with or without binding to their receptor, on cell membranes, enzymes or RNA.

Nontranscriptional Effects of Estrogens

Direct effects of estrogens not involving transcriptional processes can be inferred from actions exerted on extranuclear subcellular fractions, from influences on activity of isolated enzymes or from responses occurring in the presence of nucleic acid and protein synthesis inhibitors or so rapidly that transcriptional events can be ruled out.

Estrogens appear to bind specifically to cell membranes (51,52). Direct effects of estradiol at the cell surface are evident in brain neurons, which are very rapidly hyperpolarized by estradiol, even in the presence of cycloheximide or actinomycin D (53). Similarly, changes in Ca^{++} flux in suspensions of cells isolated from uteri of ovariectomized rats could be detected in less than 3 min after addition of estradiol (10^{-9} M) to the medium (54) and increases in ^{3}H-uridine uptake 2 min after administration of estradiol have been postulated on the basis of observed elevations of RNA labeling (55). Furthermore, estradiol has been shown to provoke increases in adenylate cyclase activity in plasma membranes isolated from human secretory endometrium (56) and changes in the binding of dopaminergic agents in membranes isolated from rat pituitary cells (57). Examples of binding and allosteric effects of estradiol on enzymes are found in studies with isolated tyrosine hydroxylase (58) and nucleoside-nucleotide phosphotransferase C (59). Estrogens may also have posttranscriptional effects, participating in the processing and transport of mRNA as suggested by the interaction of the estrogen-receptor complex with the 80S ribonucleoprotein particle (60) and by other actions reviewed by Spelsberg et al. (61).

Experiments from our laboratory yielded results that may be interpreted to suggest a direct action of estradiol on prostaglandin synthase not involving the activation of estrogen receptors, in spite of the observed antagonism of 4-hydroxytamoxifen on the estradiol stimulation of $PGF_{2\alpha}$ output by endometrial fragments (32). In these experiments, fragments of endometrial tissue were divided in several dishes containing Ham's F10 medium supplemented with 10% charcoal-treated calf serum and kept for a preincubation period of 2 to 8 h at either 37 or 40°C, followed by an incubation period of 1 or 2 days at 37°C in the presence or absence of estradiol (10^{-8} M). Levels of estrogen receptor, measured with the hydroxylapatite method (62) after exposure of the tissue to 40°C, were significantly reduced in comparison to the levels in tissue kept at 37°C, in some cases to one-tenth of the original value and to levels as low as 5 fmol/mg protein (32). Whenever tested, these levels remained lowered even after 2 or 3 days of incubation at 37°C. Interestingly, fragments derived

278

from the same tissue and containing either higher or lower estrogen receptor levels after preincubation at 37 or 40°C, respectively, responded about equally to the stimulatory effect of estradiol on $PGF_{2\alpha}$ output (32). Furthermore, a similar lack of correlation between estrogen receptor levels and effects of estradiol on $PGF_{2\alpha}$ production was noted during incubations of endometrial adenocarcinoma specimens with estrogen receptor levels ranging from undetectable to 500 fmol/mg cytosol protein.

Interpretation of Estrogen Receptor Measurements

The measurement of estrogen receptor levels in specimens of endometrial adenocarcinoma can be flawed by a variety of errors, conceptual as well as technical. Conceptually, it is important to have a clear definition of what a receptor is since specific binding of the ligand or immunoreaction with specific antibodies do not necessarily reveal the functional aspect of the detected protein(s). Heterogeneity of high affinity binders has been demonstrated in human endometrium (63) and endometrial adenocarcinoma cells (see below). They are characterized by affinity constants for estradiol of less than 1 nM and between 1-10 nM; no differences in their functionality as mediators of the estrogenic effects have been shown. Distinction between these different binders can only be achieved by performing analysis of each sample at various concentrations of substrate. No information on whether one or more of these binders are detectable using immunocytochemical methods is available. Furthermore, data on estrogen receptor levels determined by ligand binding cannot be truly evaluated unless accompanied by histologic information on the cellular homogeneity of the tissue analyzed since specimens of primary endometrial tumors may include myometrial tissue, necrotic portions, large numbers of lymphocytes and extracellular protein.

Another limitation of the value of estrogen receptor measurements is evident from cases in which the presence of receptors is not associated with responsiveness to the hormone. An example of such a situation is provided by the finding that 2 endometrial adenocarcinoma cell lines, one responsive (Ishikawa) and the other unresponsive (HEC-50) to estrogens, have binding sites of equal affinity constants for estradiol (Table 5) but differ in their reactivity with the monoclonal antibody JS 34/32 (65) raised against the calf uterine estradiol receptor (Fig. 4), and in their binding to DNA (Kassan S and Gurpide E, unpublished).

Tests Based on In Vitro Responses to Hormones

It follows from the preceding considerations that in vitro tests based on responsiveness of tumor samples to estrogen or progestins might go beyond revealing the presence of hormone-specific binders to indicate the functional status of receptors. Actually, several sensitive in vitro tests applicable to endometrial tumors are available, although they have

Table 5. Saturation analysis of estradiol specific binding in cytosol of estrogen responsive (Ishikawa) and unresponsive (HEC-50) endometrial adenocarcinoma cells (64).

Cell line	Number of experiments	Dissoc. constant Mean (nM) + SE	No. of binding sites Mean (fmol/mg prot±SE)
Ishikawa	4	0.58 ± 0.14	7.8 ± 3.1
HEC-50	4	0.65 ± 0.21	5.8 ± 2.1

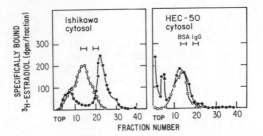

Fig. 4. Effects of JS 34/32 monoclonal antibody against estrogen receptor on sedimentation of specific estradiol binders on 0.4
M KCl-glycerol gradients. S Kassan and E
Gurpide (unpublished).

not been subjected to experimental correlation with in vivo responses to
treatment (66).

Effects of estrogen can be evaluated by incubating tumor fragments
with estradiol at 10^{-8} M concentration and measuring the output of $PGF_{2\alpha}$ or
PGE_2, as described in previous publications (28-30). From experience
acquired by performing many incubations with fragments of normal endometrium and primary tumors, we consider that a 50% increase in output over
control values is significant, provided that samples used for RIA include
duplicate dishes and measurements are made in replicates at different
dilutions. Effects of progestins could be examined in this test by
observing the antiestrogenic action of progesterone (10^{-7}-10^{-6}M) added to
the medium. In responsive tissues, progestins lower the basal output of
$PGF_{2\alpha}$ or PGE_2 and counteract the stimulatory effects of estrogens when
added as a mixture to the culture medium (28,29,67).

Responsiveness to progestins can also be tested by evaluating their
effects on glycogen accumulation, evident from the formation of sub- or
supranuclear vesicles recognizable histologically by eosin-hematoxylin
staining or a diastase-sensitive PAS reaction (68). A reliable in vivo
test for responsiveness to progestins involves the radiometric determination of estradiol 17β-dehydrogenase activity, which has been shown to be
specifically stimulated by progestins in normal endometrium (69,70) and
endometrial adenocarcinoma (69,71).

Regulation of Estrogen Receptor Levels

The pattern of changes in concentration of estrogen receptor in the
normal endometrium observed during the menstrual cycle, namely high levels
during the follicular phase and a marked decline after ovulation (72,73),
suggested that progesterone might be responsible for downregulation of
the estrogen receptor, as had been previously noted in rodents. In vivo
experiments have confirmed this hypothesis and demonstrated its applicability to responsive endometrial adenocarcinoma, as described in a
previous review (16).

Studies on the estrogen binding capacity of cells from an endometrial
cancer line, carried out in our laboratories, revealed an influence of
cyclic nucleotides on estrogen binders. When sodium molybdate at 20 mM
concentration was added to cells of the HEC-1 line, established by H.
Kuramoto (74), specific binding of ^{3}H-estradiol increased. This increase
was not due to the stabilization of the binding molecule since the same
effect was obtained when the molybdate was added before or after homogenization of the cells and was lost when plasma membranes were removed

from the homogenate by centrifugation (75). Following up this observation, effects of cyclic nucleotides, whose formation depends on membrane-bound cyclases, were tested in cytosol. It was found that the presence of ATP was necessary to obtain these effects, an observation that suggests the involvement of phosphorylation, both in the action of cGMP and cAMP (76).

Interestingly, good correlations were found between intracellular cGMP/cAMP ratios and estrogen binding in cells whose binding capacity change during culture (16). A potential application of these effects, which still are not understood mechanistically, is suggested by the ability of cGMP to augment specific binding levels for ^{3}H-estradiol when added to cytosol of some endometrial tumors with undetectable receptor levels (77). Furthermore, an enhancing effect of dibutyryl-cGMP on responses to estradiol was detected when the stimulation of alkaline phosphatase was studied in Ishikawa cells (25).

CONCLUSIONS

Endometrial tissue is very responsive to estrogens and progestins in vivo and, to some extent, in vitro. Responsiveness is maintained in some primary and metastatic tumors. End points to evaluate responsiveness to estrogens include enhancement of prostaglandins, peroxidase activity, progesterone receptor levels and tritiated thymidine incorporation; progesterone action end points include inhibition of prostaglandin output, increases in 17β hydroxysteroid dehydrogenase or isocitric dehydrogenase activities, and glycogen accumulation.

Availability of a human endometrial adenocarcinoma cell line (Ishikawa) responsive to estrogens is providing useful information on characteristics of endometrial tumors. For instance, an estrogen unresponsive endometrial cell line (HEC-50) and the Ishikawa cells possess the same set of high affinity, specific binding sites but only the estrogen-responsive line reacts with an antibody recognizing the estrogen binders.

The finding that estradiol can influence proliferation of Ishikawa cells in serum-free medium and provoke the resumption of proliferation when added to cultures at plateau densities strongly suggests effects of estradiol on the production of growth factors acting as autocrine regulators of endometrial cancer cell proliferation.

ACKNOWLEDGMENT

This investigation was supported by HPH Grant Number CA-15648, awarded by the National Cancer Institute, DHHS.

REFERENCES

1. MacMahon B. Risk factors for endometrial cancer. Gynecol Oncol 1974; 2:122-9.
2. Gusberg SB. Hormone-dependence of endometrial cancer. Obstet Gynecol 1967; 30:287-93.
3. Ziel HK, Finkle WD. Increased risk of endometrial carcinoma among users of conjugated estrogens. N Engl J Med 1975; 293:1167-70.
4. Smith DC, Prentice R, Thompson DJ, Hermann WL. Association of exogenous estrogen and endometrial carcinoma. N Engl J Med 1975; 293:1164-7.
5. Mack T, Pike MC, Henderson BE, et al. Estrogens and endometrial

cancer in a retirement community. New Engl J Med 1976; 294:1262-7.

6. Kelly RM, Baker WH. The role of progesterone in human endometrial cancer. Cancer Res 1965; 25:1190-2.

7. Reifenstein EC. The treatment of advanced endometrial cancer with hydroxyprogesterone caproate. Gynecol Oncol 1974; 2:377-414.

8. Swenerton KD, White GW, Boyes DA. Treatment of advanced endometrial carcinoma with tamoxifen. N Engl J Med 1979; 301-5.

9. Ehrlich CE, Young PCM, Cleary RE. Cytoplasmic progesterone and estradiol receptors in normal, hyperplastic, and carcinomatous endometria: therapeutic implications. Am J Obstet Gynecol 1981; 141:539-46.

10. McCarty KS Jr, Barton TK, Fettler BF, Creasman WT, McCarty KS Sr. Correlation of estrogen and progesterone receptors with histologic differentiation in endometrial adenocarcinoma. Am J Pathol 1979; 96:171-83.

11. Martin PM, Rolland PH, Gammere M, Serment H, Toga M. Estradiol and progesterone receptors in normal and neoplastic endometrium: correlations between receptors, histopathological examination and clinical responses under progestin therapy. Cancer 1979; 23:321-9.

12. Benraad T, Friberg LG, Koenders AJM, Kullander S. Do estrogen and progesterone receptors (E_2R and PR) in metastasizing endometrial cancers predict the response to gestagen therapy? Acta Obstet Gynecol Scand 1980; 59:155-9.

13. Kauppila A, Janne O, Kujansuu E, Vihko R. Treatment of advanced endometrial adenocarcinoma with a combined cytotoxic therapy. Cancer 1979; 46:2162-7.

14. Martin JD, Hahnel R, McCartney AJ, Woodings TL. The effect of estrogen receptor status on survival in patients with endometrial cancer. Am J Obstet Gynecol 1983; 147:322-4.

15. Kauppila A, Kujansuv E, Vihko R. The cytosol estrogen and progestin receptors in endometrial carcinoma of patients treated with surgery, radiotherapy, and progestin. Clinical correlates. Cancer 1982; 50:2157-62.

16. Gurpide E, Fleming H, Holinka CF. Steroid receptors and responsiveness to hormones in endometrial cancer. In: Hollander V, ed. Hormonally responsive tumors. New York: Academic Press, 1985:341-65.

17. MacMahon B, Cole P, Brown J. Etiology of human breast cancer—a review. J Natl Cancer Inst 1973; 50:21-42.

18. Dickson RB, Lippman M. Estrogenic regulation of growth and polypeptide growth factor secretion in human breast carcinoma. Endocr Rev 1987; 8:29-43.

19. Zaino RJ, Satyaswaroop PG, Mortel R. Hormonal therapy of human endometrial adenocarcinoma in a nude mouse model. Cancer Res 1985; 45:539-41.

20. Lippman ME, Bolan G, Huff K. The effects of estrogens and antiestrogens on hormone-responsive human breast cancer in long term culture. Cancer Res 1976; 36:4595-601.

21. Butler WB, Kirkland WL, Gargala TL, Goran N, Kelsey WH, Berlinski PJ. Steroid stimulation of plasminogen activator production in a human breast cancer cell line (MCF7). Cancer Res 1983; 43:1637-41.

22. Soto AM, Sonnenschein C. Cell proliferation of estrogen-sensitive cells: the case for negative control. Endocr Rev 1987; 8:44-51.

23. Nishida M, Kasahare K, Kaneko M, Iwasaki H. Establishment of a new human endometrial adenocarcinoma cell line, Ishikawa cells, containing estrogen and progesterone receptors. Acta Obstet Gynaec Japonica 1985; 37:1103-11 (in Japanese).

24. Gravanis A, Gurpide E. Effects of estradiol on DNA polymerase α activity in the Ishikawa human endometrial adenocarcinoma cell line. J Clin Endocr Metab 1986; 63:356-9.

25. Holinka CF, Hata H, Kuramoto H, Gurpide E. Effects of steroid hor-

mones and antisteroids on alkaline phosphatase activity in human endometrial cancer cells (Ishikawa line). Cancer Res 1986; 46: 2771-4.

26. Holinka CF, Hata H, Kuramoto H, Gurpide E. Responses to estradiol in a human endometrial adenocarcinoma cell line (Ishikawa). J Steroid Biochem 1986; 24:85-9.

27. Holinka CF, Hata H, Gravanis A, Kuramoto H, Gurpide E. Effects of estradiol on proliferation of endometrial adenocarcinoma cells (Ishikawa line). J Steroid Biochem 1986; 25:781-6.

28. Markiewicz L, Schatz F, Barg P, Gurpide E. Prostaglandin $F_{2\alpha}$ output by human endometrium under superfusion and organ culture conditions. J Steroid Biochem 1985; 22:231-5.

29. Schatz F, Markiewicz L, Barg P, Gurpide E. In vitro effects of ovarian steroids on $PGF_{2\alpha}$ output by human endometrium and endometrial epithelial cells. J Clin Endocrinol Metab 1985; 61:361-7.

30. Gurpide E, Markiewicz L, Schatz F, Hirata F. Lipocortin output by human endometrium in vitro. J Clin Endocrinol Metab 1986; 63:162-6.

31. Schatz F, Markiewicz L, Barg P, Gurpide E. In vitro inhibition with antiestrogens or estradiol effects on $PGF_{2\alpha}$ production by human endometrium and endometrial epithelial cells. Endocrinology 1986; 118:408-12.

32. Markiewicz L, Gravanis A, Schatz F, Holinka CF, Deligdisch L, Gurpide E. Prostaglandin production by human endometrial adenocarcinoma in vitro. In: Baulieu EE, Iacobelli S, McGuire WL, eds. Endocrinology and malignancy. London: Partheon Press, 1986:420-7.

33. Brodie AMH, Wing L-Y, Goss P, Dowsett M, Coombes RC. Aromatase inhibitors and the treatment of breast cancer. J Steroid Biochem 1986; 24:91-7.

34. Markiewicz L, Gurpide E. C_{19} adrenal steroids enhance $PGF_{2\alpha}$ output by human endometrium in vitro. Am J Obstet Gynecol (submitted).

35. Hirata F, Schiffman E, Venkatasubramanian K, Salomon D, Axelrod J. A phospholipase A_2 inhibitory protein in rabbit neutrophils induced by glucocorticoids. Proc Natl Acad Sci USA 1980; 77:2533-6.

36. Davidson FF, Edward A, Dennis MP, Glenney JR Jr. Inhibition of phospholipase A_2 by "lipocortins" and calpactins. J Biol Chem 1987; 262:1698-1705.

37. Hirata F. Lipomodulin: a possible mediator of the action of glucocorticoids. In: Samuelsson B, Paoleti R, Ranwell P, eds. Prostaglandin, thromboxane and leukotriene research. New York: Raven Press, 1983:11:73-8.

38. Gurpide E. Enzymatic modulation of hormonal action at the target tissue. J Toxicol Environ Health 1978; 4:249-68.

39. Gurpide E. Metabolic influences on the actions of estrogens. Therapeutic implications. Pediatrics 1978; 62:1114-20.

40. Gurpide E, Tseng L. Factors controlling intracellular levels of estrogens in human endometrium. Gynecol Oncol 1974; 2:221-7.

41. Tseng L, Stolee A, Gurpide E. Quantitative studies on the uptake of metabolism of estrogens and progesterone by human endometrium. Endocrinology 1972; 90:390-404.

42. Tseng L. Estrogen synthesis in human endometrial epithelial glands and stromal cells. J Steroid Biochem 1984; 20:877-81.

43. Buirchell BJ, Hahnel R. Metabolism of estradiol-17β in human endometrium during the menstrual cycle. J Steroid Biochem 1975; 6:1489-94.

44. Pack BA, Tovar R, Booth E, Brooks SC. The cyclic relationship of estrogen sulfurylation to the nuclear receptor level in human endometrial curettings. J Clin Endocrinol Metab 1979; 48:420-4.

45. Tseng L, Liu HC. Stimulation of estrogen sulfurylation and arylsulfotransferase activity in human endometrium by progestin in vitro. J Clin Endocrinol Metab 1981; 418-21.

46. Tseng L, Gurpide L. Effect of estrone and progesterone on the nuclear uptake of estradiol by slices of human endometrium. Endocrinology 1973; 93:245-8.

47. Hata H, Holinka CF, Pahuja SL, Hochberg RB, Kuramoto H, Gurpide E. Estradiol metabolism in Ishikawa endometrial cancer cells. J Steroid Biochem 1987; 26:699-704.

48. Tseng L, Mazella J. Kinetic studies of human endometrial hydroxysteroid dehydrogenase. J Steroid Biochem 1981; 14:437-42.

49. Larner JM, MacLuskey NJ, Hochberg RB. The naturally occurring C-17 fatty acid esters of estradiol are long-acting estrogens. J Steroid Biochem 1985; 407-13.

50. Adams JB, Hall RT, Nott S. Esterification-deesterification of estradiol by human mammary cancer cells in culture. J Steroid Biochem 1986; 24:1159-62.

51. Szego CM. Mechanisms of hormone action: parallels in receptor-mediated signal propagation for steroid peptide effectors. Life Sci 1984; 35:2381-96.

52. Bression D, Michard M, Le Dafniet M, Pagesy P, Peillon F. Evidence for a specific estradiol binding site on rat pituitary membranes. Endocrinology 1986; 119:1048-51.

53. Nabekura J, Oomura Y, Minami T, Mizuno Y, Fukuda A. Mechanism of the rapid effect of 17β-estradiol on medial amygdala neurons. Science 1986; 233:226-8.

54. Pietras RJ, Szego CM. Endometrial cell calcium and oestradiol action. Nature 1975; 253:357-9.

55. Means AR, Hamilton TH. Early estrogen action: concomitant stimulations within two minutes of nuclear synthesis and uptake of RNA precursor by the uterus. Proc Natl Acad Sci 1966; 56:1594-8.

56. Bergamini CM, Pansini F, Bettochi S Jr, et al. Hormonal sensitivity of adenylate cyclase from human endometrium: modulation by estradiol. J Steroid Biochem 1985; 22:299-303.

57. Bression D, Brandi AM, Pagesy P, et al. In vitro and in vivo antagonistic regulation of the rat pituitary domperidone binding sites: correlation with ovarian steroid regulation of the dopaminergic inhibition of prolactin secretion in vitro. Endocrinology 1985; 116:1905-11.

58. McCarty KS Jr, Wortman J, Stowers S, Lubahn DB, McCarty KS Sr, Siegler HF. Sex steroid receptor analysis in human melanoma. Cancer 1980; 46:1463-70.

59. Lenger K. Allosteric effects of cortisol, estradiol, progesterone and of the DNA-sequences poly d(A-T) and poly d(C-G) on the adenosine and thymidine phosphorylation of the nuclear nucleoside-nucleotide phosphotransferase C. Int J Biochem 1983; 15:1241-8.

60. Liang T, Liao S. Association of the uterine 17β-estradiol-receptor complex with ribonucleoprotein in vitro and in vivo. J Biol Chem 1974; 15:4671-8.

61. Spelsberg TC, Ruh T, Goldberger A, Horton M, Hora J, Singh R. Nuclear acceptor sites for steroid hormone receptors: comparisons of steroid and antisteroids. In: Pasqualini J, Raynaud JP, eds. Antiestrogens. Oxford: Pergamon Press (in press).

62. Clark JH, Peck EJ Jr. Female sex steroids. Receptors and functions. In: Monographs on endocrinology; vol 14. Berlin-Heidelberg-New York: Springer-Verlag, 1979.

63. Smith RG, Clarke SG, Zalta E, Taylor RN. Two estrogens in reproductive tissue. J Steroid Biochem 1979; 10:31-5.

64. Mechanick JI, Peskin CS. Resolution of steroid binding heterogeneity by Fourier-derived affinity spectrum analysis (FASA). Anal Biochem 1986; 157:221-35.

65. Moncharmont B, Su J-L, Parikh I. Monoclonal antibodies against estrogen receptor interaction with different forms and functions of the receptor. Biochem 1982; 21:6916-21.

66. Gurpide E. In vitro effects of steroids on human endometrium. In: Genazzani AR, Volpe A, Faccinetti F, eds. Gynecological endocrinol-

ogy. Lanes UK: The Parthenon Group, 1987:569-75.

67. Abel MH, Baird DT. The effect of 17β-estradiol and progesterone on prostaglandin production by human endometrium maintained in organ culture. Endocrinology 1980; 106:1599-606.

68. Holinka CF, Deligdisch L, Gurpide E. Histological evaluation of in vitro responses of endometrial adenocarcinoma to progestins and their relation to progesterone levels. Cancer Res 1984; 44:293-6.

69. Tseng L, Gurpide E. Induction of human endometrial estradiol dehydrogenase by progestins. Endocrinology 1975; 825-33.

70. Whitehead MI, Townsend PT, Pryse-Davis J, Ryder TA, King RJB. Effects of estrogens and progestins on the biochemistry and morphology of the postmenopausal endometrium. N Engl Med 1981; 305:1599-1605.

71. Pollow K, Boquoi E, Lubbert H, Pollow B. Effect of gestagen therapy upon 17β-hydroxysteroid dehydrogenase in human endometrium and endometrial carcinoma. J Endocrinol 1975; 67:131-2.

72. Bayard F, Damilano S, Robel P, Baulieu EE. Cytoplasmic and nuclear estradiol and progesterone receptors in human endometrium. J Clin Endocrinol Metab 1981; 46:635-48.

73. Pollow K, Schmidt-Gollwitzer M, Pollow B. Progesterone- and estradiol-binding proteins from normal human endometrium and endometrial carcinoma: a comparative study. In: Wittliff JL, Dapunt O, eds. Steroid receptors and hormone-dependent neoplasia. New York: Masson, 1980:69-94.

74. Kuramoto H, Tamura S, Notake Y. Establishment of a cell line of human endometrial adenocarcinoma in vitro. Am J Obstet Gynecol 1972; 114:1012-9.

75. Fleming H, Blumenthal R, Gurpide E. Effect of cyclic nucleotides on estradiol binding in human endometrium. Endocrinology 1982; 111:1671-7.

76. Fleming H, Blumenthal R, Gurpide E. Rapid changes in specific estrogen binding elicited by guanosine-3',5'-cyclic monophosphate of cAMP in cytosol from human endometrial cells. Proc Natl Acad Sci USA 1983; 80:2486-90.

77. Gurpide E, Blumenthal R, Fleming H. Regulation of estrogen receptor levels in endometrial cancer cells. In: Gurpide E, Calandra R, Levy C, Soto RJ, eds. Hormones and cancer. New York: Alan R Liss, 1984:145-65.

21

STRUCTURAL FEATURES AND CLINICAL SIGNIFICANCE OF ESTROGEN RECEPTORS

James L. Wittliff,[1] Joseph C. Allegra,[2]
Thomas G. Day, Jr.,[3] and Salman M. Hyder[1]

Hormone Receptor Laboratory, and Departments of
Biochemistry,[1] Medicine[2] and Obstetrics and Gynecology[3]
and J. G. Brown Cancer Center
University of Louisville, Louisville, KY 40292

INTRODUCTION

An important question in molecular endocrinology is how structurally simple molecules, such as the steroid hormones, initiate the myriad of effects in a wide variety of target organs via their receptor proteins. It is generally accepted that a prerequisite for responsiveness to a steroid hormone stimulus is a cellular protein termed the steroid hormone receptor or steroid binding protein. These receptor proteins have been found in concentrations ranging from 50–50,000 sites per target cell but are virtually absent in nontarget cells. A biologically important property is the association of a steroid hormone with its characteristic receptor protein in a manner exhibiting both high affinity and ligand specificity.

Our understanding of the sequence of events which follows the interaction of the steroid hormone with a target cell evolved from the original "two-step" mechanism suggested independently by Gorski and co-workers (1) and by Jensen and colleagues (2) in the late 1960s. More recent contributions from these two groups using either monoclonal antibodies to the estrogen receptor (3) or enucleated cells (4) suggest that the receptor proteins are essentially associated with nuclear components although the exact location is still debated. Furthermore, the manner in which the steroid hormone-receptor complexes are involved in regulating the synthesis of DNA, RNA and specific proteins is unknown.

Since the late 1960s, our laboratory, first at the University of Rochester in New York and later at the University of Louisville, has pursued the relationship between the structural features of these steroid hormone receptor proteins and the mechanism by which they recognize their steroid hormone ligands (5–10). Furthermore, we have investigated the chemistry of hormone receptor complexes and the reactions which initiate the complicated cascade of intracellular events leading to alterations in macromolecular synthesis in target organs such as the breast and uterus. Complementary to these fundamental studies has been our clinical research in establishing the relationship between the presence of the steroid hormone receptors in tumor biopsies in breast and endometrial carcinoma and patient's response to endocrine therapy.

287

Previously our laboratory proposed that the estrogen receptor molecule is a complex composed of one or more subunits of similar size but differing in ionic properties (11-13). This suggestion is analogous in some respect to the proposed structure of the progesterone receptor of the chick oviduct (14,15). Our observations by sucrose density gradient centrifugation analysis of both 4-5S and 8-9S forms of the estrogen receptor in human breast cancer could be attributed to the unequal production of one of the constituents of the macromolecular complex (11,13) or to their interconversion. A multidimensional analysis of the receptor by a combination of size, shape, and charge mediated methods of separation would investigate this hypothesis. A choice for this type of analysis might involve PAGE except that the receptor-estradiol-17β complex is highly susceptible to loss of radioactive ligand under these conditions. Two-dimensional analysis on O'Farrell gels (i.e., isoelectric focusing followed by PAGE separation) recently has been employed for a similar exploration of the glucocorticoid receptor (16) employing a nondissociable ligand (dexamethasone mesylate).

Our laboratory has developed high performance liquid chromatography (HPLC) in the size-exclusion (HPSEC) (17), chromatofocusing (HPCF) (18), ion-exchange (HPIEC) (19) and hydrophobic interaction modes (HPHIC) (20, 21) to investigate the forms of the estrogen receptor from a variety of tissues. These technologies separate estrogen receptor forms without the use of urea or SDS (i.e., under nondenaturing conditions). These methodologies are rapid, reproducible, and exhibit high recoveries (9,2224). Madhock and Leung (25) reported a multistep analysis employing HPIEC followed by sucrose density gradient centrifugation and HPSEC in the study of rabbit uterine ER and have further substantiated our earlier proposal of receptor polymorphism.

We have used multidimensional analysis of ER from human uterus utilizing various HPLC methodologies in combination with sucrose density gradient centrifugation. In addition we employed [16α-^{125}I]iodoestradiol-17β, a ligand of high specific radioactivity (2200 Ci/mmole), which allows (a) the assay of extremely low levels of receptor (1-3 fmoles), (b) simultaneous, on-line determination of gamma radioactivity and conductivity (for HPIEC) using appropriate detectors (10,26), and (c) multistep analysis since fractions obtained from one procedure may be used directly in another. We have demonstrated the use of HPSEC and HPIEC for rapid, multidimensional assessment of ER from human uterus and endometrial carcinoma under nondenaturing conditions (27). The results indicate that estrogen receptors may be dissociated into smaller subunits of similar size but different surface charges. This approach appears useful in steroid receptor structure/function studies.

High-performance hydrophobic interaction chromatography (HPHIC) of proteins is widely gaining recognition in the rapidly growing field of high-performance liquid chromatography (HPLC) since the introduction of microparticular rigid packing materials (28,29). Among the various modes of HPLC such as reversed-phase (RPLC), HPIEC, HPSEC and HPCF, HPHIC represents the mildest means of separating protein molecules with complete retention of their biological activity. This fact, coupled with recoveries of these biopolymers of almost 100%, indicates that HPHIC is a favorable choice of methods for separating such complex molecules (20,21, 30,31). An additional feature which merits mention is that HPHIC, unlike most RPLC procedures, may be performed at physiological pH.

HPHIC relies on the interaction of hydrophobic patches, present in the protein, with the stationary phases. Hydrophobic patches usually are present in the interior of the molecule and therefore must be exposed. This is achieved by promoting such interaction in the presence of high-ionic-strength buffers used as the initial mobile phase. The latter exposes the hydrophobic patches buried within the protein molecule. Subsequent elution of the protein is obtained by lowering the salt concentration in a gradient mode and thus selectively dissociating the proteins from the stationary phase. The least hydrophobic molecules will be eluted earlier in the separation gradient.

The recent advances in molecular biology requiring protein purification suggest that the mild conditions of HPHIC in combination with the short analysis time will make it a preferred protein separation technique. Currently, we are involved in optimizing various HPLC separation modes for characterization of labile regulatory proteins. We have previously reported that HPHIC rapidly separates steroid receptors with retention of their biological activity (21,24,32).

We have optimized conditions for HPHIC of steroid receptors, performed on a recently developed, polyether-bonded stationary phase, which is nonionic in nature (21). This appears to be a suitable column material for HPHIC of receptors, since these proteins are highly charged molecules which show retention on both ion-exchange and size-exclusion columns (33). We report further that, although ER separates into two isoforms following HPHIC, only the receptor dissociated by high salt (less hydrophobic) was eluted together with a Mg^{2+}-dependent protein kinase activity. Protein kinase activity was immunoprecipitated with monoclonal antibodies raised against the estrogen receptor.

CLINICAL METHODOLOGY AND QUALITY ASSURANCE

Current methods of assessing steroid hormone receptors in tumor biopsies employ radioligand binding procedures usually with tritium labeled steroid hormones and analogs and more recently with iodine-125 labeled ligands (8,23). The predominant assay used clinically is a multipoint titration analysis which provides a measure of the number of binding sites (specific binding capacity expressed as fmol/mg cytosol protein) and of the affinity constant of the steroid receptor complex often given as the Kd value. Procedures used in the clinical chemistry laboratory assess the presence of unoccupied binding sites in the cytosol (cell sap) of a tissue which provide only a preliminary estimate of the biological integrity of the receptor. However, since the progestin receptor (PR) appears to be a marker of estrogen action in vivo (34), presence of both receptors should reflect retention of a hormonally responsive mechanism as seen in breast cancer (Table 1). Receptor distribution profiles and levels for breast cancer (8), uterine cancer (35,36) and other clinical alterations in these organs (38) from established laboratories are useful for comparison to insure a procedure is satisfactory.

Since various programs for establishing uniformity of steroid receptors have been described elsewhere (38,39), they are mentioned briefly. As a result of reports presented at the First International Workshop on Estrogen Receptors in Breast Cancer (40), it was obvious that greater efforts must be made to establish uniformity and quality control of receptor methods. In fact, one of the conclusions drawn from the 1979 NIH Consensus Development Conference (41) was that "there is a need for quality control of steroid receptor assays." Since 1977, the Hormone Receptor Laboratory at the University of Louisville has established a reference facility for monitoring quality assurance of steroid receptors in biopsies of breast and endometrial carcinomas.

Each shipment of frozen reference powders is designed according to the specific needs of the cooperative trial groups and shipped on dry ice

Table 1. Relationship between steroid-receptor status of breast tumor and patient's objective response to endocrine therapy.[a]

Steroid receptor status[b]			
ER^+/PR^+	ER^+/PR^-	ER^-/PR^-	ER^-/PR^+
135/174 (78%)	55/164 (34%)	17/165 (10%)	5/11 (45%)

[a]NIH Consensus Development Conference on Steroid Receptors in Breast Cancer, 1979 (41).
[b]Ratio of number of patients responding to number with receptor status designated.

to the participating laboratories. More recently, we have developed lyophilized tissue powders which are being evaluated. A summary of the sequence of events transpiring in the Quality Assurance Program is given in Figure 1. Thus far, our laboratory has cooperated with the National Surgical Breast and Bowel Adjuvant Project (NSABP), Southeastern Cancer Study Group, Southwest Oncology Group, Cancer and Leukemia Group B, North Central Cancer Treatment Group and the Eastern Cooperative Oncology Group. We also collaborate with the College of American Pathologists in providing annual surveys. Currently, we have assisted more than 400 laboratories in North America and have worked with various laboratories in Europe, South America, Asia, Australia, and Africa to establish quality assurance measures.

It is essential that a laboratory utilize a daily quality control material and periodically participate in an outside quality assurance program such as those established by the clinical cooperative groups. Criteria for evaluating agreement of results have been established by committees composed of oncologists and clinical chemists. The committee contacts each laboratory in writing regarding their performance relative to that of the reference laboratory and other laboratories taking part in the clinical trial. This important information should be available to the

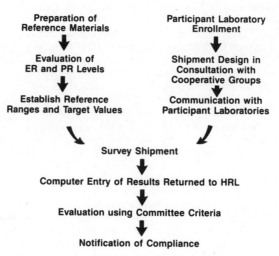

Fig. 1. Flow diagram of sequence of events which occur simultaneously in the quality assurance program. Reproduced from reference 42.

physician treating the patient. In this way, meaningful relationships between biochemical markers such as the steroid hormone receptors and clinical response to experimental therapies can be realized. An example of the success of this effort by the NSABP (43) is described.

Clinical Application in Breast Cancer

Estrogen receptors are determined routinely on biopsies of breast carcinoma and used as predictive indices of a patient's response to endocrine therapy. A multitude of reports (6,40,41) indicated that more than one-half of primary and metastatic lesions of the breast contain ten or more fmoles of ER per mg of cytosol protein. Furthermore, 50-60% of women with breast carcinomas containing ER exhibit objective remissions to endocrine manipulation of either the administrative or ablative type (41). These data suggest that more than one-third of patients presumably have breast tumors with only a portion of the cellular mechanism required to respond to hormonal stimulus. Recognition of estradiol-17β by its receptor represents the first step in the intracellular cascade of events necessary to exert the physiologic action of the hormone.

Since the presence of functional ER is required for the formation of PR, there should be a direct relationship between these two receptors in responsive cells. The majority of the breast tumors containing both receptors would be assumed to retain hormonal responsiveness. A summary of results presented at the Consensus Development Conference (41) suggests this proposal is reasonable. The presence of the progestin receptor is now accepted as a marker that the estrogen response mechanism is intact (34). When a tumor biopsy contained both ER and PR (Table 1), 78% of patients experienced objective remissions to endocrine manipulation (8,41). If only ER was present, a 34% response rate was observed while only 10% of patients responded to endocrine manipulation if neither receptor was present in the breast tumor. In North America, this value drops to 3% possibly due to increased emphasis on quality assurance programs (39,42). Surprisingly, 5 of 11 patients responded objectively to hormone therapy, although each had breast tumors containing only the PR. We found that there was no significant difference in properties of PR appearing in either the presence or absence of ER (44). Thus, if there is a relationship between ER and PR in responsive tumors, expression of ER^-/PR^+ status may be related to the endocrine milieu of the patient. These latter data suggest that PR may be particularly important in the selection of premenopausal patients for endocrine manipulation (45). Clark et al. (46) showed PR was a strong prognostic index. Thus, both receptors may be considered predictive indices of breast cancer patients' response to hormone therapy.

The NSABP initiated a prospectively randomized clinical trial for women with primary operable breast cancer and positive axillary nodes in 1977 (43). 1891 patients were randomized to receive L-phenylalanine mustard and 5-flurouracil (PF) either with or without tamoxifen (T). The median follow-up time was 3 years in an interim report (43). Patients >50 years of age with either 1-3 or >3 positive axillary nodes had a markedly longer disease-free survival on PFT than those receiving PF adjuvant therapy. The effectiveness of PFT (curve with T) was related to tumor levels of steroid receptors (Fig. 2). PF alone is indicated by open squares. Patients >50 years old with both tumor ER and PR levels of >10 fmole displayed the greatest benefit in disease-free survival from PFT. Patients <50 years with tumor ER and PR levels <10 fmole had a poorer survival when given PFT. Those whose tumors demonstrated a high ER and a low PR also had a shorter survival on PFT. The observation of no benefit in younger patients when both receptor levels were high, but a benefit in older patients with receptor-poor tumors, indicates that the difference between the two age groups cannot be explained by the association of age with receptor content under the conditions of this study (43).

Multivariate analyses supported the conclusion that, while nodes and ER exerted strong prognostic influences in both PF and PFT-treated patients, the PR content of tumors was a stronger predictor of the effectiveness of PFT therapy than was ER content. This suggested a heterogeneity in response to PFT therapy that was both age and PR dependent. The findings emphasized the need for accurate quantitative determinations of both the ER and PR content of tumors. The data indicated that T should not be administered with PF to patients under 60 years of age with PR-poor tumors and, finally, they suggested that prolonged administration of tamoxifen may be clinically useful (47).

ENDOMETRIAL CANCER AND HORMONAL RECRUITMENT THERAPY

Progestin administration has been used routinely in the treatment of endometrial carcinoma with a <30% response rate. To improve patient selection, a number of studies have shown that PR content correlates well with response to progestin therapy. A comprehensive study by Creasman et al. (35) showed that ER, PR as well as combined ER/PR status were significant independent prognostic factors, replacing histologic assessment of glandular or nuclear differentiation. Thus, ER and PR content of endometrial cancer permits an improved prediction of prognosis and appears helpful in predicting responses to therapy at the time of a future recurrence. Furthermore, these and other studies (36) provided a basis for examining the use of antiestrogen and progestin therapies in uterine carcinoma.

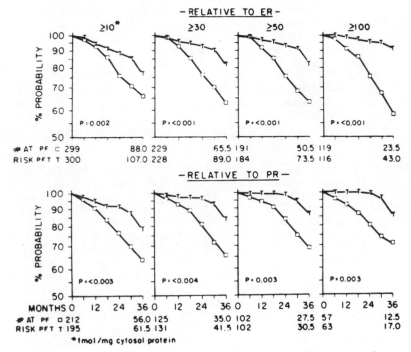

Fig. 2. Disease-free survival of patients 50 years of age or older. Reproduced from reference 43.

A pilot study conducted by Swenerton et al. (48) to assess the efficacy of tamoxifen in advanced endometrial carcinoma demonstrated response in several patients. Furthermore, there was a suggestion that cross-resistance did not occur between progestins and tamoxifen. Such treatment showed remarkably little toxicity which was a particular advantage in this group of patients who are often elderly and contributes to their unsuitability for intensive combination chemotherapy. Finally, Mortel et al. (49) reported that short-term administration of the antiestrogen, tamoxifen, led to increased PR in 11 of 15 endometrial carcinomas including 4 which were initially PR$^-$. The ability of tamoxifen to increase PR, coupled with its cytotoxicity via the antiestrogen mechanism, makes the combination of tamoxifen with a progestational agent a scientifically sound therapeutic approach. Operationally, we have described hormonal recruitment therapy as the use of hormone-related drugs or antihormones to recruit (induce) cells to a therapeutically sensitive state.

Our hypothesis was that sustained or intermittent use of tamoxifen (a) induces PR in tumors, (b) increases the duration of response to progestin therapy by hormonally sensitive tumors, and (c) increases the absolute number of progestin responsive patients by induction of PR in tumors which were initially PR$^-$. The treatment protocol is shown in Figure 3 (36). Thus far, 54 patients have been treated. An example of tamoxifen's influence on ER and PR is shown in Table 2. Note that in addition to the induction of PR in most grade 2 carcinomas, tamoxifen occasionally increased ER to very high levels. As shown in Table 3, tamoxifen increased the incidence of PR from 48% to 80%, indicating this aspect of our hypothesis was correct. As expected, short-term tamoxifen administration decreased ER incidence from 54% to 41% after 5 days of therapy. Since the trial is ongoing, clinical response data are still being collected. Our study suggests tamoxifen improves the candidacy of many patients for progestin treatment who previously would have been given nonhormonal therapies.

POLYMORPHISM OF STEROID HORMONE RECEPTORS

Steroid hormones associate specifically with several proteins in extracts of endocrine target organs. However, the origin and composition of these multiple forms of receptors (termed isoforms) and their biological significance is germane to an understanding of steroid hormone action. We are proponents of the view that many of these are distinct physiologic species of ER in breast tissues (7-10). In contrast, the 8S and 4S isoforms of estrogen receptors identified on sucrose gradients (6,8) may be artifacts from alterations of the "native" species. Presumably, this would occur during homogenization, prolonged incubation, and centrifugation. However, to our knowledge, no one has provided conclusive evidence of the "native" state of the ER in target cells. The functional

Day 1   Initial Biopsy   - ER and PR
    ↓   - Histologic Grade
                           - Begin Tamoxifen
                              (10/mg P.O. B.I.D.)
Day 5   Discontinue Tamoxifen

    ↓

Day 6   Post-Tam Biopsy   - ER and PR
                           - Begin Medroxy-progesterone
                              Acetate (250/mg I$_M$ q week)

Fig. 3.   Combination hormonal therapy in advanced endometrial carcinoma. Adapted from reference 36.

Table 2. Alterations in estrogen and progesterone receptors in histologic grade 2 endometrial carcinoma after tamoxifen.*

Progesterone receptors (fmol/mg cytosol protein)		Estrogen receptors (fmol/mg cytosol protein)	
Biopsy		Biopsy	
Initial biopsy	After tamoxifen	Initial biopsy	After tamoxifen
316	1242	182	7405
UD	15	UD	714
UD	57	8	UD
14	306	14	UD
40	1415	38	19
UD	40	UD	UD
28	138	67	20
63	88	58	4
10	134	UD	UD
137	35	71	27
2293	638	258	114

*Adapted from reference 36.

unit of receptor, however, appears to be a 65 kDa protein molecule consisting of three distinct regions, the N-terminal region of unknown function, the DNA binding region and the C-terminal ligand binding domain (50).

HIGH PERFORMANCE LIQUID CHROMATOGRAPHY

To circumvent the problem of prolonged manipulation of receptor preparations, high performance liquid chromatography was adapted in HPSEC, HPIEC, HPCF and HPHIC modes for rapid separation of isoforms of these receptors (9,10,51). Receptor isoforms are defined as protein components in target cells which exhibit discreet ligand binding affinity and specificity for a single class of steroid hormones (e.g., estrogens) and may be identified and separated based upon characteristics of size, shape, surface ionic charge and hydrophobicity. With respect for the contributions of other investigators who have either developed or applied techniques and instruments for steroid hormone receptor determinations, this paper is largely an account of the Hormone Receptor Laboratory at the University of Louisville.

Table 3. Tamoxifen induction of progestin receptors in endometrial carcinoma.

Treatment	Receptor Presence (>10 fmol/mcp)	
	Progestin	Estrogen
Pre-Tamoxifen	26/54 (48%)	29/54 (54%)
Post-Tamoxifen	43/54 (80%)	22/54 (41%)

The configuration of the Altex (Beckman) HPLC set-up with in-line technology used in our laboratory is shown in Figure 4. Briefly, a two-pump system is used for HPIEC, HPCF and HPHIC with UV detector, pH meter (Pharmacia), conductivity meter (Bio-Rad), and gamma radioactivity detector (Beckman) in-line before fraction collection. All chromatography is performed in a Puffer-Hubbard cold box at 3-4°C to minimize ligand-receptor dissociation and receptor denaturation. HPSEC is conducted isocratically. Pre- and postcolumn derivatization and fluorescence may also be employed with this arrangement.

Safety precautions must be taken when using any human tissue due to the potential biohazard of infectious organisms, such as hepatitis and AIDS. Furthermore, extra care must be emphasized regarding the handling of radioactive material. Finally, common sense measures are exercised in the thorough cleaning of the HPLC apparatus after a day of experimentation due to the corrosive effects of the salts employed and their potential for inducing undesired changes in the receptor protein's characteristics.

Labeling of Receptor Complexes with Radioactive Steroids

All procedures such as the multipoint titration assay, sucrose density gradient centrifugation and HPLC were carried out at 0-4°C. Human

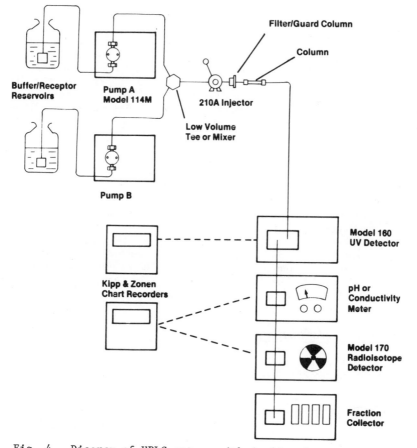

Fig. 4. Diagram of HPLC set-up with in-line instrumentation used to separate and identify steroid receptor isoforms. Reproduced from reference 33.

breast and uterine cancer as well as noncancerous uteri were used as sources of sex hormone receptors. A thorough discussion of buffers and other conditions and methods of preparation related to receptor characterization are given in recent reviews of our investigations (9,10,23, 33,51).

Since most receptors are present in cytosol in very low amounts, their detection depends upon the formation of complex with its specific ligand, the steroid hormone or analog. Cytosols for studies of ER were incubated at 4°C for 4 h with either [^{3}H]estradiol-17β or [16α-^{125}I]-iodoestradiol-17β in the presence (nonspecific binding) or absence (total binding) of a 200-fold molar excess of an unlabeled competitor, such as diethylstilbestrol. For identification of PR, the ligands, [^{3}H]R5020, [^{3}H]ORG-2058 and [^{125}I]iodovinyl-nortestosterone were employed. Specific binding capacity was expressed as femtomoles of steroid bound per milligram of cytosol protein.

High Performance Hydrophobic Interaction Chromatography

High-performance hydrophobic interaction chromatography (HPHIC) of proteins is widely gaining recognition in the growing field of HPLC since the introduction of microparticular rigid supports and the production of recombinant proteins. Among the various modes of HPLC, HPHIC represents the mildest means of separating protein molecules with complete retention of their biological activity (24). HPHIC relies on the interaction of hydrophobic patches present in the protein with the stationary phases which must be exposed. This fact, coupled with recoveries of these biopolymers of almost 100%, indicates HPHIC is a favorable choice of separating such complex molecules. An additional feature which merits mention is that HPHIC, unlike most RPLC procedures may be performed at physiological pH. A representative profile of estrogen receptor isoforms is shown in Figure 5. Note the polymorphism of this receptor. Treatment of receptors with RNase suggests that RNA is not an integral part of receptor and is not the cause of this heterogeneity. We have reported our results on optimizing conditions for HPHIC of steroid receptors performed on a recently developed, polyether bonded stationary phase which is nonionic in nature (33). This appears to be a better support for HPHIC of receptors since these proteins are highly charged molecules which show retention on both ion-exchange and size-exclusion columns (51). We have further shown that incorporation of sodium molybdate in the mobile phase leads to elution of receptor which is less hydrophobic in nature (52). Still two components are observed, one of which (least hydrophobic) appears to be associated with HSP 90 (Dr. David Toft, personal communication). The most hydrophobic species of the receptor (obtained in the absence of molybdate) appears to contact the stationary phase of the column through its DNA binding domain of the receptor and appears a monomeric protein as judged by further analysis on size exclusion columns (53,54).

High Performance Size Exclusion Chromatography (HPSEC)

Most experiments employed TSK2000 SW, TSK3000 SW and TSK4000 SW columns manufactured by Toya Soda (supplied by Altex/Beckman). The TSK3000 SW column quickly separated ER isoforms in cytosol from target organs (Figures 5 C-D and Figure 6). We have separated receptor isoforms in cytosols from human breast carcinomas and uteri as well as from calf uterus, lactating mammary glands of rats and rabbit endometrial carcinoma (17,23). The principal size isoforms in the breast cancer exhibited Stokes radii of 60A and 29-32A similar to those of human uterus. The principal estrogen receptor isoform in lactating mammary gland also gave a Stokes radius of 60A although there was evidence of receptor heterogeneity by HPCF (18). In contrast, the Stokes radius of the estrogen receptor in rabbit endometrial carcinoma was 71A (22). To extend the versatility of the HPSEC columns, we recommend they be used in series with various combinations (e.g., TSK4000 SW, then TSK3000 SW) to accommodate the receptor in question (16,23).

Preparations of monoclonal antibodies of the IgG class interact specifically with the estrogen receptor of various species (55,56). The receptor is not precipitated, but alters the sedimentation behavior of the receptor on sucrose density gradient centrifugation. In particular, the D547 preparation (provided courtesy of Drs. E. V. Jensen and G. L. Greene, University of Chicago) associated with 4S isoforms of the estrogen receptor from human breast cancer, which were extracted, then adjusted to 400 mM KC1. The resulting complex could be detected easily on sucrose density gradients as a large molecular weight species. A similar shift in size was detected on the TSK4000 SW column (10). Interestingly, in addition to the expected high molecular weight complex of antibody and receptor, other complexes of greater size were detected. It was also noted that a portion of the 4S species did not react with D547 monoclonal antibody. Recent

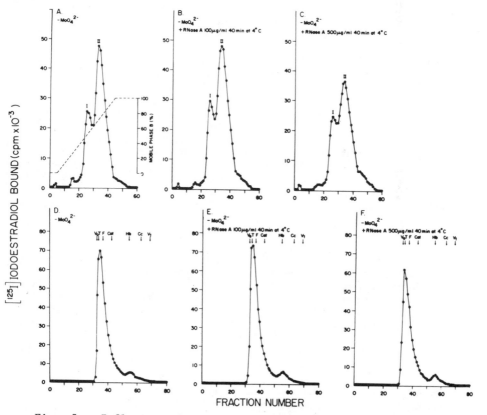

Fig. 5. Influence of RNase A on the size and hydrophobic properties of estrogen receptors from human breast cancer. Cytosol was prepared in P_{10}EDG and labeled with [^{125}I]iodoestradiol. Aliquots were then treated with different concentrations of RNase A as indicated on figure panel. Following removal of free steroid from the cytosol, samples were injected onto either the hydrophobic (A-C) or the size-exclusion columns. Receptor was then eluted with buffers indicated on the figures (D-F). Reproduced from reference 53.

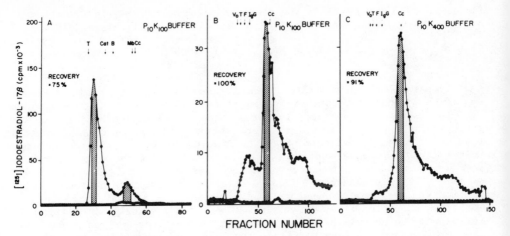

Fig. 6. Separation of estrogen receptor isoforms from human uteri (A) endometrial carcinomas (B, C) by HPSEC. Cytosols were incubated with 2-3 nM [^{125}I]iodoestradiol in the absence (•) or presence (o) of 250-fold excess of diethylstilbestrol. Estrogen receptors were eluted from a TSK3000 SW column with either $P_{10}K_{100}$ EDGK (C) buffer. The HPSEC system was calibrated with a series of marker proteins; thyroglobulin (T), ferritin (F), globulin (IgG) and cytochrome c (Cc). V_0 represents the void volume as determined using blue dextran. Reproduced from reference 27.

research has shown the H222 monoclonal antibody from the Abbott EIA kit reacts with only a portion of the estrogen receptor isoforms using HPIEC (57). From studies in our laboratory (58) and those of others (59-62), we suggest that caution must be observed in using monoclonal antibodies in clinical tests such as the enzyme immunoassay of estrogen receptors, since certain antigenic determinants may be either unrecognized or inaccessible. The demonstration that steroid receptors exhibit polymorphism, predicts a battery of monoclonal antibodies will be necessary to measure estrogen receptors in a clinically valid fashion.

We have also utilized HPSEC to study the size of isoforms of the progestin receptor (63) in human uterus and breast carcinoma. Both 30 cm TSK3000 SW as well as longer 60 cm columns have been employed. On the shorter column, receptor-bound ligand appeared as two peaks, using either [^{3}H]R5020 or [^{3}H]ORG-2058. The primary peak associating with R5020 represented the majority (>70%) of specific binding applied to the column. Recoveries on the 30 cm TSK3000 SW columns were consistently 87 to 93%. Column calibration with marker proteins suggested this component to be a very large species of >80 A.

The HPSEC mode for the analysis of estrogen receptors in human tumor samples represents a clinical application which is rapidly evolving. Quantification is essential since the levels of estrogen receptor have prognostic value in the determination of hormonal responsiveness. Our laboratory (7,8,64) and others (46,65) have proposed that the distribution of receptor isoforms has clinical significance as well. Clearly, if HPSEC analyses provide quantitative and qualitative information on hormone receptors in human tumors, it will find wide application in the clinical laboratory due to its speed. In this regard, we (9,10,26) suggested that an automated system employing high performance ion-exchange chromatography (HPIEC) could be useful in the determination of the profile of receptor

298

isoforms. The relationship of receptor isoform profiles ("fractionated receptors") to ultimate responsiveness has yet to be established (66).

High Performance Ion Exchange Chromatography (HPIEC)

HPIEC is one of the most effective modes for the study of receptor isoforms (19,26). The resolution of isoforms and their high recovery provide an excellent means of characterizing receptors for structure/ function relationships. Briefly, a portion (150-200 µl) of incubate, cleared of unbound ligand, was applied with a chromatograph equipped with anion exchange columns. Each column was equilibrated previously with low ionic strength phosphate buffer. A wash (30 min) of the column with buffer was followed by elution with a linear gradient of potassium phosphate at pH 7.4 which approaches 500 mM at a previously set time after gradient initiation. Subsequently the column was returned to starting conditions. We have compared the use of the SynChropak AX-500 and AX-1000 columns in the HPIEC mode using human uterus and breast cancer, lactating mammary gland of the rat and endometrial carcinoma of the rabbit (19).

A representative separation profile of estrogen receptor isoforms from human breast cancer is shown in Figure 7. A major isoform eluted at 190 mM phosphate while others were observed at 52 to 100 mM phosphate. Isoforms eluting at 100 and 200 mM phosphate have been observed in cytosols from mammary gland of the rat and human uterus (19). The isoforms in the cytosol of endometrial cancer of the rabbit exhibited a 50 mM species and 175 mM component when separated on HPIEC (22).

As shown in Figure 8 D, when the 30A component from normal uterus was separated under similar conditions but within 15 min of its elution from the TSK-3000SW column, a profile similar to that observed with a transfer time of 150 min was recorded. In this case, the predominant species were eluted by the wash buffer and at 50-70 mM phosphate. Similar results were observed when the 30A isoform in cytosol from endometrial carcinoma (Fig. 6 B) was further characterized by HPIEC (Fig. 9 A). The presence of 400 mM KCl in the elution buffer of the size exclusion step also gave predominantly a 30A component (Fig. 6 C) which apparently contained two ionic isoforms as characterized by HPIEC (Fig. 9 B). It was concluded (27) that regardless of the size of the estrogen receptor isoforms (i.e., 30A or 60A), as identified by HPSEC, each of these is composed of at least two subunits with different surface charge properties. The latter was readily characterized by HPIEC with the AX-1000 column.

Studies with the partially purified 60A isoform suggest that a factor(s) which may stabilize its ionic properties has either been removed or changed in concentration. This would alter the equilibrium in such a way that the isoform eluting at 180 mM phosphate would be converted to binding components exhibiting lower negative surface charges. It appears this conversion is not the result of proteolysis since the initial studies indicate that inhibition of trypsin-like proteases which are known to alter the sedimentation properties of estrogen receptors, did not change the ionic properties (67). These data also suggest that consideration of time for the analysis of the higher molecular weight isoform (approximately 60A) is very important in the interpretation of the molecular composition of the estrogen receptor. The results also support the idea that both the 60A and 30A species compared the manual and on-line profiles of 1-10 fmol of total receptor-bound radioactivity from human breast cancer and uterine tissue separated by HPIEC (26). Measurements obtained manually were comparable to the continuous tracings and gave virtually identical profiles. The presence of different ionic isoforms of the receptor in breast and uterine tissues revealed by this rapid format with HPIEC allows the comparison required of clinical studies (Fig. 7).

Chromatofocusing is a technique which separates proteins based upon their surface charge properties using a column which is essentially a weak ion-exchanger (10,18,22). Free steroid or the ligand-labeled cytosols are applied to anion-exchange columns. Protein elution is carried out using

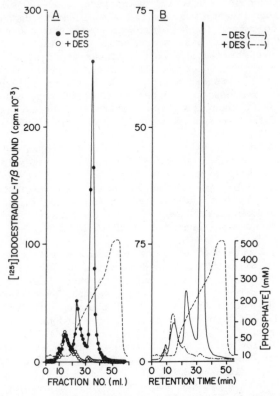

Fig. 7. HPIEC separation of ionic isoforms of estrogen receptors from human breast cancer. Cytosol was labeled for 2 h with 5 nM [^{125}I]iodoestradiol-17β in the presence or absence of a 200-fold excess diethylstilbestrol (DES). Elution of the AX-1000 column was performed on 200 µl of cytosol (7.4 mg/ml) cleared of unbound ligand at 1.0 ml/min using a gradient of potassium phosphate at pH 7.4 (---). A, 1 ml fractions were collected and radioactivity measured manually with a gamma counter; B, radioactivity recorded continuously using an on-line Model 170 radioisotope detector with a conductivity flow cell. Total binding is indicated by o in A and by —— in B, and nonspecific binding is indicated by ● in A by — - — - — in B. Recovery of radioactivity from the column was 97% for the total bound curve determined by counting a 10 µl aliquot before sample injection. Specific binding was 167 fmol receptor/mg cytosol protein determined by multi-point titration analysis. Reproduced from reference 26.

Altex Model 112 pumps and the absorption profile of the eluate is monitored at 280 nm with a spectrophotometer equipped with an in-line flow cell. pH is also measured in-line or manually as shown in Figure 10.

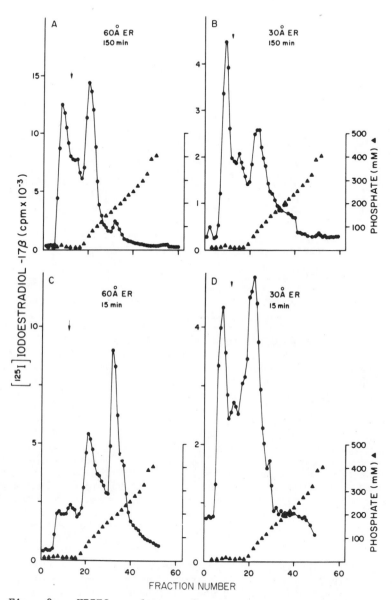

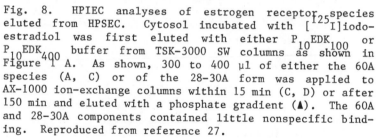

Fig. 8. HPIEC analyses of estrogen receptor species eluted from HPSEC. Cytosol incubated with [^{125}I]iodoestradiol was first eluted with either $P_{10}EDK_{100}$ or $P_{10}EDK_{400}$ buffer from TSK-3000 SW columns as shown in Figure 1 A. As shown, 300 to 400 µl of either the 60A species (A, C) or of the 28–30A form was applied to AX-1000 ion-exchange columns within 15 min (C, D) or after 150 min and eluted with a phosphate gradient (▲). The 60A and 28–30A components contained little nonspecific binding. Reproduced from reference 27.

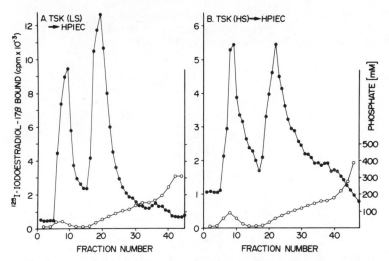

Fig. 9. Representative profile of HPIEC analyses of human uterine estrogen receptor eluted from HPSEC. One to two ml of the 28-30A species from low salt (A) or high salt (B) elution of TSK-3000 SW columns were adjusted to 100 mM KCl and applied to an AX-1000 column and eluted with a phosphate gradient (o). Reproduced from reference 27.

Two different column equilibration and elution programs have been used depending upon the initial buffer conditions of the receptor preparations (18). The columns are first equilibrated to the starting pH (slightly above the desired upper limit) using a common cationic buffer. We have used 25 mM Tris-HCl containing 1 mM dithiothreitol and 20% (v/v) glycerol adjusted to pH 8.1-8.3 at 0°C or a similar phosphate buffer (63). For chromatofocusing molybdate-stabilized receptor components, 10 mM sodium molybdate is included in the column equilibration buffer. Cytosols prepared in homogenization buffer were eluted with a 30:70 mixture of polybuffers 96 and 74 adjusted to between pH 4.0 and 5.0 at 0-4°C. Our first experiments with estrogen receptor indicated that the SynChrom columns formed a stable pH gradient with the polybuffers, and that a number of cytosolic proteins were well resolved within the gradient (18). We were concerned that the initial (i.e., "loading") peak may be composed of unresolved species, namely, that certain proteins would be excluded based upon size and charge properties. However, HPCF of labeled estrogen receptors from human uterus (Fig. 10) showed that isoforms were not eluted in the loading peak but were recovered in the gradient when the AX-500 column was employed. Similar results were observed when estrogen receptors in lactating mammary gland of the rat were separated (19).

HPCF of progestin receptors was accomplished primarily on the AX-500 column as described previously (63). Even in the presence of 10 mM molybdate, the column appeared to strip some labeled-steroid from the receptor. However, a second peak appeared at a pH of 5.6-6.1 which contained specifically bound steroid. The results presented with [3H]R5020 were virtually identical to those observed when [3H]ORG-2058 was used as ligand (63). Thus, based on pH, the progestin receptor isoform focused at a pI value of 5.6-6.1 regardless of the ligand used in contrast to the HPSEC profiles. The origin and significance of progestin receptor polymorphism remains obscure. Although certain components may represent distinct physiological species, proteolytic cleavage may occur with a labile receptor. Dougherty et al. (68) identified two 8S forms of the progesterone receptor from chick oviduct. Interestingly, each form contained a 90,000 molecular

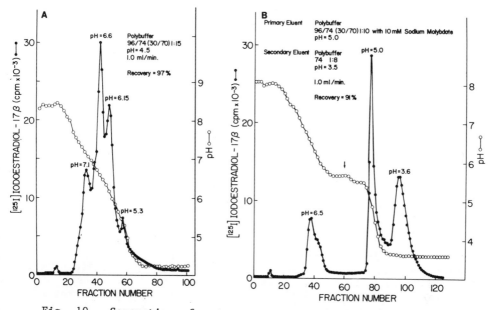

Fig. 10. Separation of estrogen receptor isoforms from human uterus in the presence or absence of molybdate by HPCF. A, cytosol was incubated with [¹²⁵I]iodoestradiol-17β in the presence or absence of excess diethylstilbestrol. Receptor activity (●) was eluted from the AX-500 column with a mixture of polybuffers 96 and 74 adjusted to pH 4.5. B, cytosol was prepared in buffer containing 10 mM molybdate and incubated with [¹²⁵]iodoestradiol-17β as described earlier. The primary eluant was a mixture of polybuffers 96 and 74 containing 10 mM sodium molybdate and adjusted to pH 5.0. The secondary eluant (arrow) was polybuffer 74 (no molybdate) adjusted to pH 3.5. Specific profile (●) showed the presence of acidic isoforms. Reproduced from reference 18.

weight (MW) component which did not associate with progestin and either a 75,000 or 110,000 MW steroid binding species. Various combinations of these components could give rise to considerable size heterogeneity as we (63) and others (69) have observed with receptors from human uterus.

One advantage of HPCF is that stabilizing agents such as sodium molybdate may be included in the buffer systems. Molybdate has several useful properties, including the preservation (stabilization) of larger forms of the receptor and the ability to block receptor activation. Thus, molybdate is a valuable tool in correlating the interrelationships between receptor isoform structure and biologic function.

STRUCTURAL FEATURES OF THE ESTROGEN RECEPTOR

Numerous workers in the field of estrogen receptors favor a model which contains a single type of subunit. Apparently, the dimer is the species most likely to occur at physiologic ionic strength (10). Regardless of the ionic strength of the environment in vitro, it is assumed that no more than four types of components are possible as depicted. These include the meroreceptor (3.5 S) which is presumed to arise due to proteolytic cleavage of higher molecular weight species.

We employed a monoclonal antibody that Greene and co-workers (55) produced against estrogen receptor from the MCF-7 human breast cancer cell line and demonstrated that immunopurified isoforms of the estrogen receptor from extracts of these cells were associated with both protein kinase (Fig. 11) and phospholipid kinase activities (70). Although unexpected, these enzyme activities were easily ascertained in vitro on femotmolar quantities of the receptors by virtue of the fact that the isoform-monoclonal antibody complexes were immobilized on a single polystyrene bead (58). A further novel use was that the receptor could be associated with [^{125}]iodoestradiol-17β and easily measured in a gamma counter by placing the bead coated with labeled receptor into the counting well. The receptor directed an autophosphorylation reaction requiring ATP rather than GTP as the phosphoryl donor (Fig. 11) and was highly dependent on the presence of Mg2+. Only estrogen receptor positive cell lines (MCF-7) exhibited the protein kinase activity; estrogen receptor negative breast cancer cell lines such as the MDA and the T-47D showed minimal or no activity (70).

Several groups have implicated steroid receptor phosphorylation as a possible regulatory mechanism that alters the binding capacity of these molecules (71). Furthermore, many protein-hormone receptors, growth factors, and oncogenic transforming products contain autophosphorylating activities as well as exhibit the ability to phosphorylate exogenous substrates. Exciting observations that two oncogenic products, p68v-ros (72) pp60v-src (73), contained phospholipid kinase activity has brought new insight in the phosphate transfer reaction related to tumorigenesis.

Our evidence that immunopurified estrogen receptor directs autophosphorylating activity and phosphorylates phosphoinositides (70) leads us to postulate a mechanism by which steroid hormone receptors may share similar properties with oncogene products as recently discussed by Sluyser and Mester (74). It should be mentioned, however, that the kinase activity exhibited by estrogen receptor molecules from MCF-7 breast cancer cells is a serine-type kinase (75) in contrast to the tyrosine kinase mode exhibited by most of the oncogenic transforming products (76). Of course, considerable work is needed to establish a relationship between steroid hormone receptors and the synthesis of oncogenic products. However, these results suggest that the steroid binding site of the estrogen receptor represents only a portion of a more complex regulatory molecule.

As discussed above, current reports from our laboratory have demonstrated a Mg2+-dependent protein kinase activity, associated with immunopurified ER from human breast cancer cells (MCF-7) (70). It was shown that receptors eluted by HPIEC retained this kinase activity(75). We investigated whether retention of kinase activity was also possible following HPHIC. Figure 12 A illustrates a typical isoform chromatogram of ER, separated from rat uteri and used for analysis of protein kinase activity associated with ER. These separations resulted in a 5- to 20-fold purification for each isoform, depending upon the relative proportion present. In this experiment, both components were purified approximately 15-fold following a single pass (21). To demonstrate protein kinase activity, fractions from the receptor peaks (No. 22 and No. 28) and two control points at Fractions 12 and 50 were incubated directly with polystyrene beads, linked to D547 monoclonal antibodies against ER (Abbott ER-EIA kit). A separate bead was incubated with nonfractionated receptor in P$_{10}$EDG buffer for each experiment. After an overnight incubation, these antibodies were washed and then one bead was analyzed for ER content by the EIA procedure and the other was used for protein kinase assay with phosvitin as the exogenous substrate. Histones were also used successfully as substrates. Figure 12 B is an autoradiogram demonstrating that only the ER eluted in Fraction 22 immunoprecipitated with monoclonal

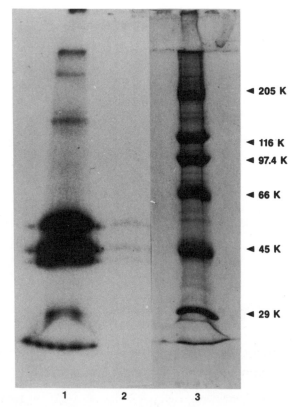

Fig. 11. Nucleotide dependence of estrogen receptor autophosphorylation activity from MCF-7 cells. ER was purified from MCF-7 cytosol using the one-step procedure with immobilized monoclonal antibody. The immunocomplexes were washed extensively with dH_2O and detergent-containing buffer before incubation of bound receptor with either 10 μCi $[y-^{32}P]$-ATP or $[y-^{32}P]$-GTP. Reactions were terminated by removal of the reaction medium and the $[^{32}P]$-labeled polypeptides were solubilized and separated on 7.5% polyacrylamide-SDS gel electrophoresis. The slab gels were dried and autoradiography performed for 16 h at 25°C. Lane 1: MCF-7 MAb receptor complex incubated with $[y-^{32}P]$-ATP as substrate showing the presence of phosphorylated proteins with molecular weights of 57, 47 and 43 kilodaltons. Lane 2: same as lane 1 but $(y-^{32}P]$-GTP was used as substrate. Note absence of phosphorylation activity. Lane 3 shows the corresponding molecular weight standards. Numbers on the right indicate the position of molecular weight standards in kilodaltons. Reproduced from reference 70.

antibody D547, exhibited protein kinase activity. Importantly, no reaction was observed when the monoclonal antibody was allowed to interact with Fraction 12, where most of the proteins were eluted.

Unlike previous studies with human breast cancer cells (70), we have not been able to demonstrate autophosphorylating activity of ER from rat

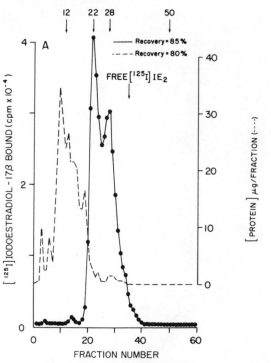

Fig. 12. Protein kinase activity associated with ER isoforms, separated by HPHIC. (A) Rat uterine cytosol was
subjected to chromatography on the CAA-HIC column. (●)
Total cpm/fraction; (---) protein profile, as determined
by the Bradford procedure. For clarity, the nonspecific
binding profile, which was virtually undetectable, is
omitted. (B) Fractions 12, 22, 28, and 50 from the HPHIC-
separated sample (shown in A) were directly incubated with
monoclonal antibody (D547), which was coated on polystyrene beads. A nonfractionated control sample was also
incubated with the monoclonal antibody complex bead.
Following an 18-h incubation and subsequent washing, one
bead was analyzed for ER content (mass) by an EIA procedure and the second bead was tested for protein kinase
activity. The recep- tor content associated with the
monoclonal antibody in fmol/bead was 0 in fraction 12, 1.4
in fraction 22, 2.1 in fraction 28, and 0 in fraction 50.
The control bead contained 7 fmol of receptor from the
unfractionated cytosol in this representative experiment.
Reproduced from reference 21.

uterus. In the present experiments (Fig. 12) both isoforms were purified
to the same extent (approximately 15- to 16-fold) and yet only Isoform I
(Peak I) exhibited protein kinase activity. This exciting finding
suggests that putative regulatory components are associated with these ER
isoforms to a different extent, which may be due to varied affinities.
The protein kinase activity associated with purified Isoform I may even be
an intrinsic property of the receptor molecule. Extensive investigation
is required to resolve this question. Several investigations of other
steroid hormone receptors suggest that phosphorylation/dephosphorylation
reactions play an important role in the activity of these regulatory
proteins (77-80).

Our data using ion-exchange chromatography, isoelectric focusing, and more recently, high performance liquid chromatography (8-10,13,23), are more consistent with the model of protein polymorphism (10). In this model, the molecular heterogeneity of the estrogen receptor arises due to the various possible combinations of two unlike subunits. It is unclear presently which are the so-called "native" forms and which are proteolytic fragments retaining the ligand-binding domain in HPLC profiles of these receptors. These differences in separation characteristics may be due to a variety of physiologic reasons including phosphorylation, protein-protein interaction such as subunit association-dissociation and possible protein-nucleic acid association. We have preliminary evidence that a high molecular weight component ($\geq$400,000 daltons) exists in cytosol from studies with molybdate using [^{125}I]iodoestradiol-17β and HPLC. This binding protein may be a precursor of the functional estrogen receptor. The high affinity of estrogen receptors (ER) for the monoclonal antibody D547 Spγ and for the ligand, diethylstilbestrol (DES) suggested that they may prove useful as an efficient absorbant for the purification of ER.

Affinity resins were synthesized using epoxy-buffer. After associa-tion with the affinity column, proteins were eluted with 50 mM borate buffer, pH 11.5 (with MAb-agarose) and SDS-PAGE sample buffer (with DES-agarose). After elution, proteins were visualized on SDS-PAGE by silver stain and receptor related peptides by Western blotting employing the MAb D547 Spγ. Two estrogen receptor related proteins (MW = 50,000 and 65,000) were observed after immunoaffinity chromatography (81). The ratio of the immunoblot intensities showed considerable variation from prepara-tion to preparation. When DES-agarose was employed, a much improved separation was attained in less time (1.5 vs. 30 h for immunoaffinity separation). One major ER-related protein was observed (MW = 65,000). These results suggest that the existence of the 50 kDa ER protein may be a preparational artifact. In spite of the variability of immunoaffinity preparations, stabilization of the 65 kDa protein using appropriate protease inhibitors and the fast DES-agarose affinity separation, suggest this is the major size isoform. This is also predicted based upon the sequence of the cloned gene (50). Affinity eluant from ^{32}P-labeled uterine proteins applied to the DES-affinity column displayed a 65 kDa ^{32}P-labeled protein after SDS-PAGE electrophoresis (81). The significance of this observation is being evaluated, since a variety of receptor components have been separated based on size, ionic charge, and hydropho-bicity as described previously by our laboratory. It appears that recep-tor polymorphism arises in part from posttranslational modification such as phosphorylation and from association with nonreceptor components such as the heat shock proteins or protein kinases.

Our current research is directed toward an understanding of the interrelationships of the various molecular species or isoforms of steroid hormone receptors and their role in target cell response. HPLC and [^{125}I]iodoestradiol-17β provide the means to explore these receptor proteins at a molecular level which was not possible five years ago. Although the biological significance of receptor polymorphism is not well understood currently, there are important physiological implications which include the utility of receptor isoform profiles as new markers of endocrine responsive tissues in the clinical setting.

ACKNOWLEDGMENTS

Studies from the authors' laboratory have been supported in part by USPHS grants CA-19657, CA-34211, CA-32102, CA-25224, CA-42154 and CA-31946 from the National Cancer Institute and by grants from the American Cancer Society (PDT-210 and BC-514B) and Phi Beta Psi Sorority. The important contributions of numerous co-workers during the past decade are acknowledged, particularly those of Drs. R. D. Wiehle, G. E. Hofmann, A. Fuchs, M. Lonsdorfer, T. W. Hutchens, N. A. Shahabi, A. van der Walt, D. M. Boyle, A. Baldi, D. W. Brandt, L. Myatt, W. Mujaji, N. Sato, Y. J. He, C. Lee, and S. S. Jung. The authors also express their deepest appreciation to Mitzie Wittliff for assistance with the clinical and reference laboratory studies, and to Ms. Linda K. Sanders for her assistance in the preparation of this typescript.

REFERENCES

1. Gorski J, Toft D, Shyamala G, Smith D, Notides A. Hormone receptors: studies on the interaction of estrogen with the uterus. Recent Prog Horm Res 1968; 24:45-80.

2. Jensen EV, Suzuku T, Kawashima T, Stumpf WE, Jungblut PW, DeSombre ER. A two-step mechanism for the interaction of estradiol with rat uterus. Proc Natl Acad Sci USA 1968; 59:632-9.

3. King WJ, Greene GL. Monoclonal antibodies localize oestrogen receptor in the nuclei of target cells. Nature 1984; 307:745-7.

4. Welshons WV, Lieberman ME, Gorski J. Nuclear localization of unoccupied oestrogen receptors. Nature 1984; 307:747-9.

5. Wittliff JL, Hilf R, Brooks WF Jr, Savlov ED, Hall TC, Orlando RA. Specific estrogen-binding capacity of the cytoplasmic receptor in normal and neoplastic tissues of humans. Cancer Res 1972; 32:1983-92.

6. Wittliff JL. Specific receptor of the steroid hormones in breast cancer. Semin Oncol 1974; 1:109-18.

7. Wittliff JL, Lewko WM, Park DC, Kute TE, Baker DT Jr, Kane LN. Steroid binding proteins of mammary tissues and their clinical significance in breast cancer. In: McGuire WL, ed. Hormones, receptors, and breast cancer. New York: Raven Press, 1978:325-59.

8. Wittliff JL. Steroid hormone receptors in breast cancer. Cancer 1984; 53:630-43.

9. Wittliff JL. Separation and characterization of isoforms of steroid hormone receptors using high-performance liquid chromatography. In: Moudgil VK, ed. Molecular mechanisms of steroid hormone action. Berlin: Walter de Gruyter and Company, 1985:791-813.

10. Wittliff JL. HPLC steroid-hormone receptors. LC-GC Magazine of Liquid and Gas Chromatography, Aster Publishing Co, 1986; 4(11):1092-106.

11. Wittliff JL, Beatty BW, Savlov ED, Patterson WB, Cooper RA Jr. Estrogen receptors and hormone dependency in human breast cancer. In: St Arneault A, Band, Israel L, eds. Recent results in cancer research; vol 57. Berlin: Springer-Verlag, 1976:59-77.

12. Kute TE, Heidemann P, Wittliff JL. Molecular heterogeneity of cytosolic forms of estrogen receptors from human breast tumors. Cancer Res 1978; 38:4307-13.

13. Wittliff JL, Feldhoff PA, Fuchs A, Wiehle RD. Polymorphism of estrogen receptors in human breast cancer. In: Soto R, DeNicola AF, Blaquier JA, eds. Physiopathology of endocrine diseases and mechanisms of hormone action. New York: Alan R Liss, Inc., 1981:375-96.

14. Schrader WT, Kuhn RW, O'Malley BW. Progesterone binding components of chick oviduct. XIII. Receptor B subunit protein purified to apparent homogeneity from laying hen oviducts. J Biol Chem 1977; 252:299-307.

15. Schrader WT, Birnbaumer ME, Hughes MR, Weigel NL, Grody WW, O'Malley BW. Studies on the structure and function of the chicken progesterone receptor. Recent Prog Horm Res 1981; 37:583-633.

16. Cidlowski JA, DeLorenzo TM, Susek RE. Nuclear binding and biological activity of dexamethasone mesylate in human cells. 7th Intl Congr Endocr Abs 1984:277.

17. Wiehle RD, Hofmann GE, Fuchs A, Wittliff JL. High performance size exclusion chromatography as a rapid method for the separation of steroid hormone receptors. J Chromatogr 1984; 307:39–51.
18. Hutchens TW, Wiehle RD, Shahabi NA, Wittliff JL. Rapid analysis of estrogen receptor heterogeneity by chromatofocusing with high performance liquid chromatography. J Chromatogr 1983; 266:115–28.
19. Wiehle RD, Wittliff JL. Isoforms of estrogen receptors by high performance ion exchange chromatography. J Chromatogr 1984; 297: 313–26.
20. Hyder SM, Wiehle RD, Brandt DW, Wittliff JL. High-performance hydrophobic interaction chromatography of steroid hormone receptors. J Chromatogr 1985; 327:237–46.
21. Hyder SM, Sato N, Wittliff JL. Characterization of estrogen receptors and associated protein kinase activity by high-performance hydrophobic-interaction chromatography. J Chromatogr 1987; 397:251–67.
22. Shahabi NS, Hutchens TW, Wittliff JL, Halmo SD, Kirk ME, Nisker JA. Physiocochemical characterization of estrogen receptors from a rabbit endometrial carcinoma model. In: Raynaud JP, Bresciani F, King RJB, Lippman ME, eds. Progress in cancer research and therapy. New York: Raven Press, 1984:63–71.
23. Wittliff JL, Wiehle RD. Analytical methods for steroid hormone receptors and their quality assurance. In: Hollander VP, ed. Hormonally responsive tumors. New York: Academic Press, Inc., 1985:383–428.
24. Hyder SM, Wittliff JL. High-performance hydrophobic interaction chromatography of a labile regulatory protein: the estrogen receptor. BioChromatography 1987; 2(3):121–30.
25. Madhock TC, Leung BS. Characterization of uterine estrogen receptors by size-exclusion and ion-exchange high-performance liquid chromatography. Biochem Biophys Res Commun 1983; 115:988–94.
26. Boyle DM, Wiehle RD, Shahabi NA, Wittliff JL. A rapid high-resolution procedure for assessment of estrogen receptor heterogeneity in clinical samples. J Chromatogr 1985, 327:369–76.
27. Shahabi NA, Hyder SM, Wiehle RD, Wittliff JL. HPLC analysis of estrogen receptor by a multidimensional approach. J Steroid Biochem 1986; 24:1151–7.
28. Gooding KM. High-performance liquid chromatography of proteins—a current look at the state of the techniques. BioChromatography 1986; 1:34.
29. Kato Y, Kitamura T, Hashimoto T. New resin-based hydrophilic support for high-performance hydrophobic interaction chromatography. J Chromatogr 1986; 360: 260–5.
30. Gooding DL, Schmuck MN, Gooding KM. Analysis of proteins with new, mildly hydrophobic high-performance liquid chromatography. J Chromatogr 1984; 296:107–14.
31. Fausnaugh JL, Pfannkoch E, Gupta S, Regnier FE. High-performance hydrophobic interaction chromatography of proteins. Anal Biochem 1984; 137:464–72.
32. Hyder SM, Wittliff JL. High-performance hydrophobic-interaction chromatography. In: Ausubel F, Brent R, Kingston R, Moore D, Smith JA. Current protocols in molecular biology. Greene Publishing Associates, 1987:10.15.1–8.
33. Wittliff JL, Shahabi NA, Hyder SM, van der Walt A, Myatt L, Boyle D, He YJ. High-performance liquid chromatography as a means of characterizing isoforms of steroid hormone receptor proteins. In: L'Italien J, ed. Modern methods in protein chemistry. New York: Plenum Press (in press).
34. Horwitz KG, McGuire WL, Pearson OH, Segaloff A. Predicting response to endocrine therapy in human breast cancer: a hypothesis. Science 1975; 189:726–7.

35. Creasman WT, et al. Influence of cytoplasmic steroid receptor content on prognosis of early stage endometrial carcinoma. Am J Obstet Gynecol 1984; 151:922-32.

36. Carlson JA, Allegra JC, Day TG Jr, Wittliff JL. Tamoxifen and endometrial carcinoma alterations in estrogen and progesterone receptors in untreated patients and combination hormonal therapy in advanced neoplasia. Am J Obstet Gynecol 1984;149:149-54.

37. van der Walt LA, Sanfilippo JS, Siegel JE, Wittliff JL. Estrogen and progestin receptors in human uterus: reference ranges of clinical conditions. Clin Physiol Biochem 1986; 4:217-28.

38. Sarfaty GA, Nash AR, Keighty DD, eds. Estrogen receptor assays in breast cancer: laboratory discrepancies and quality assurance. New York: Masson Publishing USA, Inc., 1981.

39. Wittliff JL, Durant JR, Fisher B. Methods of steroid receptor analyses and their quality control in the clinical laboratory. In: Soto R, DeNicola AF, Blaquier JA, eds. Physiopathology of endocrine diseases and mechanisms of hormone action. New York: Alan R Liss, Inc., 1981:397-411.

40. McGuire WL, Carbone PO, Vollmer EP, eds. Estrogen receptors in human breast cancer. New York: Raven Press, 1975.

41. Anonymous. Proceedings of the NIH consensus development conference on steroid receptors in breast cancer. Cancer 1980; 46(12):2759-963.

42. Wittliff TH, Isenhour JL, Ross DE, Hogancamp WE, Wittliff JL. Quality assurance programs for predictive tests used in cooperative clinical trials of breast and endometrial cancer. Proc 15th Intl Congr Chemotherapy, Landsberg, W Germany: Ecomed Verlagsgesellschaft mbH (in press).

43. Fisher B, Redmond C, Brown A, et al. Influence of tumor estrogen and progesterone receptor levels on the response to tamoxifen and chemotherapy in primary breast cancer. J Clin Oncol 1983; 1:227-41.

44. Hyder SM, Kohrs FP, Wittliff JL. Progestin receptors from tissues either exhibiting or lacking estrogen response mechanisms. J Chromatogr 1987; 397:269-78.

45. Bland KL, Fuchs A, Wittliff JL. Menopausal status as a factor in the distribution of estrogen and progestin receptors in breast cancer. Surgical Forum 1981; 32:410-2.

46. Clark GM, McGuire WL, Hubay CA, Pearson OH, Marshall JS. Progesterone receptors as a prognostic factor in stage II breast cancer. N Engl J Med 1983; 309:1343-7.

47. Fisher B, Brown A, Wolmark N, et al. Prolonging tamoxifen therapy for primary breast cancer. Ann Intern Med 1987; 106(5):649-54.

48. Swenerton KD, Shaw D, et al. Treatment of advanced endometrial carcinoma with tamoxifen. N Engl J Med 1979; 301: 105-9.

49. Mortel R, Levy C, Wolff JP, Nicolas JC, Robel P, Baulieu EE. Female sex steroid receptors in postmenopausal endometrial carcinoma and biochemical response to an antiestrogen. Cancer Res 1981; 41:1140.

50. Greene S, Walter P, Kumar V, Krust A, Burnest JM, Argos P, Chambon P. Human oestrogen receptor cDNA: sequence expression and homology to v-erb A. Nature 1986; 320:134.

51. Wittliff JL, Wiehle RD, Shahabi NA, van der Walt LA, Hyder SM. HPLC as a means of characterizing the polymorphism of steroid hormone receptors. In: Venter JC, Harrison LC, series eds; Kerlavage A, vol ed. Receptor biochemistry and methodology (in press).

52. Hyder SM, Sato N, Hogancamp WE, Wittliff JL. High-performance hydrophobic interaction chromatography of estrogen receptor and an ATP/MG2+ dependent protein kinases(s): detection of two molecular forms of ER in the presence and absence of sodium molybdate. J Steroid Biochem (in press).

53. Hyder SM, Wittliff JL. High performance hydrophobic interaction chromatography as a means of identifying estrogen receptors expres-

sing different binding domains. J Chromatogr (in press).

54. Hyder SM, Wittliff JL. Molecular organization of estrogen receptor (ER) from human breast cancer as determined by high-performance hydrophobic interaction chromatography (HPHIC) [Abstract]. 70th Endocr Soc Meeting (submitted).

55. Greene GL, Fitche FW, Jensen EV. Monoclonal antibodies to estrophilin: probes for the study of estrogen receptors. Proc Natl Acad Sci USA 1980; 77:157-61.

56. Greene GL, Sobel NB, King WJ, Jensen EV. Immunochemical studies of estrogen receptors. J Steroid Biochem 1984; 20:51-6.

57. Brandt DW, Wittliff JL. Assessment of estrogen receptor monoclonal antibody interaction by HPLC. J Chromatogr 1987; 397:287-97.

58. Sato N, Hyder SM, Chang L, Thais A, Wittliff JL. Interaction of estrogen receptor isoforms with immobilized monoclonal antibodies. J Chromatogr 1986; 359:475-87

59. Mirecki DM, Jordan VC. Steroid hormone receptors and human breast cancer. Lab Med 1985; 16(5):287-94.

60. Nakao M, Sato B, Koga M, et al. Identification of immunoassayable estrogen receptor lacing hormone binding ability in tamoxifen-treated rat uterus. Biochem Biophys Res Commun 1985; 132:336-42.

61. Raam S, Vrabel DM. Evaluation of an enzyme immunoassay kit for estrogen receptor measurements. Clin Chem 1986; 32:1496-502.

62. Anonymous. Collective papers from symposium on estrogen receptor determination with monoclonal antibodies. Cancer Res 1986; 46 (suppl):4231S-313S.

63. van der Walt LA, Wittliff JL. Assessment of progestin receptor polymorphism by various synthetic ligands using HPLC. J Steroid Biochem 1986; 24:377-82.

64. Wittliff JL, Savlov ED. Estrogen-binding capacity of cytoplasmic forms of the estrogen receptor in human breast cancer. In: McGuire WL, Carbone PO, Vollmer EP, eds. Estrogen receptors in human breast cancer. New York: Raven Press, 1975:73-91.

65. McCarty KS Jr, Cox C, Silva JS, et al. Comparison of sex steroid receptor analyses and carcinoembryonic antigen with clinical response to hormone therapy. Cancer 1980; 46:2846-50.

66. Wittliff JL. Clinical analyses of steroid hormone receptors. In: Pesce P, Kaplan L, eds. Clinical chemistry—methods. New York: CV Mosby Publishers, Inc., 1987:767-95.

67. Hyder SM, Wiehle RD, Wittliff JL. Alterations in estrogen receptor isoforms in the mammary gland and uterus of the rat during differentiation. Comp Biochem Physiol (in press).

68. Dougherty JJ, Puri RK, Toft DO. Polypeptide components of two chick oviduct progesterone receptor. J Biol Chem 1984; 259:8004-16.

69. Heubner A, Manzy B, Grill H. High performance and ion-exchange chromatography and chromatofocusing of the human uterine progesterone receptor: its application to the identification of 21-[^{3}H]dehydro ORG-2058 labeled receptor. J Chromatogr 1984; 297:301-11.

70. Baldi A, Boyle DM, Wittliff JL. Estrogen receptor is associated with protein and phospholipid kinase activities. Biochem Biophys Res Commun 1986; 135:597-606.

71. Auricchio F, Migliaccio A, Castoria G. Dephosphorylation of oestradiol nuclear receptor in vitro. Biochem J 1981; 198:699.

72. Macara IG, Marinetti GV, Balduzzi PC. Transforming protein of avian sarcoma virus UR2 is associated with phosphatidylinositol kinase activity: possible role in tumorigenesis. Proc Natl Acad Sci 1984; 81:2728-32.

73. Sugimoto Y, Whitman M, Cantly LC, Erikson RL. Evidence that the Rous sarcoma virus transforming gene product phosphorylates phosphatidylinositol and Diacylglycerol. Proc Natl Acad Sci 1984; 81:2117-21.

74. Sluysser M, Mester J. Oncogenes homologous to steroid receptors? Nature 1985; 315:546.

75. Baldi A, Boyle DM, Wittliff JL. Unpublished data.
76. Hunter T, Cooper, JA. Protein-tyrosine kinases. Ann Rev Biochem 1985; 54:897
77. Weigel NL, Tash JS, Means AR, Schrader WT, O'Malley BW. Phosphorylation of hen progesterone receptor by cAMP dependent protein kinase. Biochem Biophys Res Commun 1981; 102:513-9.
78. Dougherty JJ, Puri RK, Toft DO. Phosphorylation in vivo of chicken oviduct progesterone receptor. J Biol Chem 1982; 257:14226-30.
79. Housley PR, Pratt WB. Direct demonstration of glucocorticoid receptor phosphorylation by intact L-cells. J Biol Chem 1983; 258:4630-5.
80. Singh WB, Moudgil VK. Protein kinase activity of purified rat liver glucocorticoid receptor. Biochem Biophys Res Commun 1984; 125:1067-73.
81. Brandt DW, Wittliff JL. Characterization of estrogen receptor proteins from rat uterus using immunoaffinity and ligand affinity chromatography. Protein Soc Abs 1987:52.

22

THE ROLE OF THE RAS ONCOGENE IN HUMAN MAMMARY CANCER

Edward P. Gelmann, Connie Agnor, and Marc E. Lippman

Medical Breast Cancer Section
National Cancer Institute
Bethesda, MD 20892

INTRODUCTION

The cellular homologues, termed proto-oncogenes, of transforming genes transduced or activated by transforming retroviruses have been implicated in the etiology of a number of human cancers. Several specific mechanisms have been proposed in which proto-oncogenes cause cellular transformation. These mechanisms include point mutation (1-3), gene truncation (4), transcriptional activation (5), gene rearrangement (6,7), and gene amplification (8-10). More than 20 proto-oncogenes have been identified and fall into five general categories: (1) growth factors (e.g., sis [11] and perhaps int-2 [12]); (2) growth factor and hormone receptors (e.g., erbB [13], fms [14], and erbA [15]); (3) intracellular tyrosine (e.g., src [16]) and serine (e.g., mos [17]) kinases; (4) nuclear-associated oncogenes (e.g., fos [18], myc [19], and myb [20]); and, (5) G-protein-like molecules (e.g., ras [21]).

This discussion will focus on the ras gene family and, in particular, its putative role in the etiology of human breast cancer. First we will review the current understanding of ras gene structure and function. Next we will discuss the evidence collected from tumor and patient material which has suggested an association between ras genes and breast cancer. Lastly, we will review our own and others' work with experimental model systems for breast cancer tumorigenesis and the role ras plays in these tumorigenesis models.

RAS GENES: A REVIEW

Members of the ras Gene Family

There are at least 4 distinct ras genes in the human genome. These code for proteins whose amino-termini and specific internal regions are highly conserved among the group, and whose carboxy-terminal ends are more variable. The 4 well-characterized human genes are ras^H on chromosome 11 (22,23), ras^K on chromosome 12 (22,23), ras^N on chromosome 1 (24), and ras^R on chromosome 19 (25). The ras genes have similar exon structures, suggesting that they arose from the same ancestral precursor.

RAS genes are present throughout evolution as evidenced in yeast (26-28) and Dictyostelium discoidium (29). The structure of the yeast RAS genes also show preservation of amino-terminal homology with other members of the $\underline{ras}$ gene family and divergence at the extreme carboxy-terminal end (30). Yeast has 2 genes, $\underline{RAS1}$ and $\underline{RAS2}$, both of which apparently play the same role in the activation of yeast adenylate cyclase (31,32). Either gene may be deleted from yeast without any apparent consequences to the organism. It appears that the deletion of both $\underline{RAS}$ genes is a lethal maneuver. However, the human $\underline{ras}^H$ proto-oncogene can complement a yeast which has had both $\underline{RAS}$ alleles deleted (33,34). Despite the structural conservation of $\underline{ras}$, its function has evolved somewhat since $\underline{ras}$ p21 in higher organisms does not interact directly with adenylate cyclase (35).

Structure and Activity of the ras p21 Protein

Detailed studies of the structure-activity relationships of various peptide domains of the $\underline{ras}$ p21 protein have been done using the $\underline{ras}^H$ gene. We will confine the following discussion to data obtained with $\underline{ras}^H$ unless stated otherwise. It should be borne in mind that many of the conclusions from experiments done with $\underline{ras}^H$ can be extended to $\underline{ras}^K$ and to $\underline{ras}^N$ based on their close structural homology. Much less is known about $\underline{ras}^N$, which has been characterized only recently.

The $\underline{ras}$ p21 is a 189 amino-acid, 21,000 d protein which binds GTP. The protein is made as a precursor, undergoes posttranslational modification (36), and in its mature form is palmitylated and bound to the inner surface of the plasma membrane (37,38). All $\underline{ras}$ p21 proteins have a cysteine residue at position 186 (Cys^{186}) which is essential for both membrane association and biological activity (39). A phosphoryl binding region, which is characteristic of many nucleotide binding proteins, is located at residues 10-16 of the $\underline{ras}$ protein (40). Within this domain is the Gly^{12} which is the most frequent substitution site for transforming mutations of $\underline{ras}$ genes. The substitution of any amino acid, except proline, will serve to activate the transforming capability of $\underline{ras}$ p21 (41).

Amino acids 116-119 define the region which determines guanine specificity (42). Mutations at Asn^{116} affect GTP binding and hydrolysis. Some of these mutations also affect the transforming ability of $\underline{ras}$ p21, but other Asn^{116} mutations are not transforming, even though GTP hydrolysis ia markedly diminished (43).

It has been proposed that the region 27-42 is the region where the $\underline{ras}$ protein interacts with its target (44,45). This target molecule is, as yet, unknown. The 27-42 region is conserved among $\underline{ras}$ proteins from higher organisms, but not well conserved in yeast and Dictyostelium discoidium. Since $\underline{ras}$ p21 function differs between yeast, where $\underline{RAS}$ p21 activates adenylate cyclase, and higher organisms, where $\underline{ras}$ p21 does not directly interact with adenylate cyclase, it has been suggested by D. Lowy that the 27-42 region may be responsible for this difference in function. Mutations in this region can affect the transforming capability of a v-$\underline{ras}^H$ gene (D. Lowy, personal communication).

V-$\underline{ras}^K$, the transforming gene of the Kirsten murine sarcoma virus, v-$\underline{ras}^H$ the transforming gene of the Harvey murine sarcoma virus, and many naturally occurring human tumors have been found to contain $\underline{ras}$ genes with mutations substituting for amino acids Gly^{12} or Gln^{61} (1-3, 46-48). These mutations markedly enhance the activity of $\underline{ras}$ genes when assayed by in vitro transformation. A limited number of other mutations may also confer transforming capacity to normal $\underline{ras}$ genes (49). It was first believed that transformation-activating mutations also caused a reduction in the ability of the mutant $\underline{ras}$ p21 to hydrolyze GTP (50-53). However, some $\underline{ras}$ gene mutations enhance transforming activity despite the maintenance of normal GTP hydrolysis activity. G. Cooper's group has suggested that the rate of GDP-GTP exchange from ras p21 binding is related to the ras p21 transforming activity in those mutant proteins which have normal GTPase activity (personal communication). McCormick and co-workers have found that nucleotide hydrolysis in Xenopus oocytes or in the presence of oocyte extracts does correlate with transforming capacity. This result has led them to hypothesize that the transforming mutations affect interactions of ras p21 with cellular factors which influence the rate of GTP hydrolysis by ras p21 (F. McCormick et al., personal communication). There is a consensus, however, that ras p21 is able to interact with its target only when bound with GTP. Whatever mechanism stabilizes that binding may enhance transformation.

RAS STRUCTURE AND EXPRESSION IN HUMAN BREAST CANCER

Activated ras oncogenes have been detected in a number of human tumors as assayed by the transformation of NIH/3T3 cells, such that they lose contact inhibition and can form tumors in nude mice. Ras activation may be achieved by point mutation or by enhanced gene expression (54). Point mutations in ras genes have been detected in a wide variety of human cancers. Breast cancer has been underrepresented on this list. No breast carcinoma has been found to have a point mutation of the ras^H proto-oncogene. A cell line from a carcinosarcoma, HS578T, contains an Asp^{12} mutation (55).

Although ras^K mutations in breast cancer have not been reported in the literature to date, this will probably change with the use of oligonu-cleotide-specific probes to detect ras^K mutations. The ras^K proto-oncogene extends over 40 kb and as a result is inefficiently integrated intact in gene transfer experiments (56). Oligonucleotide-specific probes can distinguish between normal and mutated regions of the ras^K gene by Southern analysis, obviating the need for a successful gene transfer of the intact ras^K gene. Mutated ras^N genes have not been identified in breast cancer.

High levels of ras proto-oncogene expression also can transform NIH/3T3 cells and cause them to become tumorigenic, both to an albeit lesser degree than with the mutated ras genes (54). In the face of largely negative data for ras mutations in breast cancer, attention has been focused on the levels of expression of ras p21 in tumor specimens and cultured cells.

ras p21 Expression in Breast Cancer Tissues and Cell Lines

Since inappropriate expression of the ras gene could be important for the malignant phenotype, Spandidos and Agnantis examined breast tumor tissue and adjacent normal tissue for the expression of the c-ras^H gene (57). In 12/12 tumors there was an apparent four- to fifteenfold increase in c-ras^H mRNA compared with adjacent normal tissue as determined by dot blot analysis. For comparison, the expression of c-sis was also examined and found not to differ between the tumor and normal tissues. Northern blot analysis of a number of RNA samples in this series did not dem-onstrate the differences as clearly as the dot blot data. A follow-up study by the same group sought to correlate the amount of c-ras^H gene expression with clinical parameters, but the paper lacked rigorous statis-tical analysis to support the contention that elevated c-ras expression correlated with more advanced histologic grades (58).

Another group examined the expression of the ras p21 protein in breast cancer tissues, benign breast tumors, and normal mammary gland

(59). p21 levels were determined by Western blotting analysis to be elevated in 7/7 hormone-responsive breast cancer specimens and in 5/6 hormone-independent tumors. Normal breast tissue and 3 fibroadenomas had very low or undetectable levels of p21. Using a photoaffinity label, the authors showed that the elevated levels of p21 were accompanied by a high GTPase activity. Ras p21 expression was also examined in paraffin-embedded sections of benign and malignant breast tissue by immunohisto-chemical staining with monoclonal antibodies prepared against p21 peptides (60). The antibodies clearly identified malignant mammary cells in 19 of 30 samples, but did not show binding to most of the benign tissues tested, of which only 3 of 21 were positive.

In a more recent study, high levels of expression of _ras_ p21 were detected using protein blotting and immunostaining in a variety of fresh human tumor specimens, including gastrointestinal, ovarian, lung, liver, kidney, lymph node, as well as breast (61). The antibodies used in these experiments had been raised against peptides, two of which were designed to share homology with ras^{K} and ras^{N} and one of which was specific for ras^{H}. Eight of 10 breast cancer samples reacted with one or the other cross-reactive anti-p21 sera, but none reacted with the specific anti-p21 ras^{H} serum. The conclusion that breast tissues express p21 species different from ras^{H} is a novel finding. Specific data to the contrary were obtained in a Northern blot analysis of mRNA from 22 invasive ductal carcinomas among which 16 expressed c-ras^{H}, but c-ras^{K} and ras^{N} were expressed at low levels or not at all (62). There is no explanation for the discrepancy between this report and other published data.

A more comprehensive study of _ras_ p21 expression in mammary tissues reinforced many of the earlier presumptions about the role of normal _ras_ genes in breast neoplasia (63). In agreement with other reports, _ras_ p21 expression was found by immunohistochemistry to be elevated in invasive mammary carcinoma. In hyperplastic lesions, p21 expression was lower than in malignant lesions. p21 expression in mammary cancers was heterogeneous among primary and neoplastic lesions. Although there was a trend toward higher expression in postmenopausal patients than in premenopausal patients, there was no correlation of p21 expression with estrogen receptor status. Among 18 patients with hyperplastic lesions who had been followed for up to 15 years, p21 expression tended to decrease slightly over time. Of the 18 mammary hyperplasia patients, the 5 who developed carcinoma had significantly higher levels of p21 expression at the time of first biopsy than the 13 patients who did not develop carcinoma. The authors concluded that p21 expression may contribute to the establishment of cancer, but probably was not essential for its maintenance.

Structure of the ras Gene in Human Breast Cancer

Lidereau and co-workers identified common and rare c-ras^{H} alleles by means of restriction fragment length polymorphism (RFLP) analysis of Southern blots with human tumor DNA (64). Four common and 16 rare alleles were identified in the study population which included breast cancer patients and normal controls. The distribution of common and rare alleles differed significantly between the groups of normal controls and breast cancer patients. Common RFLPs represented 91% of the normals' ras^{H} alleles and 59% of the breast cancer patients' ras^{H} alleles. Among the 104 breast cancer patients in this survey, the frequency of having two of the common alleles was markedly diminished.

The state of the c-ras^{H} gene in breast cancers has also been examined with respect to genomic structure and allelic exclusion. Southern anal-ysis of DNA from 104 breast cancer samples failed to disclose any in-stances of rearrangement or amplification of c-ras^{H} (62). However, the

$c-ras^H$ gene has been shown to have frequent BamHI restriction fragment length polymorphisms (RFLP). Among 51 patients who were heterozygous for these polymorphic sites, 14 exhibited allelic exclusion of one of the two ras alleles in the tumor tissue. Loss of an allele did not alter p21 expression. Although allelic exclusion did correlate significantly with advanced histologic grade, lack of hormone receptors, and subsequent occurrence of distant metastases, such a correlation in the face of negative protein expression data may reflect general chromosomal instability which may coincide with a more undifferentiated tumor.

There is very little data on the roles of other members of the ras family of oncogenes in human breast cancer. One cell line, MCF-7, has been found to have an amplified ras^N gene (65). The extent of ras^N amplification in different substrains of these cells correlates with the level of ras^N mRNA. However, a survey of other human mammary carcinoma cell lines and of several fresh tissues showed no evidence that ras^N amplification was a general phenomenon in breast cancer.

EXPERIMENTAL STUDIES IMPLICATING RAS GENES IN MAMMARY TUMORIGENESIS

The elucidation of differences in ras gene structure or expression in tumor tissues serves to focus our attention on the kind of genetic abnormalities which appear to be associated with breast cancer. An important test of the hypothetical role which ras gene activation plays in mammary carcinogenesis is the recapitulation of this role in an experimental model system. Three experimental approaches have been employed to address this issue. One has been carcinogen-induced mammary tumorigenesis in the sexually mature rat. A second has been the construction of transgenic mouse strains carrying an oncogene driven by a promoter preferentially expressed in mammary cells. The third has been the alteration of in vitro growth and tumorigenic properties of mammary epithelial and carcinoma cells by DNA transfer of ras oncogenes.

Ras^H Gene Activation in Carcinogen-Induced Rat Mammary Carcinomas

It had been shown that exposure of mature Buffalo (Buf/N) rats to nitroso-methylurea (NMU) resulted in the formation of mammary carcinomas in approximately 90% of the animals after a latency period of 60 days. This carcinogenic effect was hormonally dependent. Female rats castrated before carcinogen exposure did not develop tumors. However, castration after exposure to NMU does not affect the incidence of tumorigenesis although the number of carcinomas per animal decreased and the latency period was extended (66). In this model, tumorigenesis required both hormonal influences end carcinogenic insult. Even after the successful initiation of tumor formation, optimal tumor development required the presence of estrogenic hormones.

To study the details of NMU carcinogenesis at the genetic level, Sukumar et al. modified the original carcinogenesis protocol to use only a single dose of NMU (67). The exposure to the alkylating agent was very brief since NMU is highly reactive and disappears rapidly after injection. All the mammary carcinomas which developed after a 6- to 12-month latency period contained DNA which scored positive in an NIH/3T3 transformation assay. Subsequent cloning of the transforming gene and sequence analysis disclosed that a G -> A transition at nucleotide 35 was responsible for the transforming activation of the $c-ras^H$ gene. This mutation resulted in the coding of a glutamine residue at amino acid 12 of the ras p21.

Subsequent analysis of all the NMU-induced tumors using oligonucleotide sequence-specific hybridization revealed that all the tumors contained the same G -> A transition at nucleotide 35 of the c-ras^H gene. Thus, a single mutation induced by an alkylating agent appeared to participate in 100% of the NMU-induced mammary carcinomas.

In contrast to the position 12 mutations caused by NMU, a different result was obtained when 7,12-dimethyl-benz(a)anthracene (DMBA) was used as a carcinogen in rats (68). DMBA forms adducts with deoxyadenosine and deoxyguanosine residues which lead to excision repair. Analysis of tumor DNA from DMBA-induced mammary carcinomas showed that all the tumors had A -> T transversions at codon 61 and none had mutations of codon 12.

These studies provided a direct correlation between chemical carcinogens, the specific mutations they induced in the c-ras^H gene, and mammary carcinomas. It is still not clear whether the carcinogen-induced ras gene mutations were necessary or sufficient for carcinogenesis in the mature female rat. However, the circumstantial evidence of an 83% incidence of ras gene mutations in the carcinomas tested make a cogent argument that ras did play a role in the development of these tumors. Were this the case, then physiologic hormone-dependent proliferation provided a sufficient environment for the induction of malignancy by mutational activation of a single oncogene. Even though ras gene mutations have not been associated with most human breast cancers, it is important to understand the action of the mutated ras gene and the role it plays in this carcinogenesis model. That understanding may serve to highlight analogous gene action which is important for human mammary carcinogenesis.

RAS GENE-INDUCED MAMMARY CARCINOGENESIS IN TRANSGENIC MICE

The production of transgenic mice that faithfully express foreign genes has generated enthusiasm to study oncogene regulation in vivo. Coupling an oncogene to a promoter whose action is tissue-specific allows the targeting of potential oncogenic effects to the tissue in question, since the information responsible for cell type-specific expression is often located in the promoter region of a gene.

To this end constructs of the mouse mammary tumor virus (MMTV) long terminal repeat (LTR), which contains a steroid hormone-inducible promoter (69), were fused to the c-myc gene and used as a transgene (70). Of 13 strains of transgenic mice which carried different fusions of promoter and c-myc depending on the extent of normal c-myc promoter which was deleted, 2 strains with substantial c-myc promoter deletions developed spontaneous mammary adenocarcinomas. There was no obvious effect of the transgene during early or pubertal development in the mice. Tumors appeared only after females had experienced two or three pregnancies.

Subsequently, transgenic mice were constructed using an MMTV-v-ras^H fusion construct (71). These mice developed hyperplasia of the Harderian gland, an apocrine lacrimal organ located in the murine orbit, and later demonstrated malignancies of mammary, salivary, and lymphoid tissue. The appearance of malignant tumors was stochastic, apparently requiring other somatic events for the expression of the malignant phenotype. The results with the MMTV-v-ras^H construct have been independently reproduced by P. Jolicoeur, who has found a similar predisposition of the MMTV-v-ras^H transgenic mice to form tumors of apocrine organs, including breasts and salivary glands (personal communication).

Female mice arising from F_1 crosses of the MMTV-v-ras^H mice with the MMTV-c-myc mice developed mammary tumors earlier after puberty and with a higher frequency than either of the parental transgenic strains (71).

318

Thus, the expression of 2 oncogenes accelerated and improved the efficiency of tumor formation.

The whey acidic protein (Wap) promoter region has also been fused to a mutated c-$\underline{ras}^H$ gene and used as a transgene (72). Wap is expressed selectively in mammary epithelial cells in response to lactogenic hormones. Therefore, the promoter conferred mammary specificity to the expression of the oncogene. After a long latency period (9-12 months), mammary and salivary gland tumors developed in the transgenic mice. These were also the two tissues which expressed the transgene.

Transgenic experiments suggest that a mutated $\underline{ras}^H$ oncogene can contribute to the development of mammary carcinoma, but expression of the oncogenic transgene must be accompanied by other somatic events to generate tumors. Even the addition of a second activated oncogene did not guarantee the formation of carcinomas in 100% of progeny animals.

THE ROLE OF RAS IN THE IN VITRO TUMORIGENESIS OF THE MCF-7 HUMAN MAMMARY CARCINOMA CELL LINE

MCF-7 human breast cancer cells are estrogen-dependent in that they require estrogen supplementation for efficient in vitro growth. For tumor formation in the nude mouse, the cells are absolutely dependent on physiological estrogen levels. Estrogen-treated cells secrete peptide growth factors, including a factor related to tumor-derived growth factor alpha (TGF alpha) (73), insulin-like growth factor-I (IGF-I) (74), platelet-derived growth factor (PDGF) (75), an epithelial cell colony stimulating factor (76), mammary-derived growth factor (77), and autocrine motility factor (78). Production of many of these factors is responsive to estrogen supplementation in the cell growth medium.

Serum-free conditioned tissue culture medium from the estradiol-treated MCF-7 cells, when concentrated and delivered to nude mice via surgically implanted minipumps, conferred limited reconstitution of the tumor model without any estrogen supplementation in animals (79). When supported with conditioned medium supplementation instead of estrogen, MCF-7 cell implants in the mice grew to tumors of limited size and then regressed. Peptide growth factor secretion appeared to be an important element in mediating estradiol-induced tumorigenesis in that the growth-promoting activity of the concentrated conditioned medium is abrogated by heating or trypsin treatment. Furthermore, infusions of EGF and/or IGF-I also produce limited tumor growth.

Whereas hormone-dependent breast cancer cells responded to estrogen with growth factor production which accompanied alterations in growth properties, hormone-independent breast cancer cells constitutively produce a number of the same growth factors. To try to clarify whether the hormone-independent state was phenotypically similar to the hormone-induced state, Kasid et al. constructed an estrogen-independent MCF-7 cell line by transfecting with v-$\underline{ras}^H$ DNA (80). The resultant MCF-7$_{ras}$ cells expressed the mutant $\underline{ras}$ p21 protein, had a shorter doubling time in vitro than the parental MCF-7 cells, were resistant to growth inhibitory effects of antiestrogens, and formed tumors in nude mice independent of exogenous estrogen supplementation.

This new hormone-independent cell line exhibited constitutive secretion of the identical peptide growth factors whose production was stimulated by estrogen in the parental MCF-7 cells (81). Moreover, tumor implants of the MCF-7$_{ras}$ cells were able to support limited growth of MCF-7 cell implants in a nude mouse distant from the site of the MCF-7$_{ras}$

319

cells in the absence of estrogen. This implied that the secreted growth factors from the MCF-7$_{ras}$ cells supported limited tumor growth similar to the growth effects of conditioned medium from estrogen-treated MCF-7 cells. The MCF-7$_{ras}$ cells retained the expression of estrogen receptors and their function remained intact as evidenced by estrogen induction of progesterone receptor. In this derivative cell line, the introduction of a single mutated oncogene resulted in growth alterations which bypassed the hormone control of tumorigenesis phenotype without abrogating the hormone-response mechanism.

One of the properties necessary for manifestation of the malignant phenotype is the ability to invade through a basement membrane. Tumors usually exhibit the ability to invade locally through tissue planes. Ultimately, most clinical tumors generate distant metastases which result from the remote clonal outgrowth of a cell which has migrated away from the primary neoplasm, invaded through the basement membrane of a vessel in two directions, and seeded in another tissue. One step in this process is invasion, which can be assayed independently by an in vitro assay. Cells can be scored for their ability to penetrate an artificial basement membrane and migrate through a barrier. Both estrogen treatment and $\underline{ras}^H$ transfection induce a marked increase in the invasive potential of MCF-7 cells in this assay (82).

The v-$\underline{ras}^H$ gene used to generate the MCF-7$_{ras}$ cells differs in its protein product at 2 amino acids, Arg^{12} and Thr^{59} from the human proto-oncogene. Both these amino acid residues confer lower GTPase activity to p21 than the corresponding Gly^{12} and Ala^{59} in the human c-$\underline{ras}$ p21. Although the v-$\underline{ras}$ transfection demonstrated the potency of an activated $\underline{ras}$ gene for inducing the malignant phenotype in MCF-7 cells, the v-$\underline{ras}$ p21 was not representative of the $\underline{ras}$ protein directly relevant for human breast cancer. Therefore, a number of other transfected cell lines were isolated which expressed high levels of human c-$\underline{ras}$ p21, p21 (Arg^{12}), p21 (Thr^{59}), as well as v-$\underline{ras}$ p21 (Arg^{12}, Thr^{59}). Tumorigenesis experiments with these cell lines have shown that only the v-$\underline{ras}$ p21 (Arg^{12}, Thr^{59}) permitted an increase in estrogen-independent tumorigenicity. Moreover, reminiscent of the enhancement of in vitro invasive potential demonstrated by the MCF-7$_{ras}$ cells, the v-$\underline{ras}$ transfected lines were highly metastatic from heterografts in nude mice.

The interaction between the $\underline{ras}$ oncogene and MCF-7 cells has provided a useful model for the study of malignant progression in these cells. V-$\underline{ras}^H$ transfection provides an alternative to estrogen stimulation to achieve efficient tumorigenesis in nude mice. Moreover, v-$\underline{ras}^H$ transfection confer metastatic capabilities to MCF-7 cells which had not previously been demonstrated. However, the inactivity of point mutants of human c-$\underline{ras}^H$ and of high levels of proto-oncogene $\underline{ras}^H$ p21 in supporting tumorigenesis indicate that this cell line will not provide data to support the observations associating high levels of $\underline{ras}$ p21 expression and breast tumors. It remains to be seen whether other model systems will provide the direct evidence needed to substantiate the belief that a human $\underline{ras}$ proto-oncogene plays a role in the etiology of breast cancer.

REFERENCES

1. Dhar R, Ellis R, Shih TY, et al. Nucleotide sequence of the p21 transforming protein of Harvey murine sarcoma virus. Science 1982; 217:934-6.
2. Reddy EP, Reynolds RK, Santos E, Barbacid M. A point mutation is responsible for the acquisition of transforming properties by the T24 human bladder carcinoma oncogene. Nature 1982; 300:149-52.

3. Capon DJ, Chen EY, Levinson AD, Seeburg PH, Goeddel DV. Complete nucleotide sequence of the T24 human bladder carcinoma oncogene and its normal homologue. Nature 1983; 302:33-7.

4. Leder P, Battey J, Lenoir G, et al. Translocations among antibody genes in human cancer. Science 1983; 222:765-71.

5. Nishikura K, ar-Rushdi A, Erikson J, Watt R, Rovera G, Croce C. Differential expression of the normal and of the translocated human c-myc oncogenes in B cells. Proc Natl Acad Sci USA 1983; 80:4822-6.

6. Shtivelman E, Lifshitz B, Gale RP, Canaani E. Fused transcript of abl and bcr genes in chronic myelogenous leukemia. Nature 1985; 315:550-4.

7. Bakhshi A, Jensen JP, Goldman P, et al. Cloning the chromosomal breakpoint of t(14;18) human lymphomas: clustering around JH on chromosome 14 and near a transcriptional unit on 18. Cell 1985; 41:899-906.

8. Dalla Favera R, Wong-Staal F, Gallo RC. Onc gene amplification in promyelocytic leukaemia cell line HL-60 and primary leukaemic cells of the same patient. Nature 1982; 299:61-3.

9. Alitalo K, Schwab M, Lin C, Varmus H, Bishop J. Homogeneously staining chromosomal regions contain amplified copies of an abundantly expressed cellular oncogene (c-myc) in malignant neuroendocrine cells from a human colon carcinoma. Proc Natl Acad Sci USA 1982; 80:1707-11.

10. Schwab M, Ellison J, Busch M, Rosenau W, Varmus H, Bishop JM. Enhanced expression of the human gene N-myc consequent to amplification of DNA may contribute to malignant progression of neuroblastoma. Proc Natl Acad Sci USA 1984; 81:4940-4.

11. Waterfield MD, Scrace G, Whittle N, et al. Platelet-derived growth factor is structurally related to the putative transforming protein of simian sarcoma virus. Nature 1983; 304:35-9.

12. Dickson C, Peters G. Potential oncogene product related to growth factors. Nature 1987; 326:833.

13. Downward J, Yarden Y, Mayes E, et al. Close similarity of epidermal growth factor receptor and v-erb-B oncogene protein sequences. Nature 1984; 307:521-7.

14. Sherr CJ, Rettenmeier CW, Sacca R, Roussel MF, Look AT, Stanley ER. The c-fms proto-oncogene product is related to the receptor for the mononuclear phagocytic growth factor, CSF-1. Cell 1985; 41:665-76.

15. Sap J, Munoz A, Damm K, et al. The c-erb-A protein is a high-affinity receptor for thyroid hormone. Nature 1986; 324:635-40.

16. Sefton BM, Hunter T, Beemon E, Eckhart W. Evidence that the phosphorylation of tyrosine is essential for transformation by Rous sarcoma virus. Cell 1980; 20:807-16.

17. Blair DG, Oskarsson MK, Seth A, et al. Analysis of the transforming potential of the human homolog of mos. Cell 1986; 46:785-94.

18. Sambucetti LC, Curran T. The fos protein complex is associated with DNA in isolated nuclei and binds to DNA cellulose. Science 1986; 234:1417-9.

19. Persson H, Leder P. Nuclear localization and DNA binding properties of a protein expressed by human c-myc oncogene. Science 1984; 225:718-21.

20. Klempnauer K-H, Symonds G, Evan GI, Bishop JM. Subcellular localization of proteins encoded by oncogenes of avian myeloblastosis virus and avian leukemia virus E26 and by the chicken c-myb gene. Cell 1984; 37:537-47.

21. Hurley JB, Simon MI, Teplow DB, Robishaw JD, Gilman AG. Homologies between signal transducing G proteins and ras gene products. Science 1984; 226:860-2.

22. O'Brien SJ, Nash WG, Goodwin JL, Lowy DR, Chang EH. Dispersion of the ras family of transforming genes to four different chromosomes in man. Nature 1983; 302:839-42.

23. Ryan J, Barker PE, Shimizu K, Wigler M, Ruddle F. Chromosomal assignment of a family of human oncogenes. Proc Natl Acad Sci USA 1983; 80:4460-3.

24. Hall A, Marshall CJ, Spurr NK, Weiss RA. Identification of transforming gene in two human sarcoma cell lines as a new member of the ras family located on chromosome 1. Nature 1983; 303:396-400.

25. Lowe DG, Capon DJ, Delwart E, Sakaguchi A, Naylor SL, Goeddel DV. Structure of the human and murine R-ras genes, novel genes closely related to ras proto-oncogenes. Cell 1987; 48:137-46.

26. Kataoka T, Powers S, McGill C, et al. Genetic analysis of yeast RAS1 and RAS2 genes. Cell 1984; 37:437-45.

27. Defeo-Jones D, Scolnick E, Koller R, Dhar R. ras-Related gene sequences identified and isolated from Saccharomyces cerevisiae. Nature 1983; 306:707-9.

28. Tatchell K, Chaleff D, Defeo-Jones D, Scolnick E. Requirement of either of a pair of ras-related genes of Saccharomyses cerevisiae for spore viability. Nature 1984; 309:523-7.

29. Reymond CD, Gomer RH, Mehdy MC, Firtel RA. Developmental regulation of a Dictyostelium gene encoding a protein homologous to mammalian ras protein. Cell 1984; 39:141-8.

30. Powers S, Kataoka T, Fasano O, et al. Genes in S. cerevisiae encoding proteins with domains homologous to the mammalian ras proteins. Cell 1984; 36:607-12.

31. Broek D, Samily N, Fasano O, et al. Differential activation of yeast adenylate cyclase by wild-type and mutant ras proteins. Cell 1985; 41:763-9.

32. Toda T, Uno I, Ishikawa T, et al. In yeast, RAS proteins are controlling elements of adenylate cyclase. Cell 1985; 40:27-36.

33. Defeo-Jones D, Tatchell K, Robinson LC, et al. Mammalian and yeast ras gene products: biological function in their heterologous systems. Science 1985; 228:179-84.

34. Kataoka T, Powers S, Cameron S, et al. Functional homology of mammalian and yeast RAS genes. Cell 1985; 40:19-26.

35. Becker SK, Hattori S, Shih TY. The ras oncogene product p21 is not a regulatory component of adenylate cyclase. Nature 1985; 317:71-2.

36. Shih TY, Weeks MO, Gruss P, Dhar R, Oroszlan S, Scolnick E. Identification of a precursor in the biosynthesis of the p21 transforming protein of Harvey murine sarcoma virus. J Virol 1982; 42:253-61.

37. Willingham MC, Pastan I, Shih TY, Scolnick EM. Localization of the src gene product of the Harvey strain of MSV to plasma membrane of transformed cells by electron microscopic immunocytochemistry. Cell 1980; 19:1005-14.

38. Sefton BM, Trowbridge IS, Cooper JA, Scolnick EM. The transforming proteins of Rous sarcoma virus, Harvey sarcoma virus and Abelson virus contain tightly bound lipid. Cell 1982; 31:465-74.

39. Willumsen BM, Christensen A, Hubbert NL, Papageorge AG, Lowy DR. The p21 ras c-terminus is required for transformation and membrane association. Nature 1984; 310:583-6.

40. Dever TE, Glynias MJ, Merrick WC. GTP-binding domain: three consensus sequence elements with distinct spacing. Proc Natl Acad Sci USA 1987; 84:1814-8.

41. Nishikura K, ar-Rushdi A, Erikson J, Watt R, Rovera G, Croce C. Differential expression of the normal and of the translocated human c-myc oncogenes in B cells. Proc Natl Acad Sci USA 1983; 80:4822-6.

42. McCormick F, Clark BFC, la Cour TFM, Kjeldgaard M, Norskov-Lauritsen L, Nyborg J. A model for the tertiary structure of p21, the product of the ras oncogene. Science 1985; 230:78-82.

43. Walter M, Clark SG, Levinson AD. The oncogenic activation of human p21 ras by a novel mechanism. Science 1986; 233:649-52.

44. Sigal IS, Gibbs JB, D'Alonzo JS, Scolnick EM. Identification of effector residues and a neutralizing epitope of Ha-ras encoded p21. Proc Natl Acad Sci USA 1986; 83:4725-9.

45. Willumsen BM, Papageorge A, Kung H-F, et al. Mutational analysis of the ras catalytic domain. Mol Cell Biol 1986; 6:2646–54.

46. Yuasa Y, Srivastava SK, Dunn CY, Rhim JS, Reddy EP, Aaronson SA. Acquisition of transforming properties by alternative point mutations within c-bas/has human proto-oncogene. Nature 1983; 303:775–9.

47. Perucho M, Goldfarb M, Shimizu K, Lama C, Fogh J, Wigler M. Human tumor-derived cell lines contain common and different transforming genes. Cell 1981; 27:467–76.

48. Der C, Finkel T, Cooper GM. Biological and biochemical properties of human rasH genes mutated at codon 61. Cell 1986; 44:167–76.

49. Fasano O, Aldrich T, Tamanoi F, Taparowsky E, Furth M, Wigler M. Analysis of the transforming potential of the human H-ras gene by random mutagenesis. Proc Natl Acad Sci USA 1984; 81:4008–12.

50. McGrath JP, Capon D, Goeddel DV, Levinson AD. Comparative biochemical properties of normal and activated human ras p21 protein. Nature 1984; 310:644–9.

51. Gibbs JB, Sigal IS, Poe M, Scolnick EM. Intrinsic GTPase activity distinguishes normal and oncogenic ras p21 molecules. Proc Natl Acad Sci USA 1984; 81:5704–8.

52. Manne V, Bekesi E, Kung H-F. Ha-ras proteins exhibit GTPase activity: point mutations that activate Ha-ras gene products result in decreased GTPase activity. Proc Natl Acad Sci USA 1985; 82:376–80.

53. Lacal JC, Srivastava SK, Anderson PS, Aaronson SA. Ras p21 proteins with high and low GTPase activity can efficiently transform NIH/3T3 cells. Cell 1986; 44:609–17.

54. Chang EH, Furth ME, Scolnick EM, Lowy DR. Tumorigenic transformation of mammalian cells induced by a normal human gene homologous to the oncogene of Harvey murine sarcoma virus. Nature 1982; 297:479–83.

55. Kraus MH, Yuasa Y, Aaronson SA. A position 12-activated H-ras oncogene in all HS578T mammary carcinosarcoma cells but not normal mammary cells of the same patient. Proc Natl Acad Sci USA 1984; 81:5384–8.

56. McGrath JP, Capon DJ, Smith DH, et al. Structure and organization of the human Ki-ras proto-oncogene and a related processed pseudogene. Nature 1983; 304:501–5.

57. Spandidos DA, Agnantis NJ. Human malignant tumours of the breast, as compared to their respective normal tissue, have elevated expression of the Harvey ras oncogene. Anticancer Res 1984; 4:269–72.

58. Agnantis NJ, Parissi P, Anagnostakis D, Spandidos DA. Comparative study of Harvey-ras oncogene expression with conventional clinicopathologic parameters of breast cancer. Oncology 1986; 43:36–9.

59. DeBortoli ME, Abou-Issa H, Haley BE, Cho-Chung YS. Amplified expression of p21 ras protein in hormone-dependent mammary carcinomas of humans and rodents. Biochem Biophys Res Commun 1985; 127:699–706.

60. Hand PH, Thor A, Wunderlich D, Muraro R, Caruso A, Schlom J. Monoclonal antibodies of predefined specificity detect activated ras gene expression in human mammary and colon carcinomas. Proc Natl Acad Sci USA 1984; 81:5227–31.

61. Tanaka T, Slamon D, Battifora H, Cline MJ. Expression of p21 ras oncoproteins in human cancers. Cancer Res 1986; 46:1465–70.

62. Theillet C, Lidereau R, Escot C, et al. Loss of a c-H-ras-1 allele and aggressive human primary breast carcinomas. Cancer Res 1986; 46:4776–81.

63. Ohuchi N, Thor A, Page DL, Hand PH, Halter S, Schlom J. Expression of the 21,000 molecular weight ras protein in a spectrum of benign and malignant human mammary tissues. Cancer Res 1986 46:2511–9.

64. Lidereau R, Escot C, Theillet C, et al. High frequency of rare alleles of the human c-Ha-ras-1 proto-oncogene in breast cancer patients. J Natl Cancer Inst 1986; 77:697–701.

65. Graham KA, Richardson CL, Minden MD, Trent JM, Buick RM. Varying

degrees of amplification of the N-ras oncogene in the human breast cancer cell line MCF-7. Cancer Res 1985; 45:2201-5.

66. Gullino P, Pettigrew HM, Grantham FH. N-nitrosomethylurea as mammary gland carcinogen in rats. J Natl Cancer Inst 1975; 54:401-14.

67. Sukumar S, Notario V, Martin-Zanca D, Barbacid M. Induction of mammary carcinomas in rats by nitrosomethylurea involves malignant activation of H-ras-1 locus by single point mutations. Nature 1983; 308:658-61.

68. Zarbl H, Sukumar S, Arthur AV, Martin-Zanca D, Barbacid M. Direct mutagenesis of Ha-ras-1 oncogenes by N-nitroso-N-methylurea during initiation of mammary carcinogenesis in rats. Nature 1985; 315: 382-5.

69. Chandler VL, Maler BA, Yamamoto KR. DNA sequences bound specifically by glucocorticoid receptor in vitro render a heterologous promoter hormone responsive in vivo. Cell 1983; 33:489-99.

70. Stewart TA, Pattengale PK, Leder P. Spontaneous mammary adenocarcinomas in transgenic mice that carry and express MTV/myc fusion genes. Cell 1984; 38:627-37.

71. Sinn E, Muller W, Pattengale P, Tepler I, Wallace R, Leder P. Coexpression of MMTV/v-Ha-ras and MMTV/c-myc genes in transgenic mice: synergistic action of oncogenes in vivo. Cell 1987; 49:465-75.

72. Andres A-C, Schonenberger C-A, Groner B, Hennighausen L, LeMeur M, Gerlinger P. Ha-ras oncogene expression directed by a milk protein gene promoter: tissue specificity, hormonal regulation, and tumor induction in transgenic mice. Proc Natl Acad Sci USA 1987; 84:1299-303.

73. Bates S, Dickson R, McManaway M, Lippman ME. Characterization of estrogen-responsive transforming activity in human breast cancer cell lines. Cancer Res 1986; 46:1703-17.

74. Huff KK, Lippman ME, Spencer EM, Kaufman D, Dickson RB. Human breast cancer cells secrete an insulin-like growth factor I-related polypeptide. Cancer Res 1986; 46:4613-9.

75. Bronzert D, Pantazis P, Antoniades H, et al. Synthesis and secretion of platelet-derived growth factor by human breast cancer cell lines. Proc Natl Acad Sci USA 1987; 84:5763-7.

76. Swain S, Dickson R, Lippman ME. Anchorage-independent epithelial colony-stimulating activity in human breast cancer cell lines. Proc Am Assoc Cancer Res 1986; 27:844.

77. Bano M, Salomon DS, Kidwell WR. Purification of a mammary-derived growth factor from human milk and mammary tumors. J Biol Chem 1986; 260:5745-52.

78. Liotta L, Mandler R, Murano G, et al. Tumor cell autocrine motility factor. Proc Natl Acad Sci USA 1986; 83:3302-6.

79. Dickson RB, McManaway ME, Lippman ME. Estrogen-induced factors of breast cancer cells partially replace estrogen to promote tumor growth. Science 1986; 232:1540-3.

80. Kasid A, Lippman ME, Papageorge AG, Lowy DR, Gelmann EP. Transfection of v-rasH DNA into MCF-7 human breast cancer cells bypasses dependence on estrogen for tumorigenicity. Science 1985; 228:725-8.

81. Dickson RB, Kasid A, Huff KK, et al. Activation of growth factor secretion in tumorigenic states of breast cancer induced by 17B-estradiol or v-Ha-ras oncogene. Proc Natl Acad Sci USA 1987; 84: 837-41.

82. Albini A, Graf J, Kitten GT, et al. 17B-estradiol regulates and v-Ha-ras transfection constitutively enhances MCF7 breast cancer cell interactions with basement membrane. Proc Natl Acad Sci USA 1986; 83:8182-6.

AUTHOR INDEX

SUBJECT INDEX

Estrogen (continued)
  receiver (continued)
    transition, conformational
      hormone-dependent, 99–109
      hormone-independent, 99–109
    unoccupied, 4–6, 11
  regulation, 209–220
    determinant of, 163–174
  tissue
    distribution of radioactive, 28
    retention, 26
  transfection, 170
  translocation model, 28
  tumor growth in vitro, 273–275
  two-step model, 28
  and uterus, interaction with, 29
Estrone, 277
Estrone sulfate, 277

5-Fluorouracil, 291
  and breast cancer, 291
Flutamide, 200, 253

Gene
  activation and estrogen, 9
  expression and
    androgen, 119–131
    estrogen, 9
  of receptor, 151–206
    and function, 151–206
    and structure, 151–206
    superfamily of, 154–156
  transcription, see Transcription
Globulin, 119
Glucocorticoid receptor, 4, 6, 9,
      35, 71–83, 102, 154–157,
      187–206
  activation, 73
  antibody against, 72
  antiphosphotyrosine, 142–145
  chymotrypsin digestion of, 75–77
  cloned, 158, 190–191
  cyanogen bromide digestion of,
      76, 77
  and dexamethasone, 39
  distribution, subcellular, 71–83
  DNA, 73–79
  domain, functional, 75–78
  elution from gel, 145
  gene
    isolation, 187–206
    promoter, 187–206
    regulation, 196–197
    sequence, 187–206
    structure, 192–194
    transcription, 194–196
  hepatic, 40, 133–138, 142–145
  in liver, see hepatic
  localization
    intracellular, 39–42
    nuclear, 42

Glucocorticoid receptor (continued)
  lymphoma cell resistance to, 74
  model is two-step, 72–73
  mutation of, 75, 163
  phosphorylated on tyrosine, 142
  prolactin gene regulation,
      negative, 167
  protein domains, three, 163
  proteolysis, limited, 74–77
  purification, 73–74
  quantitation, 79
  resistance to, by murine lymphoma
      cell, 74
  RNA, 194
  structure, 71–83
    oligomeric, 78–79
  translocation, nuclear, 41, 71,
      72
    doubtful, 41–42
  transcription factor, activated,
      166
  trypsin digestion of, 75, 77
Glucocorticosteroid, 256
β-Glucuronidase, 119, 126, 127
Growth hormone gene, 167
  regulation, 167
Guanidine hydrochloride, 235–241,
      244, 246

Harvey murine sarcoma virus, 314
Heat-shock protein (hsp90), 7–8,
      38, 91–92, 114, 251–262,
      307
  characteristics, 254
  localization, cellular, 38
  and progesterone receptor, 38–
      39
  and RU486, 256
Hinge region, 233
Histone, 235, 236, 240
Hormone
  action without hormone?, 9–10
  affinity chromatography, 254
  antihormone action, 258
  and behavior, 14
  binding assay, 189–190, 198–201
  and cancer, 271
    grading, 273
  and lordosis, 14
  regulation and receptor mod-
      ification, 99–148
  regulatory element, 256
  responsive element, 179
    listed, 179
  and reproduction, 14
  see separate hormones
Hydroxyflutamide, 200
4-Hydroxytamoxifen, 101, 222, 252,
      253, 277, 278
17β-Hydroxyoxidoreductase, 277
Hypothalamus, 266

Immunoaffinity chromatography, 113, 307
Immunoassay of protein 52K, 227-228
Immunoblotting, 112, 114
Immunocytochemistry, 53, 54, 59, 60
  of receptor, 47-70
  technique described, 48-49
Immunogold method, 178
Immunolocalization of progesterone receptor, 178-179
  nuclear, 178
Immunoprecipitation, 114, 135-136
Insulin, 15
Interaction chromatography, hydrophobic, high-performance (HPHIC), 296
125-Iodoestradiol-17β, 297, 304, 307
Ion-exchange chromatography, high-performance (HPIEC), 298, 302, 306, 307
  for estrogen receptor of breast cancer, 299-302
Ishikawa cell line, 274, 275, 277, 279

Kidney, murine, 119-131
  androgen regulated protein, 119
  and ornithine decarboxylase, 119-131
Kirsten murine sarcoma virus, 314

Leupeptin, 85, 226
Ligand-binding, 5-6
Lipocortin production, 276-277
Liquid chromatography, high-performance, 294-303
  see separate methods
Lordosis, 14, 265-269
  control has neural localization, 265-266
  and estrogen, 265-269
  and progestin, 265-269
  and sex differentiation, 267
  and testosterone, 267
Luciferase, 166
Luteal-follicular transition, 58-64

Macaca monkeys, 48, 54, 56, 58
Matrix, nuclear, 10-11
  and receptor, hormonal, 10
Menstrual cycle, artificial, 58
Mineralocorticoid receptor, human, cDNA, 188
Molybdate, 7, 8, 114, 254, 302, 303
Mouse strain, inbred, listed, 126, 127
Mouse mammary tumor virus, 154, 158, 159
Myometrium and immunocytochemistry, 50

Nafoxidine, 140
Nitrosomethylurea, carcinogenic hormone-dependent, 317
Northern
  blot analysis, 177, 178, 190, 201, 202
  hybridization, 187
Nuclease S mapping, 192-194
Nucleotide sequence of coding region, 180-183
  cDNA of progesterone receptor, 180-183
Nucleus, ventromedial, 266
  and lordosis, 266
N-terminal region, 233, 234, 255
Nucleoplast and receptor, unoccupied, 4
Nucleosome, 72

Oligonucleotide synthesis, 189
Oncogene, 13 see Proto-oncogene
Ornithine decarboxylase, 13
  amino acid sequence, 120-121
  genes, 12
  molecular weight, 120
  in kidney, 119-131
    and androgen, 119, 126
  protein, 120-121
  regulation in kidney, 119, 126
  mRNA, 122
    accumulation, androgen-regulated, 122-127
    heterogeneity of size, 122
  source, best, 120
  and testosterone, 121
  turnover rate is very fast, 121
Orthovanadate, 138
Oviduct, 53-57, 64, 67, 68, 85, 87, 91, 92, 159, 160, 254, 257
  immunocytochemistry, 52

Pansorbin, 136, 137
Partitioning behavior of receptor, 100-104
  coefficient, 100-102
  hormone-dependent, 101-103
  temperature-dependent, 103-105
Pepstatin, 85, 226
Peptide mapping, 87, 92, 94
Permeabilization of cell, 72
Peroxidase-antiperoxidase technique, 226
Phenol red, 211-216
  structure related to estrogen, 211
L-Phenylalanine mustard, 291
  and breast cancer, 291
Phenylmethylsulfonyl fluoride, 85
Phenylphosphate, 144
Phosphatase, 8, 133-140

ras-gene (continued)
  in yeast, 313–314
Rat receptor mapping in brain, 266
  see Lordosis
Receptor
  action, 179
  binding
    assay, 53, 58
    domain, 184
  chimeric, constructed, 153–155
  complex, radiolabeled, 295–296
  cysteine-rich region, 179–181
  in cytoplasm, unoccupied, 4
  gene, 11–12
    function, 151–206
    structure, 151–206
  localization, 3–5
  methodology, 288–290, 294–303
  nuclear, 11
  see separate receptors
Ribonucleic acid, see RNA
RNA, 6–7, 124, 177–178, 188–189
RNase A, 297, 298
Rous sarcoma virus, 166
RU486 (19-norsteroid), 256, 258

SDS-PAGE, 88, 134–137, 140, 143
Sex difference and lordosis, 267
Silastic implant, 58, 123, 124
Size exclusion chromatography,
        high-performance (HPSEC),
        296–299
Southern blotting, 190, 191, 201,
        203
Spironolactone, 253
Steroid hormone
  action, mechanism of, 3–4
  binding
    assay, 49
    domain, 152, 164, 233
  function, 3, 152–153, 265
  molecule
    biologically complex, 99
    chemically simple, 99
  receptor, 3–26
    action model, 26
    analysis, immunocytochemical,
        35–45
    antibody against, 35
    binding DNA, 163, 167, 233
    in breast cancer, 13
    clinical, 13
    dephosphorylation, 14
    DNA, 11–12
      binding, 163, 167, 233
    discovery of, 27
    in endometrium cancer, 13
    estrogen retention in tissue
        reported, 26
    function, 188
    hinge region, 233

Steroid hormone (continued)
  receptor (continued)
    historical, 25–31
    isoform, 293
    ligand-free, 5–6
    localization
      intracellular, 35–45
      nuclear, 3–5
      subcellular, 3–5
    modification
      covalent, 14–16
      and hormone regulation, 99–
          148
    and molybdate, 7
    N-terminus region, immunolog-
        ical, 233
    nucleus components, 10–12
    partitioning, aqueous
        two-phase, 100
    as phosphoprotein (?), 14
    phosphorylation, 13–14
    polymorphism, 293–294
    and protein kinase, 16
    RNA, 6–7
    structure, 35–96, 252–256
    theory proposed in 1879, 25
    thermolability of, 99–100
    as transducer of information,
        macromolecular, 99
    transformation, 6, 8–9, 99–100
    transhydrogenase theory, 26–27
    translocation model, 29
  responsive element, 152–153
Streptomycin filter assay, 239, 241
Sulfotransferase, 277

Tamoxifen, 13, 135, 140, 141, 210,
        222, 224, 252, 253, 291–294
  see Cis-, Hydroxy-, Trans-
Testosterone, 14, 123, 124, 127,
        267
Thyroid hormone receptor, 12, 171,
        245
Tissue preparation, 48, 49
Tissue marker, prognostic, see
        Cathepsin-D
Transcription, 151–159, 163–176,
        194–196, 199, 257
Transfection, 196–197, 234, 255
Transformation, 6–9, 13, 99–109,
        252–257
  hypothesis, 8
  listed, 13
Transhydrogenase theory, 26–27
  disproven, 27
Transhydroxytamoxifen, 210, 212–217
Transition
  conformational, 99–109
    hormone-dependent, 101–103
    temperature-dependent, 103–105